A Clinician's Guide to Traumatic Brain Injury

A Clinician's Guide to Traumatic Brain Injury

Editor: Analise Phelps

AMERICAN
MEDICAL PUBLISHERS
www.americanmedicalpublishers.com

AMERICAN
MEDICAL PUBLISHERS
www.americanmedicalpublishers.com

Cataloging-in-publication Data

A clinician's guide to traumatic brain injury / edited by Analise Phelps.
p. cm.
Includes bibliographical references and index.
ISBN 978-1-63927-843-5
1. Brain--Wounds and injuries. 2. Brain damage. 3. Brain--Wounds and injuries--Diagnosis.
4. Brain damage--Diagnosis. 5. Brain--Wounds and injuries--Treatment. 6. Brain damage--Treatment.
I. Phelps, Analise.
RD594 .C55 2023
617.481--dc23

American Medical Publishers,
41 Flatbush Avenue,
1st Floor, New York,
NY 11217, USA

ISBN 978-1-63927-843-5 (Hardback)

Contents

Preface

In my initial years as a student, I used to run to the library at every possible instance to grab a book and learn something new. Books were my primary source of knowledge and I would not have come such a long way without all that I learnt from them. Thus, when I was approached to edit this book; I became understandably nostalgic. It was an absolute honor to be considered worthy of guiding the current generation as well as those to come. I put all my knowledge and hard work into making this book most beneficial for its readers.

A traumatic brain injury (TBI) refers to a brain injury caused by an external force such as rapid acceleration-deceleration, direct impact, blast waves, or penetration by an object. It is also called intracranial injury. On the basis of the severity of injury, TBI is categorized as mild traumatic brain injury-mTBI, moderate TBI or severe TBI. An injury to the brain may affect brain function either temporarily or permanently. The mechanical force may also cause damage to the outermost membrane of brain called dura mater. TBI may lead to axonal alteration in the subcortical white matter, corpus collasum, and the brain stem. Falls, vehicle collisions, and violence are among the causes of traumatic brain injuries. The characteristics and severity of TBI are influenced by the type, direction, strength, and duration of pressures. Clinical suspicion of TBI is validated by neurological evaluation, banyan brain trauma indicator (BTI) blood test and neuroimaging techniques such as CT-scans and MRI. The treatment of TBI includes counseling, surgery, rehabilitation therapies and rest. This book is meant for students who are looking for an elaborate reference text on traumatic brain injuries. It also provides interesting topics for research which interested readers can take up. This book aims to serve as a resource guide for students and experts alike and contribute to the growth of the discipline.

I wish to thank my publisher for supporting me at every step. I would also like to thank all the authors who have contributed their researches in this book. I hope this book will be a valuable contribution to the progress of the field.

Editor

1

Attentional Processing in Traumatic Brain Injury and Posttraumatic Stress Disorder

Tobias Wensing, Jean Levasseur-Moreau, Alexander T. Sack and Shirley Fecteau

1. Introduction

The objective of this work is to review studies that examine deficits in sustained and selective attentional processing in adults diagnosed with Traumatic Brain Injury (TBI) or Posttraumatic Stress Disorder (PTSD). Deficits in these two attentional mechanisms are assumed to underlie the most prevalent behavioral consequences of TBI and PTSD and can result in deleterious consequences for an individual's everyday life.

TBI is considered a neurological condition that involves critical physical damage to brain tissue. PTSD is a psychiatric disorder that is accompanied by symptoms including intrusive re-experiencing of the traumatic event, avoidance and hyper-arousal. Individuals diagnosed with PTSD have been exposed to a traumatic event with highly threatening physical or psychological harm [1]. Consequently, the causing events underlying TBI, such as a motor vehicle accident or military assault, might also lead to a trauma that develops into a diagnosis of PTSD. Clinical reports described case studies, in which individuals showed symptoms of PTSD following a traumatic event. Moreover, neuropsychological assessments revealed that these symptoms were also accompanied by specific deficits in sustained and selective attentional processing [2] and related cognitive task performances [3]. A vast amount of literature emphasizes that impairments in cognitive processes may play a key role in several neurological and psychiatric disorders. For instance, cognitive deficits have been reported in both TBI and PTSD with considerable overlap including difficulties to concentrate, mental fatigue and hyper-arousal (see [4] for a review). Specifically, comorbid occurrence of TBI and PTSD in military personnel returning from conflicts in Afghanistan and Iraq approaches a prevalence of 50% [1]. Additionally, recent reviews on TBI and PTSD imply that the presence of TBI in an individual might accelerate subsequent development of PTSD diagnosis [4, 5]. Thus, the relationship between TBI and PTSD is pronounced in a one-way direction with PTSD occurring as a consequence of TBI, but not vice versa. This is mainly attributed to a shared causative event [4]. However, damage to critical brain tissue in TBI that is involved in emotional and cognitive processing after injury might also promote successive development of PTSD. Recent neuroimaging studies identified shared neurobiological deficits that include portions of the prefrontal cortex, as well as subcortical regions, such as the hypothalamus or pituitary gland (for a review, see [4]).

Importantly, despite potential symptomatic overlaps, TBI and PTSD require a detailed picture of cognitive deficits that underlie the most debilitating symptoms. With regards to the complex nature of attention and its prominent implication in symptoms observed in both TBI and PTSD, it appears crucial to identify and discuss similarities and differences in attentional processing, which may help to distinguish between both medical conditions. Thus, a comparison of attentional processing towards stimuli independent of emotional valence, either shared by or exclusive to TBI and PTSD, may promote specialized subsequent treatment and rehabilitation approaches.

Attentional processes have been studied for decades. However, we have yet to entirely grasp to which extent attention affects our behaviour. Attention is a central cognitive process that is considered as a precursor of a large majority of other higher cognitive functions. Although attention underlies a variety of behavioral impairments related to neurological and psychiatric disorders, its nature is rather complex and can be observed throughout numerous distinct subtypes, such as sustained attention, selective attention, and inhibition. Accordingly, these subtypes of attention are governed by the implication of different brain regions including the posterior parietal [6], inferior frontal [7], medial frontal and dorsolateral prefrontal cortex [8]. In this work, we will address processing of sustained and selective attention, since we believe that these subtypes of attention most likely resemble mechanisms, which underlie shared symptoms in TBI and PTSD, such as difficulties to concentrate or mental fatigue. Moreover, we will focus on reviewing studies, which solely implement neutral stimuli within their experimental designs. The ability to adequately process neutral stimuli is a vital cognitive requirement for coping with our environment. Deficits in this basic function may have a critical impact on an individuals' well being and even his survival.

2. Sustained attentional processing in TBI

Sustained attention (vigilance) is the ability to maintain attention for sporadic critical events during long periods of time [9]. Maintaining vigilant while performing everyday routines, such as driving a vehicle, is crucial to react to changes and unforeseen events in the environment. To date, behavioral findings on deficits in sustained attention for TBI are inconclusive. Varying findings have been reported for almost every behavioral aspect related to sustained attention, including response time (RT), accuracy, and intra-individual variability in responses (Table 1). In the studies reviewed here, RT is defined as the latency between the onset of a stimulus and the response given by a subject; accuracy mainly reflects errors in the correct execution of task instructions; intra-individual variability in responses refers to fluctuations in subjects' accuracy or RT over the course of a cognitive task.

Study	TBI (n)	Post-Trauma	Severity	Trauma Type	Cognitive Test	Main Findings
Bloomfield et al. [15]	44	71,5 Months	Mild - Severe	Combat; RTA; Falls	SART	More commission errors in "poor sleepers" group
Bonnelle et al. [18]	28	28 Months (Range: 3-73)	Mild - Severe	Combat; RTA; Falls; Sports	CRT	Decrement in RT over time; No differences in accuracy; Higher IIV
Dockree et al. [12]	29	34,81 Months	Mild - Severe	Combat; RTA; Falls; Work	SART;DART	No differences in RT; More commission errors; Higher IIV
Kim et al. [19]	18	51,1 Months	Moderate - Severe	-	VSAT	No differences in RT; No differences in accuracy
McAvinue et al. [10]	18	38,83 Months (Range: 2-132)	Mild - Severe	-	SART	No differences in RT; More commission errors
Sinclair et al. [16]	20	133 Days-13,4 Years	Mild - Severe	RTA; Falls	PVT	Slower RT; Lower accuracy; Higher IIV
Slovarp et al. [20]	9	3,6 Years	Severe	-	SAT	Slower RT; Lower hit rate; Higher IIV for TBI subgroup
Willmott et al. [14]	40	68,38 Years (Range: 12-462)	Moderate - Severe	RTA	SART	No differences in accuracy

Table 1. Summary of methodologies and main findings of studies investigating sustained attention in TBI (Note: CRT = Choice Reaction Time Task; DART = Dual-task Attention to Response Task; IIV = Intra-individual Variability; PVT = Psychomotor Vigilance Task; RT = Response Time; RTA = Road Traffic Accident; SAT = Sustained Attention Task; SART = Sustained Attention to Response Task; VSAT = Visual Sustained Attention Task; TBI = Traumatic Brain Injury; "-" indicates missing or not reported information).

McAvinue et al. [10] compared individuals with mild to severe TBI to gender-, age- and education-matched healthy individuals on a Sustained Attention to Response Task (SART; [11]). The SART is a cognitive test measuring sustained attention following the Go/NoGo paradigm. Subjects were visually presented with a series of single digits ranging from 1 to 9. Presentation of the digits is followed by a mask and subjects were subsequently asked to press a response button as accurately and fast as possible at the occurrence of every digit but "3" (for a detailed description on the SART, see [11]). To further assess the role of error awareness and feedback on task performance, McAvinue et al. [10] divided the SART into different conditions. Subjects were presented with randomized digits and asked to withhold their response as soon as the digit "3" appeared. Also, three altered versions of the original SART were implemented in this study: an "awareness" condition, requiring subjects to give a verbal report as soon as they made a commission error (i.e., pressing the response button although no target is present); a "feedback" condition in which subjects were given auditory feedback when making an error; and a "fixed" condition, in which digits were not presented randomly but in a fixed order. Overall, individuals with TBI made more commission errors than healthy controls. However, both groups showed similar RT. Moreover, results of the "awareness" condition suggest that individuals with TBI were less aware of the errors they made during the task. Also, error awareness, that is, the number of errors a subject was unaware of, was positively correlated with the number of commission errors made by individuals with TBI. Behavioral results of the "feedback" condition indicated that both groups benefited from the provided error feedback and that both groups were able to decrease their amount of commission errors to the same extent. Another study [12] combined the SART with a continuous performance task (CPT; [13]) resulting in the Dual-task Attention to Response Task (DART). In the original CPT, subjects were asked to respond via button press to random occurrences of any letter of the alphabet, except for "x" ("x"-condition). Additionally, a more demanding task required subjects to withhold response to the letter "x" only if preceded by the letter "a" ("ax"-condition). In the classical CPT, outcome measures are levels of accuracy, assessed in terms of commission and omission errors (i.e., not pressing the response button although a target is present). According to the authors, a combination of the SART and CPT would result in a cognitively more demanding task that challenges sustained attention. In the DART, subjects are required to indicate the random occurrence of grey colored digits additionally to the classical design of the SART described previously. Dockree et al. [12] compared individuals with TBI, who had mild to severe injuries, to gender-, age- and education-matched healthy subjects on both the classical SART and the newly developed DART. Compared to the SART, the cognitively more demanding DART led to an increase in commission errors for both study groups. Individuals with TBI and healthy individuals did not differ in terms of RT on both tasks. However, individuals with TBI made more commission errors and showed higher intra-individual variability in responses during both the SART and the DART. Within a series of attentional tasks, Willmott et al. [14] also used a classical SART paradigm to test sustained attention in moderate to severe TBI. This study revealed no difference between individuals TBI and healthy individuals regarding commission errors. However, individuals with TBI tended, though not statistically significant, to make more omission errors than healthy controls (i.e., missing responses to any digit but "3").

Bloomfield et al. [15] incorporated the SART in a study that compared individuals with mild to severe TBI with respect to absent or present sleeping difficulties. The authors emphasized that individuals with TBI and those with sleep disorders constantly report concentration and attentional impairments. Thus, a deficit in sustained attention might be even more pronounced in individuals with TBI suffering from sleep disorders [15]. Based on a battery of sleep measurement indices, subjects were assigned to either the "poor sleepers" or "good sleepers" group. In accordance with the authors' hypotheses, poor sleepers made more commission errors than good sleepers at the SART. Sinclair et al. [16] compared individuals with mild to severe TBI to age- and gender-matched healthy individuals on the Psychomotor Vigilance Task (PVT; [17]). The PVT is a cognitive test that requires subjects to respond as fast as possible to a randomly presented auditory target stimulus. This task was originally developed to assess sustained attention in individuals with sleep disturbances. Similar to Bloomfield et al. [15], the authors hypothesized that TBI might be accompanied by an increase in mental fatigue and sleeping difficulties. This study examined individuals with TBI that reported fatigue and sleep difficulties and compared them to a healthy control sample. Compared to controls, individuals with TBI showed increased RT, reduced accuracy and larger intra-individual response variability. However, effects were diminished or vanished completely when controlling for reported sleep disturbances and fatigue, respectively. Nonetheless, Sinclair et al. [16] accentuated the close relation between sustained attention and fatigue and sleep disturbances that could at least in part account for the observed results in this study.

A study by Bonnelle et al. [18] assessed sustained attention with a simple Choice Reaction Time task (CRT). In the CRT, subjects were asked to respond as accurately and as fast as possible to a target arrow that pointed either in the right or left direction with respective button presses. An increase in RT over the course of the task would be indicative of possible deficits in sustained attention. The examined TBI group suffered from mild to severe brain injuries. Although individuals with TBI displayed intact accuracy, they had increased RT and larger intra-individual variability compared to healthy controls. Additionally, the same group showed an increase in response speed over time with RT being significantly slower in the last third of the task assessment than in the first one. The authors proposed that this decrease in performance speed might reflect a deficit in maintaining vigilance over time and, thus, sustained attention [18].

Kim et al. [19] assessed individuals with moderate to severe TBI and healthy individuals using a Visual Sustained-Attention Task (VSAT). In the VSAT, subjects were asked to discriminate pairs of vertical lines as either of same or different size, and press a response button only if lines were equal. However, individuals with TBI and healthy controls did not statistically differ in terms of accuracy or RT, although there was a trend towards longer RT and poorer accuracy in individuals with TBI.

Another recent study by Slovarp et al. [20] focused on sustained attention processing in individuals with severe TBI. These individuals and an age-matched control group were tested on a Sustained Attention Task (SAT). Here, subjects were presented with a display of four letters with one letter appearing in the upper half and three letters arranged in a row in the lower half of the screen. The subjects' task was to indicate by button press, if the upper letter matched one of the lower letters on the same display. Outcome measures included levels of accuracy (false alarms/hit rates) and RT. Findings revealed that individuals with TBI made more errors in terms of lower hit rates and were comparably slower in giving responses. Although there was no evidence for an increase in RT variability over time on a group level, Slovarp et al. [20] observed substantial intra-individual response variability over the course of the task in a subgroup of TBI subjects.

3. Sustained attentional processing in PTSD

Deficits in sustained attention have also been reported in studies assessing individuals diagnosed with PTSD (Table 2). Vasterling et al. [21, 22] conducted different studies examining groups of Gulf and Vietnam War veterans, respectively. The researchers compared individuals, which had developed PTSD after combat with a group of PTSD-free veterans. Within a series of cognitive tasks, subjects also performed a computerized version of the CPT [13], which is assumed to measure sustained attention. The authors reported both more commission [21] and omission errors [22] on the "ax"-condition in veterans with PTSD when compared to combat-exposed individuals without PTSD. Sustained attention has also been assessed as part of a larger study on cognitive functioning in veterans of the Bosnian War [23]. Veterans diagnosed with PTSD were compared to a similarly combat-exposed but PTSD-free control group. Both groups were assessed on the SART, which has been widely used in the study of attentional deficits in individuals with TBI. Compared to controls, veterans with PTSD made more commission as well as omission errors in the SART. However, the authors did not find any differences in RT. Another study that measured sustained attention in combat-exposed individuals used the CPT in Vietnam War veterans with PTSD and trauma-free controls [24]. In this study, the CPT was presented visually as well as auditory. In addition to the visual "x"- and "ax"-conditions, subjects performed the same task while listening to letter strings presented via headphones. Task performance was measured in terms of accuracy and RT. While there were no differences between groups in the visual CPT condition, PTSD subjects made less correct responses in the auditory condition. Moreover, subjects did not differ in RT in the auditory and visual CPT. However, the authors did not report any differences in commission errors for both modalities.

Study	PTSD (n)	Control Group	Trauma Type	Cognitive Test	Main Findings
Jenkins et al. [25]	15	Trauma Survivors	Sexual Violence	CPT; PASAT	More omission errors
Koso et al. [23]	20	PTSD-free Veterans	Combat	SART	More commission and omission errors
Shucard et al. [24]	23	Healthy Controls	Combat	CPT	No differences in RT for both modalities; Auditory: lower accuracy
Stein et al. [27]	17	Healthy Controls; Trauma Survivors	Sexual Violence	PASAT	Lower scores in PTSD compared to healthy, but not trauma controls
Vasterling et al. [21]	19	PTSD-free Veterans	Combat	CPT	More commission errors
Vasterling et al. [22]	26	PTSD-free Veterans	Combat	CPT	More omission errors

Table 2. Summary of methodologies and main findings of studies investigating sustained attention in PTSD (Note: CPT = Continuous Performance Task; PASAT = Paced Auditory Serial Attention Task; PTSD = Posttraumatic Stress Disorder; SART = Sustained Attention to Response Task).

Jenkins et al. [25] assessed survivors of sexual violence with and without subsequent development of PTSD, as well as a healthy control group on several tests of cognitive functioning. In order to examine sustained attention in PTSD for both the visual and auditory modality, the authors used two different kinds of tasks. Besides the CPT for visual attention, they presented their subjects with a Paced Serial Auditory Addition Test (PASAT; [26]). Subjects were presented with auditory single digits and instructed to add each new digit to that of a directly preceding trial. Cognitive performance was measured with respect to time needed reporting a sum of digits, as well as the amount of correctly produced sums of digits. Results showed that individuals with PTSD made more omission errors at the CPT and the PASAT compared to trauma and healthy controls. Another study utilized the PASAT for measurement of auditory sustained attention in PTSD [27]. Survivors of sexual violence showed decreased PASAT overall scores compared to healthy individuals, who matched individuals with PTSD in terms of age, education and socioeconomic status. However, there was no apparent difference in accurate task performance between individuals with PTSD and a respective trauma control group.

In sum, we identified shared processing deficits in sustained attention in TBI and PTSD. Specifically, these deficits are pronounced in terms of reduced accurate task performance, while decrements in RT and variability in task performance over time seem to be associated with processing deficits in TBI only.

4. Selective attentional processing in TBI

Selective attention is the ability to focus attentional resources oriented towards a given stimulus despite the presence of distracting or competing stimuli. Difficulties in maintaining concentration and experiences of fatigue are among the most prevalent symptoms in individuals suffering from TBI. In order to cope with general tasks that involve more than one source of stimuli, it is important that individuals are able to separate task- or content-relevant from irrelevant input. Thus, selective attention is usually assessed by tasks requiring subjects to focus on relevant stimuli while ignoring irrelevant and distracting information (Table 3).

In a study by Goethals et al. [28], individuals with severe TBI completed a Stroop Colored Word Test (abbreviated as "Stroop" subsequently; [29]). In the Stroop task, subjects were presented with three different sorts of cards: the first card contained black-printed words of highly distinguishable colors ("blue", "green", "red", "yellow"); the second card depicted rectangles printed in blue, green, red or yellow color ("color-naming" condition); the last card of the Stroop task showed the same words as card one. However, words were not printed in black, but in a color that did not resemble its actual content ("incongruent" condition; i.e., the word "blue" printed in green). Performance on the first card served as a measure of reading abilities. For assessment of selective attention, subjects were compared on a Stroop interference index calculated by subtracting RT of the incongruent condition from those in the color-naming condition. Thus, deficits in selective attention would be reflected by Stroop interference indices, which largely differ from the value 0. In this study by Goethals et al. [28], impairment in Stroop performance was classified as 1 standard deviation (SD) above mean RT of a matched normative sample. Results showed that individuals with TBI showed deficits in the incongruent, but not the color-naming Stroop condition, which might indicate difficulties in selectively

Study	TBI (n)	Post-Trauma	Severity	Trauma Type	Cognitive Test	Main Findings
Belmont et al. [35]	27	3-26 Months	Severe	-	Go/NoGo-Task	Slower RT; More omission errors
Goethals et al. [28]	9	-	Severe	-	Classical Stroop-Task	Impairment on Stroop-Task
Mayer et al. [32]	22	3-20 Days	Mild	Combat; RTA; Falls	Modified Stroop-Task	No differences in RT
Ries et al. [36]	20	12-360 Months	Severe	-	Negative Priming Paradigm	Slower RT and lower accuracy; Negative priming effect on RT for degraded words
Smits et al. [31]	21	30,6 Days	Moderate - Severe	-	Modified Stroop-Task	Moderate: no differences to controls; Severe: lower accuracy on Stroop-Task
Soeda et al. [30]	5	12-84 Months	Severe	RTA	Modified Stroop-Task	No differences in accuracy
Willmott et al. [14]	40	68,38 Days (Range: 12-462)	Moderate - Severe	RTA	SAT; 2&7	Both tests: slower RT; 2&7: lower accuracy; Larger RT differences between SAT tests
Ziino et al. [33]	46	21-1153 Days	Mild - Severe	-	C-SAT	Slower RT; Lower accuracy; no differences in IIV

Table 3. Summary of methodologies and main findings of studies investigating selective attention in TBI (Note: 2&7 = Ruff 2&7 Selective Attention Task; C-SAT = Complex Selective Attention Task; IIV = intra-individual variability; RT = Response time; RTA = Road Traffic Accident; SAT = Sustained Attention Task; TBI = Traumatic Brain Injury; "-" indicates missing or not reported information).

attending towards task-relevant information and to ignore simultaneously occurring and distracting input.

Soeda et al. [30] used a modified version of the Stroop paradigm to assess selective attention in severe TBI. Unlike in the original version of the Stroop task, subjects were asked to validate congruent word and color combinations via button press. This alteration enabled the authors to directly measure levels of accuracy as well as RT. When compared to age- and education-matched healthy controls, individuals with TBI tended to make more errors, although this difference did not reach statistical significance. Another alteration of the original Stroop task has been used by Smits et al. [31], who examined selective attention in two distinct samples of individuals with moderate and severe TBI. In their "counting" Stroop task, subjects were presented with two task conditions: in the neutral condition, subjects had to respond via button press to the displayed amount of words showing animal names; in the incongruent condition, subjects had to indicate the amount of number words that have been presented on the screen, rather than their value, if the word was presented in normal letters (i.e., at the occurrence of three times the word "five", subjects should press a button for "3"). However, in this condition there were deviant trials in which the word representing a number was given in capital letters.

In that case, subjects were asked to validate the numeric value this word was representing (i.e., at the occurrence of three times the word "FIVE", subjects should press a button for "5"). Comparison to a group of healthy controls revealed that individuals with severe but not with moderate TBI made more errors in the incongruent counting Stroop task condition. Mayer et al., [32] varied the Stroop paradigm in a way as to assess selective attention across visual and auditory modalities. The task consisted of congruent and incongruent pairs of simultaneously presented visual and auditory stimuli of written out and pronounced numbers, respectively. Both visual and auditory stimuli occurred at either a high or a low frequency condition in order to induce an increase in cognitive task demands. A preceding multimodal cue instructed subjects to attend to numbers presented in one modality while ignoring the other. Congruent trials referred to identical pairs of simultaneously occurring stimuli, whereas incongruent trials comprised different numbers presented at the same time. When compared to an age- and education-matched healthy control sample, individuals with TBI showed a non-significant trend towards longer RT to incongruent auditory stimuli at high frequency. However, no other effects regarding experimental group, modality or frequency were observed.

Besides the classical or modified versions of the Stroop paradigm, several other cognitive tasks have been used to assess selective attention in TBI. Ziino et al. [33] developed a Complex Selective Attention Task (C-SAT) in order to examine individuals with mild to severe TBI and an age- and education-matched healthy control group on selective attentional processing. The C-SAT required subjects to respond to combinations of red- or green-colored letters and numbers with specific button presses (i.e., right button for green letter/red number; left button for right letter/green number). Subjects were compared on measures of accuracy by means of errors (pressing the wrong button) and misses (not pressing any button during a predefined period of time), as well as RT. The authors argued that this task is especially difficult for subjects suffering from TBI, since it requires a larger working memory load compared to rather simple selective attention tasks [33]. Individuals with TBI showed lower levels of accuracy with significantly more produced errors than healthy individuals, as well as slower RT. Both groups were also compared on variability in RT. However, there was no apparent greater response variability for individuals with TBI as a group.

Alongside a variety of other cognitive functions, Willmott et al. [14] tested selective attention in individuals with moderate to severe TBI using two different behavioral tasks: the Ruff 2 and 7 Selective Attention Test (2&7; [34]) and the Selective Attention Task (SAT; [33]). The 2&7 is a paper-and-pencil task that required subjects to manually cross out the digits "2" and "7", which were presented within a series of either letters or other digits. The procedure of the SAT was similar to that of the C-SAT reported previously [33] with the alteration that Willmott et al. [14] added a simple version to the SAT (SSAT). The difference between SSAT and C-SAT lay within its rather low cognitive demand; subjects were asked to respond with two distinct button presses if a letter or number was shown in a specific color (i.e., right button for yellow, left button for brown targets). For both tasks, subjects were measured on accuracy and RT. Results of the 2&7 revealed that individuals with TBI were less accurate and slower cancelling out digits embedded within letters, as well as within series of other digits. However, the difference between both task conditions was larger in the healthy control group. In the SAT, individuals with TBI showed slower RT than healthy individuals. Moreover, differences in RT between the SSAT and C-SAT were larger for individuals with TBI indicating that this group had problems with the more cognitively demanding version of the SAT. Belmont et al. [35] implemented a basic Go/NoGo paradigm in their study in order to assess selective attention in a sample of individuals with severe TBI. The task required subjects to respond to target letters via button press and withhold their response at the occurrence of non-targets. Performance of individuals with TBI was compared to that of gender-, age- and education-matched healthy individuals by means of accuracy, that is, the amount of omission errors, as well as RT. The authors found that individuals with TBI made more omission errors and were generally slower in responding than healthy individuals.

Ries et al. [36] used a negative priming paradigm that took into account response inhibition as part of a selective attentional process. Thus, selective attention would be reflected by both facilitation of the selected target as well as suppression of distracting information [37]. In their behavioral task, the authors presented individuals with severe TBI and healthy controls with two subsequent screens per trial, which consisted of a priming display followed by a probe display. Both displays showed two words in two different colors indicating targets and distractors. Additionally to targets or distractors, words were visually degraded in several ways and presented on 50% of the probe displays only. The other 50% of the probe displays consisted of intact word stimuli. Subjects were asked to respond to target words on the prime displays verbally by reading them out loudly. The authors hypothesized that negative priming of intact target words on priming displays would result in inhibitory difficulties on subsequent probe trials in individuals with TBI. Results showed that individuals with TBI generally had slower RT than healthy individuals. Moreover, word degradation slowed RT in both experimental groups, whereas this effect was even significantly more pronounced in individuals with TBI. For intact stimuli, there was a negative priming effect on RT for healthy individuals, but not individuals with TBI. Nonetheless, negative priming affected RT for both groups when stimuli were degraded. Also, individuals with TBI were less accurate than healthy controls. However, neither stimulus degradation nor negative priming had an effect on accuracy of both groups. Ries et al. [36] interpreted their findings as being indicative of inhibitory difficulties in individuals with severe TBI.

5. Selective attentional processing in PTSD

Interference of emotional or threat-related stimuli on attentional processing has been commonly reported in individuals diagnosed with PTSD [38-43]. A range of studies aimed to investigate if this interference could be translated to a context of stimuli with solely neutral valence as well. Problems in selecting task relevant cues while ignoring distracting information might reflect a general attentional deficit in PTSD, which could not be addressed to emotional saliency per se (Table 4).

Study	PTSD (n)	Control Group	Trauma Type	Cognitive Test	Main Findings
Bryant et al. [45]	14	Non-traumatized Controls	Interpersonal Violence; RTA	Oddball Paradigm	No differences in RT
Jenkins et al. [25]	15	Trauma Survivors	Sexual Violence	Posner Visual Selective Attention Task	No differences in RT
Vasterling et al. [21]	19	PTSD-free Veterans	Combat	Stroop-Task	No differences in Stroop Interference Scores
Vasterling et al. [22]	26	PTSD-free Veterans	Combat	Stroop-Task	No differences in Stroop Interference Scores

Table 4. Summary of methodologies and main findings of studies investigating selective attention in PTSD (Note: PTSD = Posttraumatic Stress Disorder; RT = Response time; RTA = Road Traffic Accident).

Studies on selective attention deficits in PTSD incorporating neutral stimuli are rather rare. In two consecutive studies, Vasterling et al. [21, 22] assessed selective attention in Vietnam and Gulf War veterans with PTSD and healthy controls on a Stroop task. For both studies, PTSD subjects did not show any differences to healthy individuals on Stroop interference scores. In a series of cognitive tests, Jenkins et al. [25] instructed subjects to perform the Posner Visual Selective Attention Task [44]. In this task, subjects were asked to respond to a target with a button press, which was preceded by two different sorts of cues indicating the position of the target on a computer screen. Valid cues predicted the actual later position of the target, whereas invalid cues appeared at the target's opposite location (i.e., cue on left side of the screen, subsequent target on the right side). Survivors of sexual violence with PTSD were compared to a group of survivors of similar trauma events without PTSD and a group of healthy individuals on RT measures. Results revealed no difference in RT between corresponding groups. Bryant et al. [45] used an oddball paradigm to assess selective attention in individuals with PTSD and trauma-free controls. Auditory stimuli consisted of standard and target tones differing in frequency with target tones occurring at a probability of 15% during the experiment. There was no statistical evidence for differences in RT between both groups.

Put together, TBI appears to be accompanied by deficits in selective attention. These deficits are mainly expressed in terms of reduced accuracy in cognitive tasks, as well as a general slowing in RT. However, no study on selective attention in PTSD revealed corresponding findings, which might be related to a shortage of empirical studies addressing selective attentional processing in PTSD.

6. Discussion

Results of the here reviewed studies suggest a shared processing deficit in sustained attention towards stimuli with neutral valence for TBI and PTSD (Figure 1). This attentional deficit is expressed in terms of reduced accuracy levels when cognitive task performance of individuals with TBI or PTSD is compared to that of healthy controls. In contrast to a shared deficit in accuracy for sustained attention tasks, findings on selective attention in TBI and PTSD point towards a processing deficit of neutral stimuli that is only observed in TBI. Studies assessing individuals with TBI reported reduced accuracy in task performance, as well as a general slowing in RT across different cognitive tasks, levels of severity and trauma types. However, no such corresponding findings were demonstrated in studies that assessed individuals diagnosed with PTSD on selective attention tasks. In order to understand why sustained attention tasks reveal shared attentional deficits in TBI and PTSD, but selective attention tasks do not, we have to consider several aspects that might help explaining our main findings such as the general mechanisms incorporated in execution of cognitive tasks, the subjects' states of arousal, as well as neural correlates underlying attentional processing in TBI and PTSD.

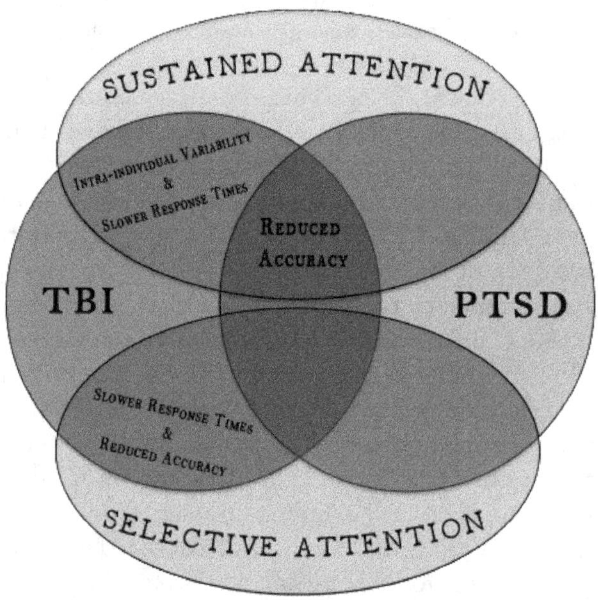

Figure 1. Schematic overview of shared and exclusive attentional processing deficits towards stimuli with neutral valence in Traumatic Brian Injury (TBI) and Posttraumatic Stress Disorder (PTSD).

6.1. The role of response inhibition

Sustained attention is mainly assessed by tasks following the Go/NoGo paradigm (i.e., SART and CPT). Here, subjects are instructed to maintain responsive to a set of targets via button press while withholding responses to a predefined and randomly occurring type of stimulus. Thus, accurate performance of a Go/NoGo-task requires subjects' ability of response inhibition. According to this rationale, we might question if a shared deficit resulting from sustained attention tasks is solely pronounced by reduced levels of accuracy, or would also reflect impairments in response inhibition. However, our findings do not support this idea. There is an obvious pattern between the here reviewed studies, which shows that studies assessing TBI and PTSD reported more commission errors only in tasks following the Go/NoGo paradigm. Commission errors are also considered false responses/alarms and occur when subjects fail to inhibit responses to a specific stimulus. However, it does not necessarily follow from these findings that a deficit in sustained attention reflects impairments in response inhibition. To the contrary, studies also reported increases in omission errors while assessing individuals with TBI and PTSD. Omission errors usually reflect missing responses to present targets and, therefore, do not require the ability to withhold responses. Additionally, other studies, which do not utilize a Go/NoGo paradigm within their cognitive tasks, report generally reduced accuracy in terms of lower hit rates towards target detection (which is similar to the concept of omission errors) in TBI and PTSD [16, 20]. Thus, it seems tempting, but unlikely that deficits in sustained attention can be simply addressed to impairments in response inhibition. Instead, there appears to be a deficit in sustained attention in terms of accuracy that is present in both TBI and PTSD.

Studies assessing selective attention point towards a processing deficit of neutral stimuli that is only observed in TBI (Figure 1). Tasks implemented in these studies follow rationales that require selection of content- and task-relevant information while inhibiting simultaneously occurring and competing sensory input (i.e., Stroop task; [28, 30-33, 36]. Thus, selective attention deficits expressed by reduced accuracy and slowing of RT might be related to an underlying impairment to inhibit distracting simultaneous information. Unlike commission errors in Go/NoGo-tasks, there is no equivalent specific accuracy measure, which might indicate an apparent deficit in response inhibition for individuals with TBI while performing selective attention tasks. It might be reasonable to assume that deficits on tasks such as the Stroop display impairments in inhibitory processes [29]. However, given that selective attention deficits have also been reported for TBI in tasks that do not require inhibition of simultaneously occurring input [14], results on these tasks do not necessarily explain selective attention deficits in individuals with TBI.

6.2. The impact of fatigue, arousal and emotion

Since neither sustained nor selective attentional processing deficits are fully explained by impairments of inhibitory mechanisms, we might argue that attentional deficits could possibly result from other phenomena that might be shared by or exclusive to TBI and PTSD. TBI has previously been associated with states of mental fatigue and sleep disturbances [46]. Two of the studies reviewed here extent this view by contrasting performance of sleep-deprived and normal sleeping individuals with TBI on a sustained attention task [15], as well as individuals with TBI and healthy individuals on a cognitive task that has been implemented in sleep studies previously [16]. Both studies propose a sustained attention deficit that is even more pronounced in the presence of sleep disturbances in individuals with TBI. Although Bloomfield et al. [15] reported more commission errors in "poor" sleepers with TBI when compared to "good" sleepers, very recent findings by Sinclair et al. [16] point towards possible floor effects of sleep difficulties in TBI. Since differences between groups in this study diminished as soon as the authors controlled for reported fatigue and sleep disturbances in their statistical analyses, it is hard to argue that these factors might exacerbate already present accuracy deficits in sustained attention for individuals with TBI. The inclusion of a healthy control group with or without sleeping difficulties in a study similar to that by Bloomfield et al. [15] might shed some light on the question in how far sleep disturbances or mental fatigue possibly influence the severity of sustained attention deficits in individuals with TBI. Sleep disturbances are also considered one of the hallmarks in PTSD [1]. However, sleep disturbances in PTSD are mainly pronounced in terms of reoccurring nightmares that resemble aspects of the experienced traumatic event. Therefore, sleep disturbances in PTSD might be rather related to mechanisms that enter the domain of memory and affective states than basic attentional processing (for a review on mechanisms of sleep disturbances in PTSD, see [47]). To our knowledge, there is only one recent study that examined the relation between attentional processing deficits and sleep disturbances in PTSD [48]. In this study, individuals with disaster-related PTSD-symptomatology were assessed on the PASAT. Behavioral outcomes, that is, the number of correct responses in the PASAT, were then related to self-reported symptom severity, including subscales of sleep disturbances. Although results revealed that deficits in sustained attention increased with symptom severity, there was no evidence for an impact of sleep disturbances on attentional processing. The authors argued that the lack of impact of sleep disturbance might be indicative of a solely attentional deficit in PTSD.

Although results from studies reviewed here are somewhat inconsistent with respect to how or if sleep disturbances and fatigue might influence performance on sustained attention tasks, we nonetheless see the urge to consider them in explaining a shared deficit for TBI and PTSD. Cognitive tasks assessing sustained attention are rather simple and modest in terms of duration. The original SART was administered over a period of 4.3 minutes [11]. Other sustained attention tasks, such as the PVT, show high validity when administered over a period of 10 minutes [17]. One might argue that tasks lasting shorter than 15 min might not be able to display the ability to maintain vigilance over time. However, we need to keep in mind that individuals with TBI, as well as those diagnosed with PTSD, might suffer from severe cognitive impairments, which could account for findings on sustained attention presented here. Symptoms of fatigue and difficulties to concentrate have been reported for both TBI and PTSD [4]. Thus, we propose that a shared deficit in sustained attentional processing might reflect a common underlying symptom in both medical conditions.

In selective attention tasks, processing deficits were observed for individuals with TBI, but not for those diagnosed with PTSD. Since deficits in selective attention for individuals with TBI are expressed in terms of decreased accuracy, as well as slower RT, we might again argue that impairments in TBI could be a possible consequence of states of fatigue. Studies reported that errors in selective attention task highly correlated with measures of self-reported fatigue [33, 35]. This effect even remained when results were controlled for mood by depression or general anxiety assessment scales. However, we did not find any apparent selective attentional processing deficits for studies on PTSD. Noteworthy, cognitive tasks assessing selective attention require larger mental effort than sustained attention tasks. Thus, selective attentional processing deficits only observed in TBI might be linked to increases in task difficulty and cognitive demands. Vice versa, an absent selective attention deficit in PTSD might reflect intact arousal, that is, a general reactivity and alertness to stimuli with neutral valence. This would be in line with symptoms of hyper-arousal, which are underlying the diagnosis of PTSD [1]. Nonetheless, the studies reviewed here did not report any facilitating effects towards stimuli for individuals with PTSD either. It seems more reasonable that states of hyper-arousal are closely related to stimuli with emotional valence. A vast amount of studies suggests that in studies on PTSD, individuals' performance on cognitive tasks is highly affected by interference of emotionally related stimuli [38-43]. Consequently, intact selective attentional processing might serve as a marker for subsequent development of hyper-arousal, and thus, would in part explain absent deficits on selective attention in individuals with PTSD reviewed here.

6.3. Neural correlates of sustained and selective attention in TBI and PTSD

It is rather difficult to draw an overall picture related to the impact of brain damage in TBI on behavioral results in this review. One major drawback in studies assessing attentional processing in TBI concerns missing reports of lesion sites in TBI. It seems quite obvious that damage to different brain regions may affect various cognitive networks and might subsequently result in a variety of behavioral and cognitive impairments. Within the studies reviewed here, only one systematically reported lesion sites for each participating individual [12]. However, given a large heterogeneity in lesion sites within the study's sample of individuals with TBI, the authors did not make any further relations between damaged brain regions and behavioral outcomes.

Regardless of challenges to make inferences of neurobiological deficits based on individual damage to the cortex, a handful of studies made an attempt to relate attentional deficits to alterations or specific states of cortical activity in individuals with TBI. Studies on attention in TBI reported deactivation of cortical areas relevant for accurate task performance [32], as well as changes in cerebral blood flow of the brain in resting state [19], that is, cortical activity and functional connectivity without stimulus-induced processing demands. The brain in resting state comprises a default mode network (DMN), which includes medial portions of the parietal, frontal and temporal cortex [49]. In individuals with TBI, studies indicate that insufficient deactivation of the DMN during cognitive tasks, as well as functional connectivity between areas incorporated in the DMN might be a neurological marker of behavioral deficits observed in sustained attention tasks [18, 32]. Similar to TBI, we identified only few studies that directly linked cortical abnormalities accompanying PTD to deficits in sustained attentional processing. Here, study results indicated that stress induced in combat-related situations might affect sustained attention task performance by a decrease in midbrain activity [50]; an effect, which seemed to diminish after multiple testing sessions, providing evidence for recovery mechanisms related to combat PTSD. However, studies examining the direct relations between attention to neutral stimuli and neural processing in PTSD are still rare. Hence, it seems quite assumptive to derive specific implementations for treatment or cognitive improvements from single study results.

Studies assessing selective attentional processing in TBI reported both decreases [30] or increases [31] in activity of the anterior cingulate cortex (ACC). Since this area is assumed to be involved in conflict monitoring [51], a mechanism essential for specific selective attention tasks such as the Stroop, decreases in task-related activity might reflect underlying impairments in cortical processing that could partially explain selective attentional processing deficits in TBI. However, studies did not distinguish between dorsal or rostral portions of the ACC. The former is assumed to be involved in general cognitive processing, whereas the latter shows responsiveness to stimuli with emotional valence, which might possibly account for these contradictory findings. Accordingly, increased activity in the ACC has been reported in studies on selective attention in PTSD [45, 52], including both dorsal and rostral portions. Thus, processing of stimuli in selective attention tasks appears to be unaffected at least in the ACC for individuals diagnosed with PTSD. Contrasting these results with decreases in ACC activity for TBI might serve as an indicator why selective attentional processing deficits were only observed in individuals with TBI.

6.4. Attentional deficits in comorbid TBI and PTSD

Historically speaking, it was long debated if TBI and PTSD could arise in a comorbid fashion, since TBI is accompanied by at least partial loss of consciousness and posttraumatic amnesia [12, 16, 19, 20, 32, 33]. According to this theory, amnesia or loss of consciousness would circumvent construction of a trauma-related memory, which is considered to facilitate PTSD-related symptoms, such as intrusive thoughts and re-experiencing. However, recent research proposed that TBI and PTSD share certain diagnostic features (for an extensive review, see [53]). As stated previously, it is assumed nowadays that TBI and PTSD occur at a prevalence rate of almost 50% [1]. Moreover, several case studies provided evidence that comorbid TBI and PTSD are not only theoretically related, but require accurate and reliable rehabilitation and treatment plans [2, 3]. Thus, we see a necessity to further explore attentional processing in populations with comorbid TBI and PTSD. To our knowledge, there is only one study that examined attentional processing in individuals with combat-related comorbid TBI and PTSD [54]. Individuals with comorbidity diagnosis were compared to two control groups, a group consisting of individuals with PTSD only and healthy controls on measures of the Attentional Network Task (ANT; [55]). The authors used the ANT to assess attentional processing on three distinct metrics, each reflecting a different aspect of attention: (1) *alerting*; (2) *orienting*; (3) *executive*. Although the ANT's theoretical framework slightly differs from other cognitive tasks reviewed in this work, we might link its alerting and executive networks to mechanisms of sustained and selective attention, respectively [54]. Study results indicated that individuals with comorbid TBI and PTSD were less accurate and slower in responding, and showed higher variability in responses compared to both the PTSD and healthy control group. Respective effects were also observable between individuals with PTSD and healthy controls, although without statistical significance. These findings were in line with several findings of attentional processing deficits described above. While there appeared to be a clear pattern for deficits in sustained and selective attention in TBI, this picture is less consistent in PTSD. Barlow-Odgen et al. [54] pointed out that none of the participating subjects had an exclusive diagnosis of TBI, but was always accompanied by PTSD. More systematic research on comorbid TBI and PTSD and even the inclusion of a group that only consists of individuals with TBI might further progress our understanding about shared and exclusive attentional processes in TBI and PTSD. Besides a considerable prevalence rate of comorbid TBI and PTSD, individuals with PTSD are very likely to meet criteria of at least one other psychiatric disorder [1]. Correspondingly, psychiatric disorders, which also occur at a high comorbidity rate with PTSD, including other anxiety disorders, depression [56] and substance abuse disorder [57], might exacerbate the impact of attentional processing in PTSD.

6.5. Implications for rehabilitation and treatment

Based on results discussed here, we believe that attentional processing deficits need to be particularly considered when developing and conducting treatment and rehabilitation programs for both TBI and PTSD. To date, cognitive training is highly recommended during TBI in a post-acute phase, including attention training and metacognitive training, but not at an acute stage [58]. Hence, results reviewed here might aid an even further detailed and specialized cognitive training, which takes into account specific deficits in sustained and selective attentional processing for individuals with TBI. Moreover, despite the concrete implementations for cognitive training, the general finding of sustained and selective attention deficits across trauma severity, the time since traumatic event and type of trauma might also affect other types of treatment approaches in TBI, such as physical and ergonomic rehabilitation programs, as well as speech or psychological therapy. Individuals with TBI consistently display difficulties to maintain attention during a cognitive task (e.g., [10, 12]). It seems reasonable that this deficit might also influence performance on other everyday situations that require the ability to stay vigilant over a specific period of time. Findings of studies reviewed here might support that adjustments of rehabilitation or training sessions to apparent impairments on sustained attention tasks could result in improvements of treatment outcome. We also think that findings of this review might especially promote treatment of comorbid TBI and PTSD or PTSD following TBI, respectively. Clinical case studies revealed that sustained and selective attentional difficulties are already tackled in intervention plans for PTSD following a traumatic accident [2]. Providing evidence that impairments in sustained attention are present in both TBI and PTSD populations and selective attention is preserved in the latter might serve as a blueprint for future treatment approaches, especially in terms of session duration and distribution over time. This might, for instance, be achieved by adjustment of intervention plans of cognitive training for shorter, but more frequent training sessions.

7. Limitations

Although we were able to shed some light on shared and rather exclusive attentional processing deficits in TBI and PTSD, there are some limitations to this review and selected studies that need to be taken into account. First of all, there is an extensive amount of literature on attentional processing in TBI using neutral stimuli. However, this is not the case for PTSD, where a vast amount of studies on attentional processing focuses on emotion-related stimuli and research and, thus, tends to neglect corresponding experimental designs that assess similar mechanisms related to stimuli with neutral valence. One might argue that this is not really surprising, since it appears more likely to find considerable differences between individuals with PTSD and control groups when emotion or even trauma-relevant content is involved. However, this tendency could lead to a publication bias that, in turn, might result in lost opportunities to identify basic cognitive mechanisms involved in the onset and development of PTSD. Another point of limitation refers to heterogeneity in study designs, which is mostly pronounced for those studies examining attentional processing in TBI. Given that most studies differ in terms of TBI severity, type of trauma, and time elapsed since traumatic events, it is unlikely to identify a pattern that might point towards possible recovery effects or impact of damage to specific brain regions. Regarding type of trauma, the same inconsistencies in etiology and causalities between studies could be observed in PTSD.

We would also like to point out that there is a rather low verge between continuous vigilant task performance, as reflected by sustained attention, and higher cognitive functions, such as working memory. Some of the studies reviewed here used cognitive tasks or alterations of task designs to recruit higher cognitive demands, which also incorporated working memory capacities [33]. We might question if accurate and fast performance on these kinds of tasks still exclusively reflects attentional processing. Regardless of mechanisms of attention, working memory deficits are a comprehensively investigated cognitive mechanism in TBI. Even within those studies presented here, tasks on working memory were part of larger setups of cognitive tasks [19, 20, 31]. Similar to performance on sustained attention tasks, results on working memory function revealed reduced accuracy levels for TBI, with task performance getting worse with an increase in working memory load [31].

We would like to emphasize that the purpose of this review was to provide improved insight on attentional processing, which might be shared by or be rather exclusive to TBI and PTSD. Thus, one might question the ecological validity of the cognitive tasks that were used throughout the studies reviewed here. Identification of overlap in potential attentional processing deficits should ultimately result in implications on how to provide suitable treatment and rehabilitation approaches. However, experimental settings assessing attention with cognitive tasks are usually highly artificial. Parsons et al. [59] made an interesting attempt towards an increased ecological setting for such tasks. The authors developed a virtual reality Stroop task that exposes individuals to an everyday-life or work-related environment. This approach might serve as one step towards more genuine experimental designs. In turn, these designs may elicit attentional processing mechanisms, which are more closely related to real-life situations for affected individuals in both TBI and PTSD. Consequently, improving the ecological validity of cognitive tasks will not only provide a more accurate picture of the underlying mechanisms in attentional processing in both medical conditions, but might also provide a more seamless translation between cognitive assessment (i.e., characterization of cognitive mechanisms or deficits) and rehabilitation approaches.

8. Conclusion

To this end, in this work we reviewed studies that assessed individuals with TBI, as well as those diagnosed with PTSD, on measures of sustained and selective attention to stimuli with neutral valence. Results of cognitive tasks measuring sustained attention suggest a shared deficit for TBI and PTSD, which is mainly characterized by a reduction in accurate task performance. Additionally, deficits in sustained attention for TBI are characterized by a general slowing in responses, as well as variability in RT and accuracy over time. In contrast to a shared accuracy deficit in sustained attention for TBI and PTSD, the studies reviewed here point towards impairments in selective attention only observed for TBI as reflected by reduced levels of accuracy and slowing in RT. However, no behavioral deficits for selective attentional processing were found in PTSD. In order to unravel such specific cognitive processing mechanisms in TBI and PTSD, we strongly encourage the conduction of future studies explicitly considering the impact of factors, such as (1) the type of traumatic event, (2) lesion severity and lesion sites in TBI, and (3) comorbid occurring TBI and PTSD on behavioral and rehabilitation outcomes. We also see a need for studies focusing on cognitive processes in PTSD to neutral rather than only emotionally loaded stimuli. Our review proposes that shared and exclusive attentional processing deficits in TBI and PTSD should be considered when developing or improving already existing post-trauma treatment approaches.

Acknowledgements

The authors would like to thank Centre Interdisciplinaire de Recherche en Réadaptation et Intégration Sociale (CIRRIS), Quebec City, Canada, the Canada Research Chair in Cognitive Neuroplasticity, Laval University, and the Faculty of Psychology and Neuroscience, Maastricht University, Maastricht, The Netherlands for supporting this work.

Author details

Tobias Wensing[1,2], Jean Levasseur-Moreau[1,3,4], Alexander T. Sack[2,5] and Shirley Fecteau[1,3,4*]

*Address all correspondence to: shirley.fecteau@fmed.ulaval.ca

1 Centre Interdisciplinaire de Recherche en Réadaptation et Intégration Sociale, Canada

2 Faculty of Psychology and Neuroscience, Maastricht University, Maastricht, The Netherlands

3 Centre de Recherche Universitaire en Santé Mentale de Québec, Quebec, Canada

4 Medical School, Laval University, Quebec, Canada

5 Maastricht Brain Imaging Center, Maastricht University, Maastricht, The Netherlands

References

[1] American Psychiatric Association. Diagnostic and statistical manual of mental disorders. 5th ed. Washington, D.C.: American Psychiatric Association; 2013.

[2] Williams WH, Evans JJ, Wilson BA. Neurorehabilitation for two cases of post-traumatic stress disorder following traumatic brain injury. Cognitive Neuropsychiatry 2003;8(1) 1–18.

[3] Ryan PB, Lee-Wilk T, Kok BC, Wilk JE. Interdisciplinary rehabilitation of mild TBI and PTSD: A case report. Brain Injury 2011;25(10) 1019–1025.

[4] Stein M, McAllister T. Exploring the convergence of posttraumatic stress disorder and mild traumatic brain injury. American Journal of Psychiatry 2009;166 768–776.

[5] McAllister TW. Neurobiological consequences of traumatic brain injury. Dialogues in Clinical Neuroscience 2011;13(3) 287-300.

[6] Corbetta M, Shulman GL. Control of goal-directed and stimulus-driven attention in the brain. Nature Reviews Neuroscience 2002;3(3) 201–215.

[7] Petersen SE, Posner MI. The Attention System of the Human Brain: 20 Years After. Annual Review of Neuroscience 2012;35(1) 73–89.

[8] Wager TD, Jonides J, Reading S. Neuroimaging studies of shifting attention: a meta-analysis. NeuroImage 2004;22(4) 1679–1693.

[9] Warm JS, Parasuraman R, Matthews G. Vigilance Requires Hard Mental Work and Is Stressful. Human Factors: The Journal of the Human Factors and Ergonomics Society 2008;50(3) 433–441.

[10] McAvinue L, O'Keeffe FM, McMackin D, Robertson IH. Impaired sustained attention and error awareness in traumatic brain injury: Implications for insight. Neuropsychological Rehabilitation 2005;15(5) 569–587.

[11] Robertson IH, Manly T, Andrade J, Baddeley BT, Yiend J. " Oops!": Performance correlates of everyday attentional failures in traumatic brain injured and normal subjects. Neuropsychologia 1997;35(6) 747-758.

[12] Dockree PM, Bellgrove MA, O'Keeffe FM, Moloney P, Aimola L, Carton S, et al. Sustained attention in traumatic brain injury (TBI) and healthy controls: enhanced sensitivity with dual-task load. Experimental Brain Research 2006;168(1-2) 218–229.

[13] Rosvold HE, Mirsky AF, Sarason I, Bransome ED Jr, Beck LH. A continuous performance test of brain damage. Journal of Consulting Psychology 1956;20(5) 343-350.

[14] Willmott C, Ponsford JL, Hocking C, Schönberger M. Factors contributing to attentional impairments after traumatic brain injury. Neuropsychology 2009;23(4) 424–432.

[15] Bloomfield IL, Espie CA, Evans JJ. Do sleep difficulties exacerbate deficits in sustained attention following traumatic brain injury? Journal of the International Neuropsychological Society 2010;16(1) 17-25.

[16] Sinclair KL, Ponsford JL, Rajaratnam SMW, Anderson C. Sustained attention following traumatic brain injury: Use of the Psychomotor Vigilance Task. Journal of Clinical and Experimental Neuropsychology 2013;35(2) 210–224.

[17] Dinges DF, Powell JW. Microcomputer analyses of performance on a portable, simple visual RT task during sustained operations. Behavior Research Methods, Instruments, & Computers 1985;17(6) 652–655.

[18] Bonnelle V, Leech R, Kinnunen KM, Ham TE, Beckmann CF, De Boissezon X, et al. Default Mode Network Connectivity Predicts Sustained Attention Deficits after Traumatic Brain Injury. Journal of Neuroscience 2011;31(38) 13442–13451.

[19] Kim J, Whyte J, Patel S, Europa E, Slattery J, Coslett HB, et al. A Perfusion fMRI Study of the Neural Correlates of Sustained-Attention and Working-Memory Deficits in Chronic Traumatic Brain Injury. Neurorehabilitation and Neural Repair 2012;26(7) 870–880.

[20] Slovarp L, Azuma T, LaPointe L. The effect of traumatic brain injury on sustained attention and working memory. Brain Injury 2012;26(1) 48–57.

[21] Vasterling JJ, Brailey K, Constans JI, Sutker PB. Attention and Memory Dysfunction in Posttraumatic Stress Disorder. Neuropsychology 1998;12(1) 125–133.

[22] Vasterling JJ, Duke LM, Brailey K, Constans JI, Allain AN, Sutker PB. Attention, learning, and memory performances and intellectual resources in Vietnam veterans: PTSD and no disorder comparisons. Neuropsychology 2002;16(1) 5–14.

[23] Koso M, Hansen S. Executive function and memory in posttraumatic stress disorder: a study of Bosnian war veterans. European Psychiatry 2006;21(3) 167–173.

[24] Shucard JL, McCabe DC, Szymanski H. An event-related potential study of attention deficits in posttraumatic stress disorder during auditory and visual Go/NoGo continuous performance tasks. Biological Psychology 2008;79(2) 223–233.

[25] Jenkins MA, Langlais PJ, Delis D, Cohen RA. Attentional Dysfunction Associated with Posttraumatic Stress Disorder Among Rape Survivors. Clinical Neuropsychology 2000;14(1) 7–12.

[26] Gronwall DMA. Paced Auditory Serial-Addition Task: A Measure of Recovery from Concussion. Perceptual and Motor Skills 1977;44 367–373.

[27] Stein MB, Kennedy CM, Twamley EW. Neuropsychological function in female victims of intimate partner violence with and without posttraumatic stress disorder. Biological Psychiatry 2002;52(11) 1079–1088.

[28] Goethals I, Audenaert K, Jacobs F, Lannoo E, Van de Wiele C, Ham H, et al. Cognitive neuroactivation using SPECT and the Stroop Colored Word Test in patients with diffuse brain injury. Journal of Neurotrauma 2004;21(8) 1059–1069.

[29] Stroop JR. Studies of interference in serial verbal reactions. Journal of Experimental Psychology 1935;18(6) 643-662.

[30] Soeda A, Nakashima T, Okumura A, Kuwata K, Shinoda J, Iwama T. Cognitive impairment after traumatic brain injury: a functional magnetic resonance imaging study using the Stroop task. Neuroradiology 2005;47(7) 501–506.

[31] Smits M, Dippel DWJ, Houston GC, Wielopolski PA, Koudstaal PJ, Hunink MGM, et al. Postconcussion syndrome after minor head injury: Brain activation of working memory and attention. Human Brain Mapping 2009;30(9) 2789–2803.

[32] Mayer AR, Yang Z, Yeo RA, Pena A, Ling JM, Mannell MV, et al. A functional MRI study of multimodal selective attention following mild traumatic brain injury. Brain Imaging and Behavior 2012;6(2) 343–354.

[33] Ziino C, Ponsford JL. Selective attention deficits and subjective fatigue following traumatic brain injury. Neuropsychology 2006;20(3) 383–390.

[34] Ruff RM, Niemann H, Allen CC, Farrow CE, Wylie T. The Ruff 2 and 7 Selective Attention test: A Neuropsychological Application. Perceptual and Motor Skills 1992;75 1311–1319.

[35] Belmont A, Agar N, Azouvi P. Subjective Fatigue, Mental Effort, and Attention Deficits After Severe Traumatic Brain Injury. Neurorehabilitation and Neural Repair 2009;23(9) 939–944.

[36] Ries M, Marks W. Selective Attention Deficits Following Severe Closed Head Injury: The Role of Inhibitory Processes. Neuropsychology 2005;19(4) 476–483.

[37] Neill WT. Inhibitory and facilitatory processes in selective attention. Journal of Experimental Psychology: Human Perception and Performance 1977;3(3) 444-450.

[38] McNally RJ, Kaspi SP, Riemann BC, Zeitlin SB. Selective processing of threat cues in posttraumatic stress disorder. Journal of Abnormal Psychology 1990;99(4) 398–402.

[39] Buckley TC, Blanchard EB, Neill WT. Information processing and PTSD: a review of the empirical literature. Clinical Psychology Review 2000;20(8) 1041–1065.

[40] Constans JI, McCloskey MS, Vasterling JJ, Brailey K, Mathews A. Suppression of Attentional Bias in PTSD. Journal of Abnormal Psychology 2004;113(2) 315–323.

[41] Bardeen JR, Orcutt HK. Attentional control as a moderator of the relationship between posttraumatic stress symptoms and attentional threat bias. Journal of Anxiety Disorders 2011;25(8) 1008–1018.

[42] El Khoury-Malhame M, Reynaud E, Soriano A, Michael K, Salgado-Pineda P, Zendjidjian X, et al. Amygdala activity correlates with attentional bias in PTSD. Neuropsychologia 2011;49(7) 1969–1973.

[43] Fani N, Tone EB, Phifer J, Norrholm SD, Bradley B, Ressler KJ, et al. Attention bias toward threat is associated with exaggerated fear expression and impaired extinction in PTSD. Psychological Medicine 2011;42(03) 533–543.

[44] Posner MI., Cohen Y. Components of visual orienting. In: Bouma H., Bonwhuis (eds.) Attention and performance X: Control of language processes. Hillsdale, N. J.: Erlbaum; 1984. p551-556.

[45] Bryant RA, Felmingham KL, Kemp AH, Barton M, Peduto AS, Rennie C, et al. Neural Networks of Information Processing in Posttraumatic Stress Disorder: A Functional Magnetic Resonance Imaging Study. Biological Psychiatry 2005;58(2) 111–118.

[46] Fichtenberg NL, Zafonte RD, Putnam S, Mann NR, Millard AE. Insomnia in a post-acute brain injury sample. Brain Injury 2002;16(3) 197–206.

[47] Germain A. Sleep disturbances as the hallmark of PTSD: where are we now? American Journal of Psychiatry 2013;170(4) 372–382.

[48] Meewisse M-L, Nijdam MJ, de Vries G-J, Gersons BPR, Kleber RJ, van der Velden PG, et al. Disaster-related posttraumatic stress symptoms and sustained attention: Evaluation of depressive symptomatology and sleep disturbances as mediators. Journal of Traumatic Stress 2005;18(4) 299–302.

[49] Raichle ME, MacLeod AM, Snyder AZ, Powers WJ, Gusnard DA, Shulman GL. A default mode of brain function. Proceedings of the National Academy of Sciences of the United States of America 2001;98(2) 676–682.

[50] van Wingen GA, Geuze E, Caan MWA, Kozicz T, Olabarriaga SD, Denys D, et al. Persistent and reversible consequences of combat stress on the mesofrontal circuit and cognition. Proceedings of the National Academy of Science 2012;109(38) 15508–15513.

[51] Botvinick M, Nystrom LE, Fissell K, Carter CS, Cohen JD. Conflict monitoring versus selection-for-action in anterior cingulate cortex. Nature 1999;402(6758) 179–181.

[52] Shin LM, Bush G, Milad MR, Lasko NB, Brohawn KH, Hughes KC, et al. Exaggerated activation of dorsal anterior cingulate cortex during cognitive interference: a monozygotic twin study of posttraumatic stress disorder. American Journal of Psychiatry 2011;168(9) 979–985.

[53] Bryant RA. Posttraumatic stress disorder and traumatic brain injury: can they co-exist? Clinical Psychology Review 2001;21(6) 931–948.

[54] Barlow-Ogden K, Poynter W. Mild traumatic brain injury and posttraumatic stress disorder: Investigation of visual attention in Operation Iraqi Freedom/Operation Enduring Freedom veterans. Journal of Rehabilitation Research and Development 2012;49(7) 1101-1114.

[55] Fan J, McCandliss BD, Sommer T, Raz A, Posner ML. Testing the Efficiency and Independence of Attentional Networks. Journal of Cognitive Neuroscience 2002;14(3) 340–347.

[56] Ginzburg K, Ein-Dor T, Solomon Z. Comorbidity of posttraumatic stress disorder, anxiety and depression: A 20-year longitudinal study of war veterans. Journal of Affective Disorders. Elsevier B.V 2010;123(1-3):249–57.

[57] Berenz EC, Coffey SF. Treatment of Co-occurring Posttraumatic Stress Disorder and Substance Use Disorders. Current Psychiatry Reports 2012;14(5):469–77.

[58] Cicerone KD, Langenbahn DM, Braden C, Malec JF, Kalmar K, Fraas M, et al. Evidence-Based Cognitive Rehabilitation: Updated Review of the Literature From 2003 Through 2008. Archives of Physical Medicine and Rehabilitation 2011;92(4) 519–530.

[59] Parsons TD, Courtney CG, Arizmendi B, Dawson ME. Virtual Reality Stroop Task for neurocognitive assessment. Studies in Health Technology and Informatics 2011;163 433–439.

2

Traumatic Brain Injuries and Sleep/ Wake Disorders

Narayan P. Verma and Arunima Verma Jayakar

1. Introduction

Traumatic brain injury (TBI) and sleep/wake disorder/s have a complex relationship [1]. A sleep disorder may make a person more prone to TBI by making him or her drowsy or inattentive and therefore more prone to fall or have an accident [2]. A sleep disorder may also make a person with concussion more prone to develop prolonged concussion or post-concussion syndrome in which symptoms last more than 3 weeks or even more than 3 months [3-7]. Likewise a sleep disorder may make them more prone to future concussions and cumulative injury. [7]

Less known and more common and recently recognized is the sleep/wake disorder caused by TBI itself, most simply termed the post traumatic sleep disorder [8-10] We discourage the use of acronym **PTSD**, however, lest it be confused with post-traumatic stress disorder. We propose the acronym **PTSLD**. This chapter is dedicated to delineating this disorder.

2. TBI

TBI is a problem of significant and increasing proportions-recently described as a silent epidemic [1]. The number of individuals with TBI is expected to climb with the return of Iraq and Afghanistan veterans back to USA. Just like atom bomb induced cancer was the signature injury of World War II and Agent Orange the signature injury of Vietnam War, TBI is the signature injury of Iraq and Afghanistan wars. [1]

Current estimates indicate that the TBI occurs in 100–400 per 100,000 people per year in North America and Europe. Men are more often affected than women. The most common age group which suffers from traumatic brain injury is 15–35 years. It is the most frequent cause of death between the ages 1-15. It accounts for one third of all injury related deaths in the USA. [8]

The TBI may result from fall, domestic violence, street violence, during birth, motor vehicle accidents, war related injuries, a work related injury or due to sports. Falls and motor vehicle accidents are the most common causes in civilian practice. In developing countries such as India with smaller land size, more population density, lax driving law enforcement and booming motor vehicle growth per capita, motor vehicle accidents are as much as 100 times more common than developed countries such as UK or USA.

TBI could be due to a blunt or a penetrating trauma. The trauma may be direct or indirect such from a nearby explosion-as many as 59 percent soldiers exposed to improvised explosive devices (IEDs) develop TBI. [1]

Contrary to popular belief a significant loss of consciousness (LOC) is not always necessary to make a diagnosis especially in so called mild TBI. Per Center of disease control (CDC), a history of clear cut LOC is seen in only less than 10 percent of patients with concussion. [8]

TBI is often described as acute, subacute and chronic-arbitrarily according to the time elapsed. It is also rated as mild, moderate or severe. Although there is no consensus, many prevailing criteria exist. The departments of defense and veterans affairs [3] have attempted to do this as follows:

	GCS	PTA	LOC
Mild	13–15	<1 day	0–30 minutes
Moderate	9–12	>1 to <7 days	>30 min to <24 hours
Severe	3–8	>7 days	>24 hours

GCS-Glasgow coma scale, **LOC**-loss of consciousness, **PTA**-post-traumatic amnesia

Table 1. Severity of traumatic brain injury

Only thing mild about **mild TBI** is the name. It accounts for 75 percent of all TBI. It may potentially be associated with significant, enduring and sometimes devastating consequences, greater likelihood of injury from a repeat concussion and long-term risk of Parkinson's disease, dementia, depression, suicide or homicide. [8] The incidence of mild TBI, also called concussion, is believed to be 6 per 1000 but this may be an underestimate. Per the center of disease control (CDC), a total of 1.4 million visits to hospitals/ER per year in USA are related to concussion/mild TBI. Additional 1.6-3.8 million never visit hospital or the ER. Mild TBI is often considered to occur when Glasgow coma score (GCS) at 24 hours after trauma is 13-15, LOC is 0-30 min and post-traumatic amnesia (PTA) is less than a day. It is often used interchangeably with the term concussion. Sports teams often use the acute concussion evaluation (ACE) questionnaire to evaluate the symptoms of concussion in the sport field.

The ACE questionnaire scores the individual on characteristics of Injury (such as severity and type of trauma, LOC, amnesia and presence or absence of seizures), presence and severity of physical symptoms (such as headache, photophobia, dizziness, nausea, blurred vision etc), cognitive symptoms (fogginess, confusion, forgetfulness, perseveration, slow cerebration, lack of concentration), emotional symptoms (irritability, sadness, emotional lability, nervousness) and sleep-related symptoms (such as insomnia, hypersomnia, drowsiness, daytime sleepiness, hyperarousal, flashbacks, nightmares), whether they are increased by exertion and how the person feels as compared to before injury on a seven point sale 0-6) and risk factors such as previous history of concussion, headaches, depression anxiety, sleep disorder or developmental disorder such as ADHD or learning disability. This may also be used for serial follow up.

The military equivalent of this scale is called MACE. A score of 25 or above is considered indicative of concussion in MACE. Symptoms persist from 3 weeks to 3 months and are called post-concussive syndrome if they persist beyond 3 months. Although it is believed that concussion results from biomechanical alterations in the brain and there is no structural damage, neuropathological and MRI data with tractography (diffuse tensor imaging or more sophisticated constrained spherical deconvolution) refute this thesis. If *conventional* neuroimaging such as head CT or MRI of the brain is abnormal, the TBI is no longer mild. However moderate to severe TBI may occur with or without abnormal conventional neuroimaging.

Moderate TBI is defined as LOC greater than 30 min but less than 24 hours, GCS 9-12 and/or PTA 1-7 days. It is variously graded by Global assessment of functioning or GAF scale [4] scored from 0-100) or some regional scales such as Rancho Los Amigos Scale [5] which assesses head injured patients on 8 levels of cognitive functioning (LOCF). The GAF score would be expected to be 51-60 with moderate TBI.

Severe TBI is defined as LOC greater than 1 day, GCS 3-8 and/or PTA greater than 7 days. Seizure occurring acutely during the head trauma does not necessarily make the TBI severe but chronic seizure disorder starting 3 months to several years after the head trauma certainly qualifies the TBI as a severe injury. Likewise macro injury, infarction, encephalomalacia, hematoma, persistent focal or lateralized neurological signs, dementia, severe personality change or new onset severe psychiatric disorder stamp an injury as severe. GAF score of 50 or below will indicate a severe head injury even when the neuroimaging is negative. There were 5.3 million people in USA living with severe TBI by 1999 [6]. The number must certainly be higher now. Severe TBI is of 2 types: closed and penetrated.

TBI may occur alone or may be associated with involvement of not just the brain but also skull, scalp, meninges, eyes, ears, sinuses and other neighborhood structures as well as injuries to neck and body.

3. TBI and sleep/wake disorders

Sleep/wake disorders may, in fact, potentially make folks more prone to TBI by making them sleepy and/or inattentive and therefore more likely to be subject of an injury or accident. A preexisting sleep disorder also makes the likelihood of concussion being prolonged and persistent. However, this chapter will mainly deal with the issue of sleep wake disorder/s caused by TBI, a far more common and as yet not well defined problem.

Sleep related problems secondary to chronic TBI have been described anecdotally or in case-report format since 1941. [11-19]. Some commonly reported disorders include hypersomnia, narcolepsy, delayed sleep phase, insomnia, fatigue, alteration of sleep-wake schedule, and movement disorders. It has been found clinically that, insomnia [20], hypersomnia [21-28] and excessive daytime sleepiness (EDS) are common [29, 30] in TBI and may at times occur in the same patient at different intervals from traumatic insult (see below). Only more recently in last 30 years, attempts have been made to explore this relationship in detail. Guilleminault et al in 1982 [13] described impaired daytime functioning and somnolence in 98 percent of all patients with TBI and further expanded their findings in year 2000, [21] extending their observations to even those with cervical whiplash and commenting on the medico-legal dilemma.

Post-traumatic sleep/wake disorders may significantly impair the rehabilitation potential of an injured individual and need to be accurately diagnosed and treated. Organized literature in this important area is sparse and fragmented. An organized account of these disorders is essential not only to improve the rehabilitation potential of these unfortunate individuals but to protect their medical coverage from auto insurers, as they encounter significant skepticism from adjusters regarding their sleep/wake issues to be causally related to their accidents and injury.

To be perfectly accurate, the sleep/wake disorder may not only result from head injury but neck and bodily injuries may cause or contribute to sleep/wake issues equally or even predominantly. [21]

The post-traumatic sleep/wake disorders may evolve, recede or be persistent after TBI. In a prospective study [31], there was found to be a high prevalence of sleep disorders (46%) and of excessive daytime sleepiness (25%) in 87 subjects at least 3 months after TBI [23]. 47% of the subjects in the aforementioned study was found to have a sleep disorder: OSA (23%), PTH (11%), narcolepsy (6%), or PLMS (7%) and 26% of the subjects had EDS [23]. In immediate post-traumatic period, hypersomnia may be common in hospitalized patients due to medications and interrupted nocturnal sleep due to pain and frequent nursing evaluations. Later on, it may be replaced by insomnia. Parasomnias may occur as well. *TBI is now known to cause nearly the entire spectrum of any or all sleep disorders and further may aggravate a pre-existing sleep/wake disorder by potential mechanisms enumerated elsewhere in this chapter.*

4. Acute TBI and sleep-related symptoms

Watson et al in 2007 [32] found in a prospective study of 514 patients that sleep related symptoms are common during acute phase of TBI. As much as 54 percent patients have daytime somnolence, more in those with more severe injury. They result in daytime somnolence which in turn may lead to poor daytime performance, altered sleep-wake schedule, heightened anxiety, and poor individual sense of well-being, insomnia, and depression. Half of these individuals are still sleepy at the end of one year. Relationship with severity or localization of head injury was disputed by Baumann et al [28] who evaluated patients prospectively as well, but their study ended at 6 months instead of one year in Watson's study.,. However, similar to Watson study, they also found that quality of life was impaired by these symptoms.. CSF hypocretin-1 was found to be significantly reduced levels in those patients with excessive daytime sleepiness (EDS) symptoms.

5. Chronic TBI and sleep related symptoms

Verma et al in 2007 [10] in a retrospective study found that sleep changes and deranged sleep architecture are common in *chronic* TBI patients, arbitrarily defined as 3 months to 2 years after head trauma.. The sleep disorders seen in this population are similar to those seen in the general population but individual percentages are higher. Hypersomnia accounted for 50 percent of all patients and insomnia and parasomnia for quarter each. Global assessment of functioning (GAF) scores correlated with some (stage N1 percentage, impaired sleep efficiency and wake during sleep), but not all (stage shifts and wake before sleep) measures of sleep disruption, indicating a complex and multifactorial pathogenesis.

6. Pathogenesis

The possible pathogenetic mechanisms of TBI causing sleep disorders include: direct brain injury, indirect brain injury, collateral damage to neck and back and resulting pain interfering with sleep, [13] weight gain (secondary to head trauma or medications used to treat head trauma or its sequelae such as posttraumatic mood, anxiety or stress disorder), pre-existing genetic propensity for narcolepsy, which may be clinically aggravated or precipitated by head-trauma [11], a pre-existing anatomical abnormality of sleep-related brain mechanisms, oropharyngeal abnormality aggravated by head trauma or resulting weight gain, anatomical abnormalities caused by head trauma such as jaw dislocation, TMJ problems, and brainstem and forebrain lesions induced by TBI.

Direct brain injury was first described by Strich in 1961 [22] as diffuse degeneration of white matter subsequently termed the diffuse axonal injury (DAI). This was later determined in animal experiments to be the consequence of inertial loading of the head by prolonged coronal angular acceleration [23] with brunt of abnormality in septum pellucidum, corpus callosum, deep gray matter and dorso-lateral pons and midbrain, areas closely associated with sleep-wake mechanisms. The biochemical basis of this injury is excitotoxicity, [24] inflammation, [25] free radicals/eicasanoids, [9] hyperglycolysis, [26] hyperglycemia, [26] and apolipoprotein E e4 synthesis. [27] These mechanisms most likely operate in sleep disorders associated with mild head injury. MRI with tractography may provide a direct evidence of such injury. It has also been hypothesized that the hypocretin system may be partly responsible for the patho-physiology of sleep wake disturbances present post TBI [28].

7. Classification: We propose the following classification of post-traumatic sleep/wake disorders

1. Post-traumatic sleep wake disorder/s-resulting from TBI
2. Post-traumatic sleep/wake disorder/s resulting from neck and/or bodily injuries
3. Post-traumatic sleep/wake disorder/s resulting from both-TBI and neck and/or bodily injuries

Each group has 2 subtypes:

Primary: This group consists of patients who never had any sleep/wake related issues what so ever prior to the accident.

Secondary: These patients have a preexisting sleep/wake disorder which is either aggravated or altered by the accident and in fact may have contributed to the occurrence of accident by making patient inattentive and therefore prone to have an accident. A pre-existing sleep disorder also makes the likelihood of an enduring concussion more as well as increases the proneness to further and cumulative deterioration after repeat concussion.

8. Clinical features

Insomnia: This is the most common consequence of the TBI. It is pretty much universal in all patients with mild TBI at least in initial stages. It is associated with headache, dizziness, mood changes, imbalance and blurred vision and flashbacks in various combinations. It usually resolves in 3 weeks to 3 months in most mild cases but sometimes may be nagging and persistent. It may be sleep onset or sleep maintenance or associated with premature awakening in the morning-the so called the " terminal" insomnia. It may be contributed to by associated anxiety and depression as shown by Verma et al [10] based on Hamilton Anxiety Scale (HAS-appendix 3) and Beck's Depression Inventory (BDI-appendix 4). Nightmares and flashbacks may also contribute. At times it reflects more serious pathology such as sleep apnea caused by TBI and/or neck or spinal injury or periodic limb movements induced by medications used to manage the patient. The medications such as topiramate, methylphenidate etc themselves may aggravate or cause insomnia. Circadian rhythm disorder may complicate insomnia or cause it either due to direct injury to the biological clock or patient's sleep hygiene suffering from frequent examinations by nurses, therapists and other workers, not going to work or office and irregular bedtime and wake up time.

Many patients with more severe head injury initially have hypersomnia due to medications, TBI itself, complicating sleep apnea or narcolepsy but later on after several months or even years develop insomnia. Same factors as listed above operate. Reverse is also true. Patients with mild TBI may develop hypersomnia/ parasomnia or narcolepsy later on even though they had insomnia to begin with. Thus the natural history of sleep/wake disorders is more complicated than the sleep/wake disorders in general as the type of disorder may switch over time.

Although, sleep studies are not generally indicated in patients with most cases of insomnia from other etiologies, the post-traumatic insomnia requires a sleep study for many reasons. It requires documentation as the adjusters frequently look for objective confirmation of subjective symptoms. Also post-traumatic insomnia may not be just pure insomnia but contributed to by sleep apnea, narcolepsy, periodic limb movements, parasomnias such as the REM behavior disorder or a circadian rhythm disorder. In addition, the insomnia may be replaced by hypersomnia or parasomnia and/or even nocturnal seizures later on. The polysomnogram (PSG) should be done with expanded EEG montage with simultaneous video-taping. Traditional investigating methods such as sleep diary, actigraphy and scales such as Hamilton anxiety scale (HAS -appendix 3) and Beck's depression inventory (BDI -appendix 4) also help in dissecting, intellectualizing and treating the issue at hand.

Hypersomnia: This is the second most common consequence. It is quite universal in acute stages of moderate to severe injury as patient is often kept intubated and sedated, on pain medications and primary brain and brainstem pathology from TBI may also contribute. Weight gain from medications to use the consequences of TBI such as antidepressants, anxiolytics or anticonvulsant medications, lack of activity, not working or going to office, being sedentary due to severe TBI and/or neck/bodily injury, overeating due to injury to satiety center of the brain may result in development of obstructive sleep apnea even when there are no oropharyngeal anatomical risk factors. Direct or indirect injury to sleep centers and breathing centers may also contribute. Lowered hypocretin levels may be operative as stated elsewhere. Neck injury may impair diaphragmatic function and add insult to injury. Associated high spinal cord injury may be devastating but cervical whiplash itself is known to cause obstructive sleep apnea [21]. Narcolepsy may be precipitated in a person who is genetically predisposed for it or even be caused by TBI, sometimes even mild TBI. After several years it may be replaced by insomnia in some patients. Hypersomnia with prolonged sleep and even Klein-Levin like syndrome might occur. The periodic limb movements (PLMs) are common either due to medications used to treat TBI or due to unknown reasons such as inactivity or complex chemical changes/alterations, not yet known. Circadian rhythm disorders may contribute. Video-polysomnography with expanded EEG montage and frequently a multiple sleep latency test (MSLT) is addition if the Epworh Sleepiness Scale (ESS-appendix 1) is 11 or more is essential for the diagnosis and should be in-lab and not portable. Actigraphy and sleep diary might help as well.

Parasomnias: These are third most common complications and often co-exist with hypersomnia or insomnia. Each patient may have more than one parasomnia. They may also develop as a remote complication of TBI. As repeated concussions are known to predispose to Parkinson's disease and Parkinson's disease is associated with or even preceded by REM behavior disorder (RBD) by as much as 3 years, this is not entirely unexpected. Sleepwalking, nocturnal eating disorder, nocturnal seizures, nocturnal enuresis either as a part of post-traumatic OSA or due to TBI itself and confusional arousals all are seen and common. In-lab video-polysomnography (video-PSG) with expanded EEG montage is essential for the documentation and diagnosis. The family may also be encouraged to use their smart phones to record these events to help in diagnosis.

9. How to approach a patient with PTSLD

Detailed history is important. One should carefully ascertain if sleep related symptoms started after TBI or preceded that. If latter, document any changes in severity of symptoms or change in symptoms. The routine scales administered in our practice are: Mini mental state examination, ACE questionnaire, Hamilton anxiety Scale (appendix 3), Beck's depression inventory (appendix 4), Epworth sleepiness Scale (appendix 1) and Berlin questionnaire (appendix 2). Careful determination of LOC, PTA and GCS is done based on hospital, ER and other previous records. Computerized psychological and neuropsychological testing (easily administered by even a medical assistant using the 'neurotrax' system) to determine the global assessment of cognitive functioning and levels of anxiety and depression is important to establish a baseline and future follow up. Physical examination should pay careful attention to the HEENT examination, TMJ, neck size, chin (prognathia, retrognathia, micrognathia), oropharyngeal examination for tonsillar size from 1-4 and Mallampati score 1-4, focal and lateralized neurological signs and cardiopulmonary examination. Sleep/wake related history should include details about snoring, witnessed pauses in breathing, bedtime, wake up time, circadian rhythm, gasping and choking in sleep, hypnagogic hallucinations, hypnapompic hallucinations, nightmares, nocturnal incontinence, seizures, sleep walking and acting out of dreams, any falls from bed, restless legs and periodic limb movements (by asking questions such as do you have creepy crawling sensation in your limbs and feet which improve by movement). Wakefulness should be evaluated for alertness, drowsiness, dozing, napping, daydreaming and automatic behaviors. The ESS (appendix 1) is helpful in quantitating sleepiness and Berlin questionnaire (appendix 2) about the probability of sleep related breathing disorder. Sometimes the sleepiness scales are not reliable in patients with severe head injury. Caregiver's input is needed in those situations. Current medication list is critical.

Ancillary tests include an MRI of the head with tractography (diffuse tensor imaging or preferably constrained spherical deconvolution), EEG, an overnight in lab video-PSG with an expanded EEG montage and a 5 nap daytime multiple sleep latency test (MSLT) if ESS is greater than 10. A seven day sleep diary and actigraphy is obtained in those with insomnia or circadian rhythm issues. CSF hypocretin levels may be useful.

Initial follow up visits are monthly for 3 months and then 3 monthly times two. Six monthly visits are obtained after that. Annual ancillary evaluation is more limited and defined by patient's clinical symptomatology. However, sleep disorders may change their characteristics during the course and re-evaluation may need to be tailored accordingly. Therefore a cook book approach is not useful. Maintenance of wakefulness test may be useful in quantitating residual daytime sleepiness.

10. PTSLD

We propose this term as an acronym for post-traumatic sleep/wake disorders to distinguish it from PTSD or post-traumatic stress disorder.

1. Post-traumatic sleep-related breathing disorder:

This is fairly common in general population affecting 2-4 percent of all adults. In patients with TBI, sleep apnea defined as apnea-hypopnea index (AHI) of 10 or greater may be present in up to 30 percent of all patients. Seventy five percent of apneas and hypopneas are obstructive in nature. This condition may present as hypersomnia, insomnia or may only be seen on laboratory evaluation as an unexpected finding. It may cause a secondary REM behavior disorder (RBD -a parasomnia) which may potentially be injurious to the patient if not recognized and treated and further compound the TBI. Mechanisms of post-traumatic sleep related breathing disorder are several. Patient may have pre-existing anatomical abnormalities which were insufficient to cause the sleep related breathing disorder prior to TBI but the occurrence of TBI provides a sufficient milieu for it to clinically manifest. Sedative medications such as clonazapam may potentiate apnea, antidepressants such as sertraline and mitrazepine and anticonvulsants such as valproic acid cause weight gain which is a known risk factor for this condition. Weight gain may also result from physical inactivity and direct damage to hypothalamic centers related to feeding and satiety. Tracheostomy, if done, during the acute management of TBI may further increase the risk especially in children by causing tracheomalacia, as seen in one child by the senior author of this chapter. In addition to known risks of this condition such as premature death, hypertension, heart attack, stroke, dementia and diabetes, this condition may impair the control of patient's seizure disorder if present. Newborns with perinatal head trauma and abused children may develop central apnea due to direct injury to the breathing centers in the brain. In general, more severe the head injury, higher the apnea hypopnea index and hypoxia are. ESS (appendix 1) may be unreliable in those with moderate to severe head injury and should not be used as a sole criterion to order or not order the sleep studies. [10] Berlin questionnaire (appendix 2) also helps in predicting the probability of sleep related breathing disorder.

2. Post-traumatic narcolepsy:

The incidence of narcolepsy in general population is about 1:2000 in the USA. Hormonal change and minor head trauma at puberty are long known to be initiating factors for narcolepsy in neurology text books as the genetic propensity of narcolepsy usually manifests clinically at or after puberty 90 percent of the time. In addition, most patients with narcolepsy remain the same throughout their lifetime. Post-traumatic narcolepsy is different in that it is far more common than general population (it is seen in up to 6-9 percent of all patients with TBI) [10, 11] and down the road, after several years in our experience, symptoms may sometimes abate and even be replaced by insomnia. Hypocretin levels are known to be reduced by TBI and may well play a pathogenetic role. New onset cataplexy might occur after TBI, increasing the risk of falls and therefore repeated TBI. Nightmares are common in TBI and careful history is needed to distinguish them from hypnagogic and hypnapompic hallucinations seen as auxiliary symptoms of narcolepsy. Occurrence of narcolepsy is not correlated with the degree of TBI.

Polysomnogram (PSG) will nearly always show some degree of sleep disruption such as increased percentage of N1, frequent awakenings, reduced sleep efficiency (less than 85 percent), reduced N3 (delta) percentage (less than 15 percent) and sometimes SOREMP (sleep onset REM period or REM sleep occurring with 15 min of sleep onset). The MSLT will show a sleep latency of 8 min or less and 2 or more SOREMPs in 5 naps. [33]

3. Post-traumatic hypersomnia.

Idiopathic hypersomnolence syndrome is long known to often follow TBI and conditions such as Guillaine Barre Syndrome (GBS) or infectious mononucleosis (IM). The PSG shows relatively normal or even improved sleep efficiency sometimes greater than 95 percent, increased or normal delta percentage, relatively few awakenings, minimal sleep disruption if any but severe daytime somnolence on MSLT with no SOREMPs. Medication effect needs to be excluded and one has to be careful not to misdiagnose 15 percent cases of narcolepsy in whom MSLT is initially negative as post-traumatic hypersomnia. The PSG features described above are helpful in distinction and there is no history of hypnagogic or hypnapompic hallucinations or cataplexy. Autonomic symptoms are sometimes present. [33]

4. Post-traumatic periodic limb movement disorder (PLMD):

These may a solitary abnormality on PSG but more often are associated with other conditions such as OSA and narcolepsy. They may have been present premorbidly but are often worsened by medications used for the treatment of TBI. They may be asymptomatic and may not require any treatment or cause significant patient insomnia or spousal discomfort and need treatment. Lower extremities are affected and sometimes only one side but upper extremities may be involved in addition or alone. Neurologic deficit such as hemiparesis or paraparesis may worsen or cause this condition. Anemia of chronic disease may compromise the serum ferritin level and may compound the issue. They are considered significant if more than 15/hour in an adult or 5/hr in a child. [33] Up to 30 percent of all patients may have this condition. [10] They may or may not report RLS in addition when awake.

5. Post-traumatic REM behavior disorder (RBD):

This condition was first described to occur in cats when lesions were created in peri-locus coeruleous area to interrupt impulses going down the ventral reticulopsinal tract to spinal motor neurons in REM sleep [10]. Similar mechanisms are operative in humans with TBI. Associated Parkinson's, alcoholism and medications may also contribute. Up to 13 percent patients show symptoms of RBD and/or show increased tone in chin EMG on PSG [10]. Patients typically act out their dreams during last third of sleep at night when REM percentage is the highest and potentially fall from bed, climb out of windows or walk out in freezing weather. It may be secondary to post-traumatic OSA and then it responds to CPAP. If not, RBD precautions and medications are necessary. It may be a precursor of Parkinsonism in patients with punch-drunk syndrome and may precede that condition by as much as 3 years. It should be distinguished from sleep walking which usually occurs during the first half of sleep and there is no dream recall. It should also be distinguished from NREM sleep related confusional arousals which are similar to night terrors.

6. Other post-traumatic parasomnias:

They include sleep paralysis, cataplexy, sleep walking, nightmares, sleep enuresis and nocturnal eating disorder. [33] All parasomnias (these plus RBD) occur in 25 percent of all patients with TBI, either by themselves on in addition to other disorders. Birth injuries to the head may be associated with head banging disorder. [16]

7. Post-traumatic insomnia:

At least one quarter of all patients with TBI have insomnia either sleep onset or sleep maintenance or a combination thereof. [10] Hamilton anxiety scores (appendix 3) are typically elevated in those with sleep onset insomnia and Beck's depression inventory scores (appendix 4) in those with sleep maintenance insomnia. Physical factors such as frequent examination by nurses and respiratory therapists during ICU stay may be the cause at least in acute TBI. Medications such as bronchodilators, anticonvulsants such as topiramate or stimulants such as methylphenidate may cause insomnia. Circadian rhythm abnormalities and not going to regular work and physical inactivity leading to frequent daytime naps may cause insomnia at night. Post traumatic sleep related breathing disorder both of obstructive type or central type may cause insomnia as well. Severe restless leg syndrome (RLS) may cause sleep onset insomnia and PLMs, sleep maintenance insomnia. Patients with post-traumatic narcolepsy may sometimes present initially as insomnia at night and only a careful history uncovers the diagnosis. For example, a patient treated by the senior author was treated for 2 years as insomnia by various physicians, until she disclosed to the author additional history of severe daytime sleepiness and napping since TBI and disturbing "nightmares" (actually hypnagogic hallucinations) with automatic behavior which prevented her from holding onto any job and not succeed in her new marriage. She responded beautifully to sodium oxybutate and was immensely grateful.

8. Post-traumatic circadian rhythm disorder:

This is a fairly common complication. The disorders include a delayed sleep phase syndrome (DSPS), irregular sleep wake cycle, advanced sleep phase syndrome (ASPS) and non-24 hour sleep wake cycle. [33] Irregular sleep wake cycle is common during the acute phase of TBI in moderate to severe cases as nurses and respiratory therapists check on the patient frequently and patient is on medications including sedatives or anesthetic agents such a propofol. It is also common in chronic TBI patients with a psychiatric disorder or blindness. Otherwise DSPS is the most common complication related to circadian rhythm abnormality in patients with TBI and a direct injury to suprachiasmatic nucleus may well be the cause. ASPS is quite frequent in elderly patients with TBI. Non-24 hour cycle is a rare complication in some patients showing a stepladder pattern on actigraphy. [33]

11. Differential diagnosis

Lack of pre-existing history of sleep related symptoms is critical for the diagnosis of the primary post-traumatic sleep disorder, although the TBI may aggravate a pre-existing sleep/

wake disorder or make it more difficult to treat. Secondary gain may need to be excluded but objective confirmation from tests as outlined above, obviates that possibility. Interviewing the family members, friends, golf buddies etc and previous medical records are helpful in determining whether the disorder is primary or secondary. Previous anatomical abnormities do not automatically exclude a primary post traumatic sleep/wake disorder as patient may have been compensated before and the TBI may have been the "last straw which broke the camel's back". Likewise, a positive HLA testing does not automatically make narcolepsy pre-existing or genetic, as head trauma, even mild or minimal is known to be the initiating factor for narcolepsy. Please refer to the international classification of sleep disorders [33] edition 3 for further help in differential diagnosis of post-traumatic sleep disorder/s from non-traumatic etiologies as detailed discussion of that would be tangential to the intent of this chapter.

Treatment : Once it is realized that TBI may cause or aggravate a pre-existing sleep/wake disorder, management is simple. It is treated like any other sleep disorder of another etiology by adding medications, reduction of medications, meditation, machines, devices or behavioral techniques. Treatment is important as it will interfere with rehabilitation potential of the patient unless addressed head on. The treatment modalities outlined below are well described in standard text books of sleep medicine and in the practice guidelines of the American Academy of Sleep Medicine [34] and would only be briefly outlined below without individually referring each modality to prevent unnecessary expansion of the reference list and dilute the intent of this chapter.

Medications and reduction of medications: Mild sleep apnea may be managed with proptriptyline. Periodic limb movements may be helped by Clonazepam, dopamine agonists, gabaergic agents, tonic water and vitamin D. Nocturnal eating disorder often responds to topiramate. REM behavior disorder responds well to Clonazepam and/or melatonin. Nocturnal seizures require anticonvulsants. Carbamazepine is most effective. Hypnagogic hallucinations and nightmares may require clonazepam, imipramine or more complex pharmacological remedies as NMDA agonists.

Reduction of medications may also help by reducing weight, decreasing excessive daytime sleepiness, lessening the aggravation of OSA or reducing PLMs. Some medications such as amitriptyline may induce or aggravate RBD in TBI patients and that might improve by this strategy. Sometimes, reducing topiramate, certain antidepressants, stimulants and wakefulness promoting agents etc may improve insomnia.

Meditation: simple meditation techniques such as Hong-Sau which do not require any special equipment or posture or more complex such techniques such as yoga exercises requiring exercise mats and lotus position may be useful at times in reducing anxiety and improving sleep onset insomnia.

Behavioral techniques: 11 principles of sleep hygiene (appendix 5), 6 Bootzin's principles (appendix 6) and cognitive behavioral therapy for insomnia (appendix 7) are often useful for the management of insomnia. In fact most enduring relief of post-traumatic insomnia comes with non-pharmacological behavioral techniques.

Patients with RBD may require padding around their beds, alarms and double locks at doors and boarding up of windows (RBD precautions). Those with nocturnal eating disorder, may need to have a lock on the refrigerator.

Phototherapy: It is useful in the treatment of post-traumatic delayed sleep phase syndrome and advanced sleep phase syndrome, non 24 hr sleep/wake cycle and insomnia caused by post-traumatic depression. Morning exposure to a standard 2500-10,000 lux lamp from a distance of about 18-24 inches for 30-60 minutes is used in all of these conditions except ASPS in which evening exposure is required. Nausea and queasiness may occur and the duration of exposure may need to be optimized upwards gradually.

Chronotherapy. It will be useful in managing circadian rhythm disorders resulting from head trauma. Advancing the bedtime by 3 hrs a day may help the treatment of DSPS over 8-10 days. It may be used alone or in conjunction with phototherapy and/or melatonin.

CPAP: Continuous positive airway pressure it is the mainstay of treatment for moderate to severe OSA. Patients may experience difficulty in using this device due to facial or TMJ injuries or chest trauma or CHF or if they are claustrophobic.

BIPAP and BIPAP-ST (NIPV)- Bi-level treatment is necessary in some of the patients who have co-morbid muscle disease or CHF. It provides a lesser pressure to facilitate exhalation in an individual with weak muscles or CHF. The inhalation pressures IPAP) are at least 2 cm of H_2O or more than the pressure for exhalation (EPAP). BIPAP-ST or NIPV provides additional protection by backing up ventilation if the respiratory rate falls below a predetermined rate such as 10/min.

Adaptive servo ventilation (ASV): is often useful when nothing else works in complex or central sleep apnea caused by TBI by overwhelming the apneas not only simply by pressure but also volume of the inhaled air and mostly obviates the need for tracheostomy except in acute stages. This device is quite expensive but well worth it as the senior author has never prescribed tracheostomy for sleep-related breathing disorder ever since this device has been commercially available. Prior to that, it was needed at least in one patient every year in our clinic.

Jaw advancement devices: may be useful in those with mild post-traumatic OSA with TMJ issues.

Ongoing follow up is essential by at least 3-6 monthly office visits and yearly sleep studies since post-traumatic sleep disorders are notorious to change during their natural history and may require altogether different treatment as the time passes by.

12. Discussion

A spectrum of sleep disorders are a common finding after the acute phase of TBI [9]. They result in daytime somnolence which in turn may lead to poor daytime performance, altered sleep-wake schedule, heightened anxiety, and poor individual sense of well-being, insomnia and depression [10] Sleep changes and deranged sleep architecture are more common in *chronic* TBI patients as compared to the general population [10]. Sleep disturbances can compromise the rehabilitation process and the ability to return to work. [20] A high index of suspicion may lead to a diagnosis and subsequent treatment of these disorders and contribute to physical and cognitive rehabilitation of these patients. [10] A proper diagnosis and greater awareness of this complication protects patient's rights for medical care under auto-insurance laws in states such as Michigan [2]. This will also be critical in the management of TBI related symptoms of returning veteran of Iraq and Afghanistan war since TBI is the signature injury of those wars and has become a silent epidemic. [1]

13. Directions for future research and efforts:

The future research and efforts should concentrate on primary prevention of TBI, better delineation of premorbid sleep/wake status by some scales (similar to those which predict premorbid IQ), early identification and accurate diagnosis of post-traumatic sleep/wake disorder, its exact impact on physical, cognitive and occupational rehabilitation, convincing the auto-insurances not to be stingy in the care of these unfortunate individuals and look at sleep/wake related complaints as a medical issue and not a malingering issue, and the US government to provide greater research and medical funds for this important medical condition.

Appendix 1. The epworth sleepiness scale

0 = no chance of dozing	
1 = slight chance of dozing	
2 = moderate chance of dozing	
3 = high chance of dozing	
SITUATION	**CHANCE OF DOZING**
Sitting and reading	________
Watching TV	________
Sitting inactive in a public place (e.g. a theater or a meeting)	________
As a passenger in a car for an hour without a break	________
Lying down to rest in the afternoon when circumstances permit	________
Sitting and talking to someone	________
Sitting quietly after a lunch without alcohol	________
In a car, while stopped for a few minutes in traffic	________

Appendix 2. Berlin questionnaire

Top of Form

1. Body Mass Index Information:

Height (in inches):

Weight (in pounds):

CATEGORY 1 QUESTIONS

2. Do you snore?

Yes **

No

I don't know

3. How loud is your snoring?

My snoring is as loud as breathing

My snoring is as loud as talking

My snoring is louder than talking **

My snoring is very loud **

4. How frequently do you snore?

Almost every day **

3-4 times per week **

1-2 times per week

1-2 times per month

Never or almost never

5. Does your snoring bother other people?

Yes **

No

6. How often have your breathing pauses been noticed?

Almost every day **

3-4 times per week **

1-2 times per week

1-2 times per month

Never or almost never

CATEGORY 2 QUESTIONS

7.Are you tired after sleeping?

Almost every day **

3-4 times per week **

1-2 times per week

1-2 times per month

Never or almost never

8. Are you tired during waketime?

Almost every day **

3-4 times per week **

1-2 times per week

1-2 times per month

Never or almost never

9. How often do you nod off or fall asleep while driving?

Almost every day **

3-4 times per week **

1-2 times per week

1-2 times per month

Never or almost never

CATEGORY 3 QUESTIONS

10. Do you have high blood pressure?

Yes **

No

I don't know

BMI (body mass index)

BMI > 30 **

Weight

BMI = -------------------- X 703

Height X Height

Weight in pounds, height in inches OR Weight in kilograms, height in meters

Berlin Scoring Results

Any answer followed by double asterisks (**) is a positive response.
Category 1 is positive with 2 or more positive responses to questions 2 through 6
Category 2 is positive with 2 or more positive responses to questions 7 through 9
Category 3 is positive with 1 or more positive responses and/or a BMI>30
2 or more positive categories indicates a high likelihood of sleep apnea

---

Bottom of Form

Appendix 3. Anxiety rating scales

1. Background
    1. Authored by Max Hamilton in 1959
    2. Public domain anxiety rating scale
2. Symptom Rating Scale (0=Not Present, 4=Disabling)
    1. Anxious Mood
        - 1.1. Worries
        - 1.2. Anticipates worst
    2. Tension
        - 2.1.Startles
        - 2.2. Cries easily
        - 2.3. Restless
        - 2.4. Trembling
    3. Fears
        - 3.1. Fear of the dark
        - 3.2. Fear of strangers
        - 3.3. Fear of being alone
        - 3.4. Fear of animal
    4. Insomnia
        - 4.1. Difficulty falling asleep or staying asleep
        - 4.2. Difficulty with Nightmares
    5. Intellectual

    - 5.1. Poor concentration
    - 5.2. Memory Impairment
- 6. Depressed Mood
    - 6.1. Decreased interest in activities
    - 6.2. Anhedonia
    - 6.3. Insomnia
- 7. Somatic Complaints: Muscular
    - 7.1. Muscle aches or pains
    - 7.2. Bruxism
- 8. Somatic Complaints: Sensory
    - 8.1. Tinnitus
    - 8.2. Blurred vision
- 9. Cardiovascular Symptoms
    - 9.1. Tachycardia
    - 9.2. Palpitations
    - 9.3. Chest Pain
    - 9.4. Sensation of feeling faint
- 10. Respiratory Symptoms
    - 10.1. Chest pressure
    - 10.2. Choking sensation
    - 10.3. Shortness of Breath
- 11. Gastrointestinal symptoms
    - 11.1. Dysphagia
    - 11.2. Nausea or Vomiting
    - 11.3. Constipation
    - 11.4. Weight loss
    - 11.5. Abdominal fullness
- 12. Genitourinary symptoms
    - 12.1. Urinary frequency or urgency
    - 12.2. Dysmenorrhea
    - 12.3. Impotence
- 13. Autonomic Symptoms
    - 13.1. Dry Mouth
    - 13.2. Flushing

        13.3. Pallor
        13.4. Sweating
    14. Behavior at Interview
        14.1. Fidgets
        14.2. Tremor
        14.3. Paces

3. Interpretation
    1. Above 14 symptoms are graded on scale
        1.1. Not present: 0
        1.2. Very severe symptoms: 4
    2. Criteria
        2.1. Mild Anxiety (minimum for Anxiolytic): 18
        2.2. Moderate Anxiety: 25
        2.3. Severe Anxiety: 30

4. Other Anxiety Scales
    1. Zung Self Rating Scale for Anxiety
    2. Beck Anxiety Scale
    3. GAD-7

Appendix 4. Beck depression inventory

1. Background
    1. Twenty-one question survey completed by patient
    2. Answers scored on 0 to 3 scale
        1.1. Minimal: 0
        1.2. Severe: 3

2. Questions
    1. Sadness
    2. Hopelessness
    3. Past failure
    4. Anhedonia
    5. Guilt
    6. Punishment
    7. Self-dislike

8. Self-blame
9. Suicidal thoughts
10. Crying
11. Agitation
12. Loss of interest in activities
13. Indecisiveness
14. Worthlessness
15. Loss of energy
16. Insomnia
17. Irritability
18. Decreased appetite
19. Diminished concentration
20. Fatigue
21. Lack of interest in sex

3. Interpretation
    1. Score <15: Mild Depression
    2. Score 15-30: Moderate Depression
    3. Score >30: Severe Depression

Resources: Beck Depression Inventory
    1. General
        1.1. Intended for use by licensed professionals only
        1.2. Copyrighted by the Psychological Corporation
    2. Available for purchase from Psychological Corporation
        2.1. http://www.psychcorp.com/

5. Reference
    1. Beck (1996) Beck Depression Inventory, Harcour

Appendix 5. Eleven principles of sleep hygiene

1. Wake up and go to bed at about the same time every night. Bedtime and wake-up time should not differ from working days to weekend nights by more than approximately an hour.
2. Avoid sleeping in on weekends to "catch up" on sleep. This makes it more likely that you will have problems falling asleep.

3. If you take naps, they should be short (no more than an hour) and scheduled in the early to midafternoon. However, if you have a problem with falling asleep at night, napping during the day may make it worse and should be avoided.
4. Spend time outside every day. Exposure to sunlight helps to keep your body's internal clock on track.
5. Exercise regularly. Exercise may help you fall asleep and sleep more deeply.
6. Use your bed for sleeping only. Don't study, read, listen to music, watch television, etc., on your bed.
7. Make the 30–60 minutes before a quiet or wind-down time. Relaxing, calm, enjoyable activities, such as reading a book or listening to calm music, help your body and mind slow down enough to let you get to sleep. Don't study, watch exciting/scary movies, exercise, or get involved in "energizing" activities just before bed.
8. Eat regular meals and don't go to bed hungry. A light snack before bed is a good idea; eating a full meal in the hour before bed is not.
9. Avoid eating or drinking products containing caffeine from dinner time on. These include caffeinated sodas, coffee, tea, and chocolate.
10. Do not use alcohol. Alcohol disrupts sleep and may cause you to awaken throughout the night.
11. Smoking disturbs sleep. Don't smoke at least one hour before bed (and preferably, not at all!).

Appendix 6. Six Bootzin's principles for stimulus control in the treatment of insomnia

1. Go to bed when sleepy.
2. Use the bed for sleeping; do not read, watch television or eat in bed.
3. If you are unable to fall asleep, get up and move to another room; stay up until you are really sleepy, then return to bed; if sleep still does not come easily, get out of bed again. The goal is to associate bed with falling asleep quickly.
4. Repeat step 3 as necessary throughout the night.
5. Set the alarm and get up at the same time every morning regardless of how much you slept through the night. This helps the body acquire a constant sleep-wake rhythm.
6. Do NOT nap during the day.

Appendix 7. Cognitve behavioral therapy for insomnia: weekly for 8-10 weeks:

Sleep hygiene-see above-appendix 5

Stimulus control-see above-appendix 6

Sleep restriction or curtailment

Relaxation, meditation, hypnosis

Reducing muscle tension and hyperarousal by biofeedback

Relapse prevention:

1. Don't compensate for sleep loss
2. Start stimulus control procedures immediately
3. Re-engage sleep restriction should the insomnia persist beyond a few days.

Author details

Narayan P. Verma[1*] and Arunima Verma Jayakar[2]

*Address all correspondence to: narayangod@aol.com

1 Oakland University William Beaumont School of Medicine, Oakland, USA

2 BG Tricounty Neurology and Sleep Clinic PC, USA

References

[1] Theodorou AA, Rice SA. Is the silent epidemic keeping patients awake? JCSM 2007;3:347-348

[2] Verma NP. Importance of traumatic brain injury. J Clin Sleep Med 2008; 4: 177.

[3] Department of Defense and Department of Veterans Affairs (2008). "Traumatic Brain Injury Task Force".http://www.cdc.gov/nchs/data/icd9/Sep08TBI.pdf

[4] 4.. Modified Global Assessment of Functioning – Revised (mGAF-R)-adapted in 2004 by the Florida DCF Functional Assessment Workgroup from the original M-GAF reported by S. Caldecott-Hazard & R.C.W. Hall, 1995

[5] Gouvier, WD, Blanton, PD.LaPorte, KK, Nepomuceno, C.. Reliability and validity of the Disability Rating Scale and the Levels of Cognitive Functioning Scale in monitor-

ing recovery from severe head injury. *Archives of Physical Medicine and Rehabilitation* 1987; 68(2), 94-97.

[6] Thurman D, Alverson C, Dunn K, Guerrero J, Sniezek J. Traumatic brain injury in the United States: a public health perspective. J Head Trauma Rehabil 1999;14(6):602-615.

[7] Faul M, Xu L, Wald MM, Coronado VG. Traumatic brain injury in the United States: emergency department visits, hospitalizations, and deaths. Atlanta (GA): Centers for Disease Control and Prevention, National Center for Injury Prevention and Control; 2010.

[8] Injury prevention and control: traumatic brain injury: http://www.cdc.gov/traumaticbraininjury/

[9] Parker F, Andrews PJD, Azouvi P, Aghakhani N, Perrouin-Verbe B. Acute Traumatic brain injury. Continuum2001;7:7–31.

[10] Verma A; Anand V; Verma NP. Sleep disorders in chronic traumatic brain injury. *J Clin Sleep Med 2007*; 3(4):357-362.

[11] Gill AW. Idiopathic and traumatic narcolepsy. Lancet 1941;1:474–6.

[12] Amico G, Pasquali F, Pittaluga E. Pickwickian-narcoleptic disorders after brain concussion. Riv Sper Freniatr Med Leg Alien Ment 1972;29:74–85.

[13] Guilleminault C, Faull K, Miles L, Van den Hoed J. Post-traumatic excessive daytime sleepiness: a review of 20 patients. Neurology. 1982;33:1584–1589.

[14] Prigatano GP, Stahl ML, Orr WC, Zeiner HK. Sleep and dreaming disturbances in closed head injury patients. J Neurol Neurosurg Psychiatry 1982;45:78–80.

[15] Parsons LC, Ver Beek D. Sleep-awake patterns following cerebral concussion. Nurs Res 1982;31:260–264.

[16] Drake ME. Jactitio nocturna after head injury. Neurology 1986;36:867–868.

[17] Patten SB, Lauderdale WM. Delayed sleep disorder after traumatic brain injury. J Am Acad Child Adolesc Psychiatry 1992;31:100–102.

[18] Biary N, Singh B, Bahou Y, al Deeb SM, Sharif H. Post-traumatic paroxysmal nocturnal hemidystonia. Mov Disord 1994; 9:98–99.

[19] Lankford DA, Wellman JJ, O'Hara C. Post-traumatic narcolepsy in mild to moderate closed head injury. Sleep. 1994;17(suppl 8):S25–S28.

[20] Ouellet MC, Savard J, Morin CM. Insomnia following traumatic brain injury: a review. Neurorehabil Neural Repair.2004;18:187–198.

[21] Guilleminault C, Yuen KM, Gulevich BA, Karadeniz D, Leger D, Philip P. Hypersomnia after head-neck trauma-a medicolegal dilemma. Neurology. 1999;54:653–659

[22] Strich SJ. Shearing of nerve fibers as a cause for brain damage due to head injury. Lancet. 1961;2:443–448.

[23] Copes WS, Champion HR, Sacco WJ. Progress in characterizing anatomic injury. J Trauma. 1990;30:1200–1207.

[24] Mody I, MacDonald JF. NMDA receptor-dependent excitotoxicity: the role of intracellular calcium release. Trends Pharmacol Sci. 1995;16:356–359.

[25] McKeating EG, Andrews PJ. Cytokines and adhesion molecules in acute brain injury. Br J Anaeth. 1998; 80:77–84.

[26] Hovda DA. Effect of hyperglycemia after cortical injury. Crit Care Med. 1997;25:1267–1268.

[27] Teasdale GM, Nicoll JR, Murray G, Fiddes M. Association of apolipoprotein E polymorphism with outcome of head injury. Lancet. 1997;350:1069–1071.

[28] BaumannCR, Werth, E, Stocker R, Ludwig S, Bassetti C L Sleep–wake disturbances 6 months after traumatic brain injury: a prospective study. *Brain 2007;130*(7), 1873-1883.

[29] Rao V, Rollings P. *Sleep disturbances following traumatic brain injury. Curr Treat Options Neurol 2002;4:77-87.*

[30] Cohen M, Oksenberg A, Snir D, Stern MJ, Groswasser Z. *Temporally related changes of sleep complaints in traumatic brain injured patients. J Neurol Neurosurg Psychiatry 1992;55:313-315.*

[31] Castriotta R. J., Wilde, MC, Lai J M, Atanasov S, Masel, BE, Kuna, S T. Prevalence and consequences of sleep disorders in traumatic brain injury. *Journ Clin Sleep Med* 2007;3(4), 349.

[32] Watson NF, Dikmen S, Machamer J, Doherty M, Temkin N. Hypersomnia following traumatic brain injury. JCSM 2007; 3:363-368.

[33] International classification of sleep disorders. Third edition (ICSD-III). http://www.aasmnet.org/library/default.aspx?id=9

[34] American Academy of Sleep Medicine-Practice guidelines. http://www.aasmnet.org/practiceguidelines.aspx

3

Heterotopic Ossification after Traumatic Brain Injury

Jesús Moreta and José Luis Martínez-de los Mozos

1. Introduction

Heterotopic ossification is defined as the formation of bone within soft tissues, most frequently muscle tissue. The heterotopic ossification of muscles, ligaments and tendons is a potential complication following trauma, elective orthopaedic surgery, severe burns and neurological injury. It should not be confused with metastatic calcification associated to hypercalcaemia or dystrophic calcification related to tumours. Although there is an uncommon hereditary disease, called fibrodysplasia ossificans progressiva, most cases result from a local trauma (major local surgery, muscular trauma, fractures) or a neurological injury. The first description of heterotopic ossification after neurological injury was by Dejerne and Ceillier [1] in 1918, in soldiers with spinal cord injuries during World War I. Fifty years later, Roberts [2] described heterotopic ossifications in the elbow after brain injury. Since these articles, several studies have been published to provide information about causes, diagnosis and treatment of this complex entity.

This chapter is meant to serve as a review and an update on the literature regarding aetiology, diagnosis and management of this severe complication after a traumatic brain injury.

2. Epidemiology, aetiology and risk factors

The true incidence rate following neurological injury is difficult to establish clearly. After spinal cord injury, the percentage varies between 16% and 53% [3-6], and after traumatic brain injury has been reported to vary between 11% and 22% [7, 8]. A genetic predisposition has been suggested due to the relationship between neurogenic heterotopic ossifications (NHO) and fibrodysplasia (or myositis) ossificans progressiva [8]. The preferred locations in both cases are the proximal limbs and axial musculature. Moreover, a local trauma could predispose an individual to developing a bony formation. The influence of an association between human leukocyte antigens (HLA) and NHO is not clear. Some authors suggest a high prevalence of HLA-B18 and HLA-B27 in patients with heterotopic ossifications, but these findings should be confirmed [9].

It has been suggested that there is a higher prevalence in younger patients (20-30 years old), which may be because neurological injuries are most frequent in this patients [10, 11]. The incidence rate in relation to gender varies in the literature and the relationship has not been shown clearly.

The development of bone in soft tissues in orthopaedic surgery is a well-known complication. This complication has been associated with total hip arthroplasty, fractures or joint dislocations (mainly in the acetabulum or the elbow) and muscular trauma. For this reason, a relationship seems to exist between local trauma and the development of heterotopic ossifications.

Although the presence of traumatic brain injury alone could be associated with the development of heterotopic bone, it is not an established predictor. Brain trauma is a constant cause but there are specific risk factors implicated, such as spasticity, diffuse axonal injury, decerebrate posture, respiratory ventilation or prolonged immobilization. In a study of patients with NHO after traumatic brain injury, Garland [11] showed that 89% of joints were in spastic limbs. Moreover, diffuse axonal injury seems to be more related than focal brain injury [12]. Therefore, the extent of neurological damage must be taken into account, due to the fact that the risk is correlated with the severity of the brain injury. Flin et al. [13] evaluated patients who suffered from comas after traumatic brain injury in an acute rehabilitation unit. They founded that decerabrate posture could predispose an individual to NHO.

Ectopic bone after a neurological injury could develop spontaneously, but there is a higher risk if a local trauma is involved [14]. In general, prolonged immobility during patients' illnesses, such as multiple fractures, burn injuries or a coma, may contribute to the formation of heterotopic ossifications. In patients with brain injuries, a relatively long period of immobilization is frequent and there is therefore an association with the formation of ectopic bone [15].

3. Pathophysiology

Early in the formation of HO, oedema with exudative infiltrate is present, followed by fibroblastic proliferation and immature connective tissue formation. Posteriorly, osteoid formation is seen with the subsequent deposition of bone matrix. Primitive osteoid is deposited as small masses in the periphery early (within the first two weeks) and osteoblasts are noted, located irregularly. Osteoblasts produce tropocollagen, which polymerizes to form collagen and secrete alkaline phosphatase, which allows calcium to precipitate and the mineralization of bone matrix. As mineralization progresses, amorphous calcium phosphate is progressively replaced by hydroxyapatite crystals. During the following weeks, the lesion matures with a centripetal pattern, and after 6-12 months an appearance of true bone is noted. The new bone is always extra-articular and can be contiguous with the skeleton but generally does not involve the periosteum [16].

Many hypotheses about the physiopathology of neurogenic myositis ossificans have been proposed. Different authors have suggested vasomotor and metabolic disorders induced by immobility, the venous stasis or the induction of enchondral ossification from muscular microtrauma. The cellular mechanism of heterotopic ossification remains unclear. It has been postulated that three conditions must be met to achieve heterotopic bone formation [10]: a stimulating event, oestrogenic precursor cells and a proper environment.

Mesenchymal stem cells are pluripotent progenitor cells with the ability to generate cartilage, muscle, tendon, fat and bone. These cells are ubiquitous in soft tissues and may be induced to differentiate into oestrogenic stem cells capable of producing osteoid. Although they play a key role, these cells alone cannot produce ossification and stimulating factors are necessary. Growth factors, such as bone morphogenetic protein, could cause the differentiation of mesenchymal stem cells in a correct environment. Overexpression of bone morphogenetic protein-4 (BMP-4) has been shown to occur in fibrous dysplasia ossificans progressiva, a genetic form of heterotopic ossification mentioned before [17]. Related to this, inhibition of BMP-4 has shown to prevent ossifications in three separate experimental models [18]. Other stimulating factors such as inteleukin-1, growth hormone, prolactin, prostaglandin E-2, basic fibroblast growth factor and insulin-like growth factor type-1 have been recognized in the formation of ectopic bone after neurological injury [19-21]. After a brain injury, it has been suggested that circulating factors in the blood stimulate heterotopic ossification, but the specific mechanism remains unclear [22-23].

As has been mentioned before, the local environment has been shown to be important. Angiogenesis plays a role through the release of angiogenesis factors and differentiation of pericytes into osteoprogenitor cells [24]. Urist et al. [19] discovered that demineralized bone matrix could cause bone formation in vascular tissue. Otherwise, when they cultured this substance in an avascular system they found the development of cartilage. Other contributing factors in the local environment include hypercalcaemia, tissue hypoxia, pH changes (alkalosis) or prolonged immobilization.

It has also been suggested that there is a relationship between the nervous system and bone metabolism. Several neuropeptides and neurotransmitters have been found in the bone tissue. Glutamate, substance P, leptin, vasoactive intestinal peptide (VIP) and catecholamines have been shown to modify osteoblastic and osteoclastic activity [25-27].

In summary, there is an interaction of systemic and local factors on mesenchymal stem cells resulting in their differentiation into osteoblasts and the formation of heterotopic ossification.

4. Location

In patients who have suffered from a spinal injury, NHO develops in sites distal to the level of the spinal cord damage. After a traumatic brain injury, a considerable percentage of patients (between 10% and 20%) could develop ossifications around different joints. In all joints, the development of NHO is typically extra-articular and occurs in the connective tissue between the muscle planes and not within the muscle itself [28]. Clinically, an NHO is defined by a limited decreased range of movement, usually accompanied with pain.

Although upper and lower extremities could be affected, the most commonly affected joint is the hip. In these patients, the most common location is inferomedial and it seems to be a role of adductor spasticity. The ossified tissues extend from the pubic symphysis to the medial or anteromedial femoral shaft and usually the femoral neurovascular bundle lies anteriorly. Other locations around the hip are the posterior part and the anterior aspect of the joint, below the anterior superior iliac spine [11]. When the location is posterior, the sciatic nerve could be involved and if the ossification develops anteriorly it may involve the femoral neurovascular structure. Gartland et al. have suggested that the anteromedial location is most frequent after spinal cord injury, whereas inferomedial, lateral and posterior planes are usually affected after brain injuries [11, 29].

The next most common sites of involvement in patients with traumatic brain injuries are the shoulders and elbows, with the knees rarely being affected. Nevertheless, knees are frequently involved in patients with spinal cord injuries. After a head injury, the ectopic bone about the elbow usually develops posteriorly from the humerus to the olecranon, and could cause ankylosis of this joint. The ulnar nerve could be affected, due to its close location [30]. Although the knee is a common location after a spinal cord injury, it is uncommon in patients with brain damage. In this case, the ectopic bone may occur in any plane, but the inferomedial aspect of the distal femur seems to be the most frequent [29, 30].

5. Diagnosis

5.1. Clinical presentation

The mean time from injury to development of HO is two or three months, but some studies have reported numbers from two weeks up to one year [31]. Thorough physical examination should be performed because this is a critical point for obtaining an early diagnosis. The onset of a heterotopic ossification may simulate an infection with erythema, warmth and swelling. Lower limb swelling may mimic deep venous thrombosis (DVT), so this entity should be ruled out. Differentiating early heterotopic ossification from lower extremity DVT is sometimes difficult, because the two entities have similar clinical presentation. Furthermore, they also can occur at the same time due to the mass effect of the ectopic bone, inciting venous compression and finally phlebitis and thrombus development.

When the passive mobility is examined there is a decreased range of motion. The examiner may identify a painful joint if the patient is conscious, but the findings described before should be checked, especially if the patient is in a coma.

Although there is no total agreement, accelerated bone healing has been reported [32]. In patients with brain injuries, it could be more callus formation but there is a different histological pattern. For this reason, some authors have suggested that this new bone may be a heterotopic ossification, because its maturation is performed from the periphery. Callus maturation after a fracture occurs from the central area [33].

5.2. Laboratory tests

The serum alkaline phosphatase level reflects osteoblastic activity and is useful for obtaining an early diagnosis, especially in patients who cannot report pain or for whom a physical examination is difficult. This marker begins to rise two or three weeks after the brain injury, and values return to normal at approximately four months [34]. A clinical judgement of this test should be done, because liver disease or associated fractures also could increase the levels. Furthermore, alkaline phosphatase titres do not correlate with peak activity or maturation of HO, so they cannot be used to get information about the evolution of the ectopic bone [35]. Nevertheless, this is a cheap and easy screening tool to detect early HO and begin with treatment. Garland (ref de libro) recommends initiating medical prophylaxis on the basis of serum alkaline phosphatase elevation if there are no fractures associated.

In a study of patients after acute spinal cord injury, the 24-hour urinary excretion of prostaglandin E_2 (PGE_2) showed an increase until the maturation of the HO [37]. In patients with brain injuries, it could also be a valuable indicator before the ectopic bone is established. Indomethacin is a PGE_2- blocking agent, which is a useful medication to prevent this [38].

5.3. Radiography

Plain radiographs are an easy and cheap method to recognize a neurogenic heterotopic ossification but it may take up to six weeks for ossification to be evident. In some cases, the HO could develop in several months (Figure 1). Anteroposterior (AP) and lateral radiographs provide enough information to establish the relationship of the HO to the joint, but further radiological techniques (CT-Scan, MTI) should be performed to get more information on the anatomy and the condition of the joint. The typical radiographic appearance of the ectopic bone is a circumferential ossification with a lucent centre [39].

In the hip, the Brooker classification could be useful, which is commonly used to describe the pattern and extent of ossification around a total hip arthroplasty. The extent of the ectopic bone correlates with the degree of functional impairment. According to this classification, there are four types:

- Type I: Islands of bone within the soft tissues.
- Type II: Bone spurs arising from the pelvis or proximal femur with 1cm or less between adjacent bone surfaces.
- Type III: Bone spurs arising from the pelvis or proximal femur with more than 1cm between adjacent bone surfaces.
- Type IV: Confluent bone bridging the pelvis and proximal femur with apparent ankylosis of the hip.

A recent classification has been introduced by Mavrogenis et al. [40] according to the anatomical location of neurogenic HO in the hip: type 1, anterior; type 2, posterior; type 3, anteromedial; type 4, circumferential. These authors suggested that this classification provides better evaluation of the prognosis after surgical excision than the Brooker classification and they found higher blood loss for patients with anteromedial (type 3) or circumferential (type 4) neurogenic ossifications. They also showed a higher risk of recurrence in patients with brain injuries.

5.4. Bone scans

Bone scans or scintigraphy are considered the most sensitive method of providing early detection of HO, with detection as early as two weeks after the onset of symptoms [39].

Bone scintigraphy using 99mTc-methylene disphosphonate provides imaging in three phases: Phase I (dynamic blood flow study), Phase II (Static study for blood pool) and Phase III (amount of radionuclide in bone). The first two phases allow early detection of incipient ossification at two or three weeks. In Phase III, this test occurs approximately one week later. The level of activity on delayed bone scans usually peaks at two months and then it decreases progressively. Scintigraphy activity returns to normal after approximately 12 months, but it may remain positive even when the ossification has become mature.

5.5. Ultrasonography (US)

This technique has been used in the early diagnosis of HO about the hip joints, showing a chaotic disruption of the normal structure of the muscle in the first stages [41]. Later, a peripherally echogenic and centrally hypoechoic finding can be identified. US has the advantage of the possibility of bedside application and it requires no radiation. Ultrasonography is also a fast and useful tool for diagnosis of DVT, which is associated with patients with spinal cord injury as we mentioned before. Nevertheless, ultrasonography is a difficult technique, which depends on the skills of the examiner.

5.6. Magnetic resonance imaging (MRI) and volumetric computed tomography (CT-Scan)

Although bone scans are considered the most sensitive method for early detection of neurogenic HO, magnetic resonance imaging (MRI) suggests changes compatible with ectopic bone formation, as soon as two days after clinical presentation, especially in the knee [42]. In this joint, MRI findings are joint effusion, thickening of the intermuscular septa and a "lacy-pattern" of the muscles vastus lateralis and medialis in fast spin-echo short time inversion-recovery (STIR) images.

Evaluation with computed tomography (CT) combined with two and three-dimensional surface reconstructions provides good differentiation and the extent of the ectopic bone. Moreover, this technique shows the relationship with the joint, determines the mineral density of the bone and can predict several intra-articular lesions. In a study performed by Carlier et al. [43], they compared the density of the HO around the hip with the iliac wing. Bone mineralisation was classified in four categories: normal (M1), mild demineralisation (M2), significant demineralisation with risk of fracture (M3) and evanescent bone with a high risk of fracture (M4). They correlated these features with surgical findings, so this is an important issue because osteoporosis underlying the ankylosis can lead to fractures, which are a difficult challenge in these patients.

If surgical treatment is required, a thorough vascular assessment should be done, because there is a relationship between the HO and surrounding neurovascular structures (femoral bundle in the hip). Therefore, helical-CT with intravenous contrast or MRI with contrast (Figure 1) should be one of the requirements of the preoperative assessment in patients undergoing surgical excision of HO.

6. Treatment and prevention

The prevention of heterotopic ossification is focused on three basic principles: disrupting the inductive signalling pathways, altering the osteoprogenitor cells or modifying the environment. Although some targets are defined in some diseases such as Progressive Osseous Heteroplasia, the target cell or target tissue in NHO remains unknown [44]. Maintaining joint motion by treating spasticity and gentle physical therapy is the goal of early treatment. When a neurogenic heterotopic ossification is suspected, the treatment should start with medical treatment and when the ectopic bone is established and symptomatic surgical resection should be considered carefully. In Figure 2, there is an algorithm, which could be useful to diagnose and treat this entity.

6.1. Physiotherapy and rehabilitation

Prevention should start with early joint mobilisation. Once the diagnosis of early ossifications is suspected, physical therapy with the help of passive exercises should be done [45]. If the patient is conscious, physiotherapy should involve an assisted range of movement exercises with gentle stretch and terminal resistance training. It is crucial to achieve a good range of motion without generating pain. Although forceful manipulation, even under anaesthesia, could be beneficial, it is advisable to avoid aggressive range-of-motion exercises because they carry the risk of causing more bone formation. This may be due to the effect of repetitive microtrauma to the joint [46].

The treatment of HO by extracorporeal shock wave has been reported. Brissot et al. [47] showed less pain and better range of motion and walking distance with this treatment. If the patient is not a suitable candidate for surgical treatment because of medical comorbidities, shock wave therapy could also be a good alternative [48].

In conclusion, physical therapy aims to preserve movement and good function, avoiding or decreasing the risk of ankylosis of the joint.

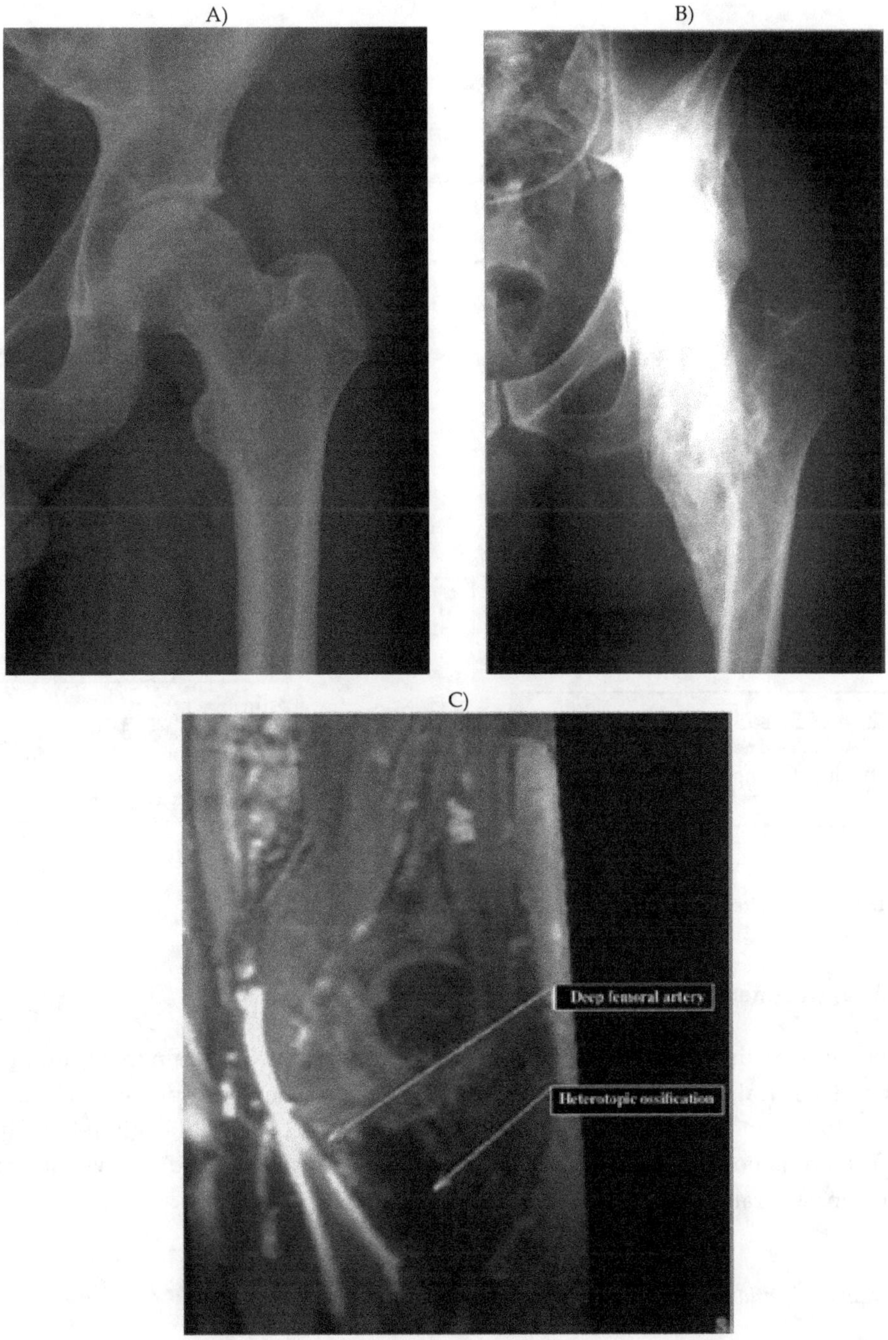

Figure 1. Neurogenic ossification in the hip in a patient after a traumatic brain injury. A) Radiograph of the left hip six months after the brain injury. B) Radiograph showing an anteromedial ossification around the hip causing severe ankylosis, 14 months after the initial injury. C) MRI enhanced with contrast showing a close relationship between the ossification and the deep femoral artery.

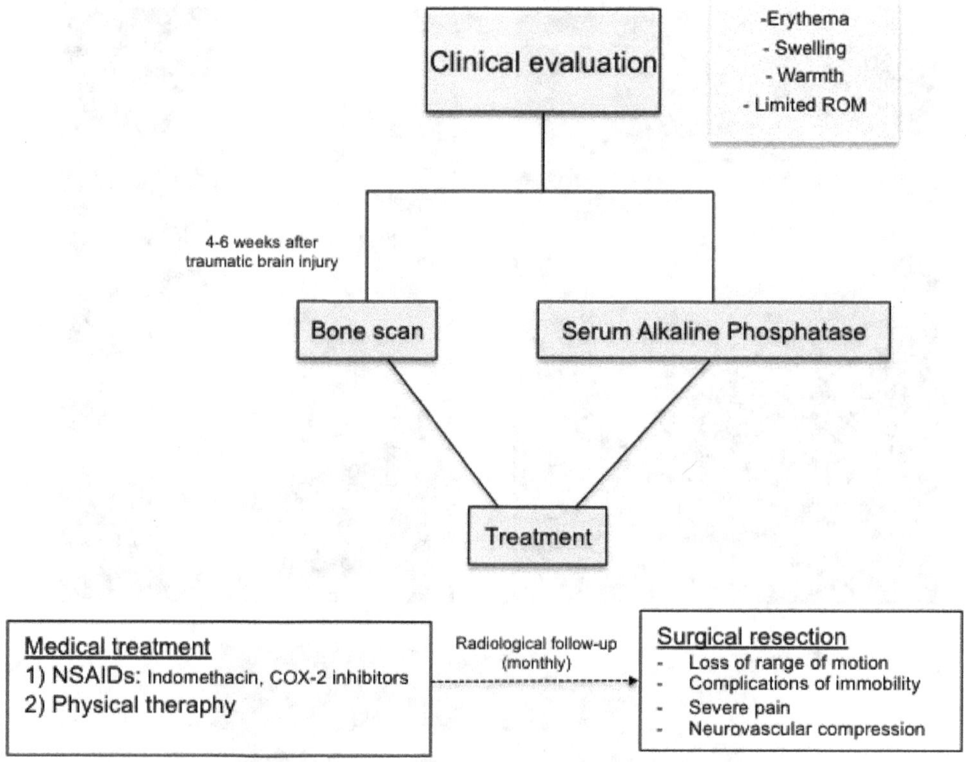

Figure 2. Diagnosis and treatment of neurogenic heterotopic ossifications

6.2. Medical treatment

Medical treatment aims to prevent the formation of HO following brain injury and to avoid recurrence if surgical excision is needed. Due to the fact that the development of HO can occur within one to two months of the initial injury, the prophylaxis should begin relatively early. Although there is no consensus on which medication should be used and when treatment should begin, several drugs have successfully been used.

Nonsteroidal anti-inflammatory drugs (NSAIDs)

These drugs have demonstrated good results in preventing heterotopic ossification after total hip arthroplasty and several studies support their use following traumatic neurological injury [49-51]. A Cochrane Review of HO formation after hip replacements performed in 2004, showed the effectiveness of prevention using NSAIDs perioperatively [52]. A direct effect of NSAIDs on the formation of heterotopic ossification has been described, due to the inhibition of the differentiation of mesenchymal cells into oestrogenic cells. There is also an indirect effect, which refers to the inhibition of bone remodelling by suppression of the prostagland unmediated inflammatory response (specifically PGE-2) [38].

Indomethacin has been considered a useful medication for heterotopic ossification prophylaxis following total hip replacement. In a randomized controlled trial, Banovac et al. [50] showed a lower incidence of early and late HO in the indomethacin group. This drug prescribed for three to six weeks in a dose of 75mg/day, within two months of the injury, may reduce the incidence of heterotopic ossification by two to three times. These same authors performed a trial to determine the effect of COX-2 selective inhibitor rofecoxib on the prevention of HO after spinal cord injury [51]. They concluded that there was a 2.5 times lower risk of developing ectopic bone. COX-2 selective inhibitors could be an attractive option because of less gastrointestinal side effects; however, rofecoxib was taken off the USA market due to elevation of cardiovascular risk. In addition, celecoxib, another selective COX-2 inhibitor, showed the same efficacy as indomethacin in the prevention of HO, but in patients with cardiovascular problems should be used cautiously. Another COX-2 inhibitor, meloxicam, did not reduce the incidence of ossification after total hip replacement compared to indomethacin [53, 54].

In conclusion, indomethacin remains the gold standard for pharmacological prevention of HO, because it is a simple and low cost option. Celecoxib could be a reasonable option in patients without cardiovascular diseases because it has shown good results with fewer gastrointestinal effects.

Bisphosphonates

Bisphosphonates have also been used in the prevention of HO. Etidronate disodium is a well-studied bisphosphonate and it seems to be effective for early ossifications [55, 56] and later phases of this disease. This medication inhibits precipitation of calcium phosphate and blocks the aggregation and mineralisation of hydroxyapatite crystals. In primary prevention, Banovac et al. [56] have suggested that the treatment should begin as soon as elevated alkaline phosphatase is diagnosed or positive findings in ultrasonography or bone scans are shown. In addition, disphosphonates could have long-term effects on prevention when the treatment is finished.

In spite of these results, some authors do not recommend bisphosphonates routinely, because additional fractures are often associated with neurological injuries and the use of bisphosphonates could impede fracture healing [57].

6.3. Radiotherapy

Radiotherapy seems to work by preventing the differentiation of mesenchymal cells into osteoblasts, which could begin the bone formation. This method has been used successfully to prevent heterotopic ossification after hip replacements [58, 59]. In a prospective, randomized study of HO after hip arthroplasty, Knelles et al. found that the best results were obtained with indomethacin and a single irradiation of 7 Gy or four sessions of 3 Gy. These and other authors have suggested that a single irradiation of 7 Gy should be useful in patients at risk, especially if administration of indomethacin is contraindicated [60].

In patients with a traumatic brain injury, radiation therapy may be given as primary (patients with high risk of developing HO) or secondary prophylaxis (those who have been diagnosed with HO and need surgical resection). Sautter-Bihl et al. [62] studied prophylaxis with radiotherapy in 36 patients with spinal cord injuries. These authors used radiotherapy as primary prophylaxis in 27 patients and as secondary prevention (after surgical resection) in 11 patients. With an average follow-up of 23.6 months, 30 of the 36 patients showed no progression of HO and improvements in rehabilitation. It has also been suggested that radiotherapy provides pain relief and decreased serum alkaline phosphatase level in a case report of a patient with HO in both hips and thighs after a brain injury [63]. In this case, the symptoms were refractory to indomethacin, so a dose of 20 Gy in ten fractions was performed.

Like other pharmacological methods of treatment, radiation therapy could affect bone healing. A study focused on HO after elbow trauma has shown that single-fraction therapy leads to an increase risk of non-union [64]. In addition, the location of HO after a total hip arthroplasty is predictable, whereas that after brain injury is difficult to predict accurately where the ectopic bone will develop [65]. For this reason, we do not recommend the routine use of radiation therapy for primary prevention of neurogenic HO, whereas it could be a good method for secondary prophylaxis.

6.4. Surgery

Surgical resection of established ossifications is the treatment of choice to facilitate rehabilitation and is the only effective procedure when the ossification is mature.

The surgery is necessary in patients with symptomatic HO and unsuccessful medical treatment, such as:

- Loss of range of motion and ankylosis with associated functional disability, such as sitting difficulties
- Complications of immobility such as pressure ulcers
- Facilitate rehabilitation and recovery of muscular atrophy secondary to prolonged immobilisation
- Difficulties of appropriate hygiene because access to the perineum or bladder care is needed
- Severe pain refractory to analgesia
- Vascular and/or nerve compression

A careful preoperative assessment is mandatory in order to avoid complications. A CT-Scan is really useful to show intra-articular pathology and the degree of osteoporosis. In addition, a CT-Scan or MRI with contrast describes the relationship with important neurovascular structures.

The timing of operative excision is controversial. Some authors recommend timetables for the best moment to remove these ossifications, but these indications have changed in recent years. Gartland recommended surgery after six months following traumatic heterotopic ossification, one year following spinal cord injury and 18 months after head injury. Another factor to take into account is the neurological condition of the patient. Severe cognitive and physical impairment have poor results from surgery with a high rate of recurrence. However, patients with good neuromuscular control before the surgical procedure have a better functional outcome [65, 66]. In the past, waiting until maturity in order to minimize the rate of recurrence after the surgical treatment was recommended. Nevertheless, recent studies do not confirm a higher rate of recurrence when the HO is excised in an earlier phase [49, 67]. In addition, a long delay before surgery leads to ankylosis, a high degree of osteoporosis and more extensive intra-articular injuries. These findings are associated with bad functional results and potential complications.

Stover et al. [5] showed that the risk of fracture was secondary to osteopenia and this complication increased with the delay in surgical treatment. Perioperative fractures are associated with grade 3 and 4 of osteopenia, according to the classification described by Carlier et al. [43], so therefore this complication could take into account with a preoperative CT-Scan. In a study of HO in 183 hips (143 patients), performed by Genet et al. [49], found 25 perioperative fractures of the femoral neck, all of which occurred in patients with ankylosed hips.

Intra-articular lesions are associated with a smaller range of motion and ankylosis. Some authors considered it to be neurotrophic arthropathy [68], but more recently Genet et al. [49] suggested that it is only ankylosis, which induces articular degradation. In addition, these authors showed that the presence of intra-articular lesions is a cause of worsening of the final results.

In general, the surgical goal is resection of a large enough amount of bone to allow improvement of the range of motion and trying to preserve the joint [49, 69]. A good knowledge of the anatomy is paramount and adequate exposure should be performed with identification of the relationship with neurovascular structures. Intraoperative neurologic monitoring with use of electromyography or somatosensory evoked potentials may be useful, especially in the hip. We use osteotomes and high-speed burrs to remove the ossifications and we frequently use fluoroscopy to check the bone removal (Figure 3). Intraoperative blood loss can be substantial so careful bleeding control should be performed and we recommend that local haemostatic agents should be available, such as bone wax and gelatine-based products. Much of the bleeding is from the osteotomized bone surfaces and is difficult to control with electrocautery. Furthermore, meticulous haemostasis and elimination of dead space decrease the risk of infection.

Wide exposure and identification of major vessels and nerves is extremely important. In many cases, the ossifications have a close relationship with important neurovascular structures and there is distortion of the normal anatomy. Therefore, there is a relatively high risk of iatrogenic injury. Especially in the hip, this complication is extremely important and sometimes life threatening, so therefore we recommend performing this surgical procedure with the assistance of a vascular surgeon [69].

There is a significant risk of recurrence and we recommend prophylaxis methods, such as physical therapy and the administration of indomethacin for two or four weeks. Although no

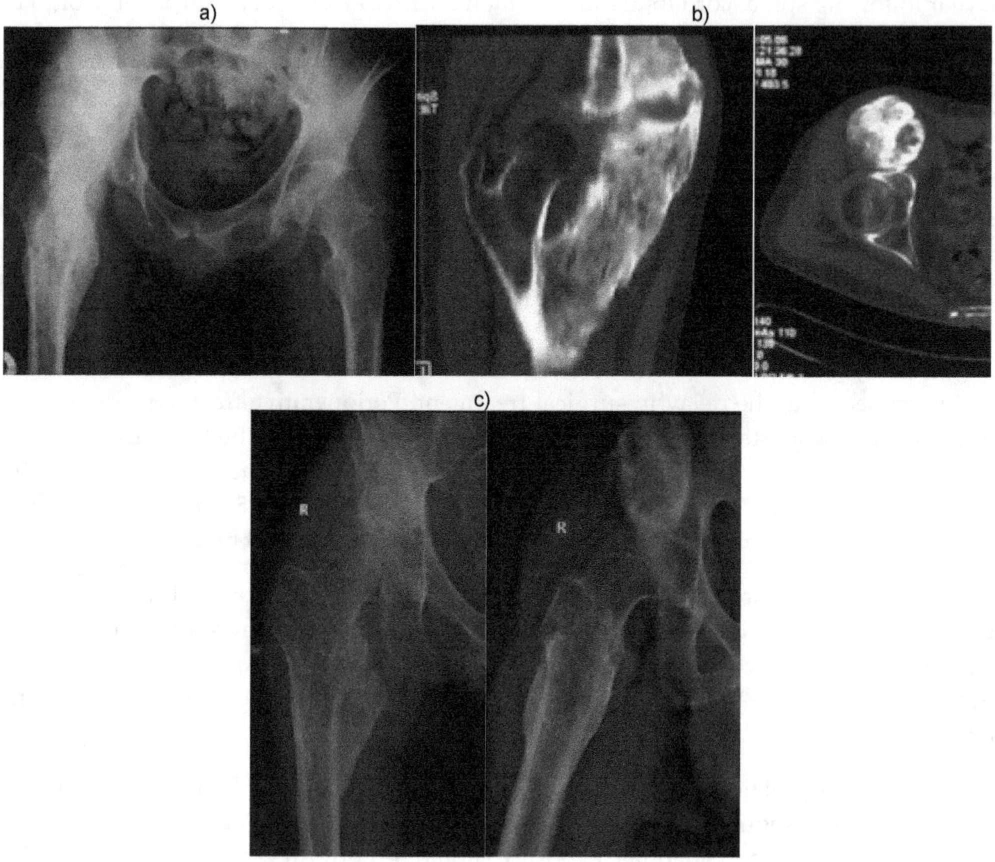

Figure 3. Heterotopic ossification in the right hip causing severe ankylosis. a) Preoperative imaging showing a huge HO from the lesser trochanter to the ilium. b) Preoperative CT-Scan showing involvement of the muscles iliopsoas, vastus medialis and vastus intermedius. b) Radiograph 12 months after surgery.

data have shown the benefit of radiotherapy or medical treatment when ossifications are mature, it is reasonable to use prophylactic treatment postoperatively aiming to prevent recurrence. [66].

7. Conclusion

Heterotopic ossifications after a brain injury present multiple challenges because of the difficult management of this disease. Although it is difficult to predict the development of NHO, it is correlated with the severity of brain damage and several risk factors have been reported. The hip is the most commonly involved joint and the clinical presentation could mimic a septic arthritis or phlebitis in the early stage (3-12 weeks after the neurological injury). Later, although the NHO could be asymptomatic, it can lead to limited range of motion and ankylosis of the affected joint. Early detection and prevention with physical therapy, NSAIDs or bisphosphonates have shown good results. Surgery is recommended when the functional status is affected and thorough preoperative planning should be done to avoid further complications. Although, there is controversy in deciding the timing of surgery, recent articles have suggested that early surgical excision decreases the likelihood of developing osteopenia and intra-articular lesions.

This entity remains a poorly understood condition, so further research in neurogenic heterotopic ossifications should help in continuing to understand pathophysiology, identify pathways and target cells and tissues to find better methods of prevention and treatment.

Acknowledgements

We gratefully acknowledge Dr. O. Sáez de Ugarte and Dr. I. Jauregui for their assistance in the preparation of the manuscript.

Author details

Jesús Moreta* and José Luis Martínez-de los Mozos

*Address all correspondence to: chusmoreta2@hotmail.com

Department of Orthopaedic Surgery and Trauma, Hospital de Galdakao-Usansolo, Galdakao, Spain

References

[1] Dejerne A, Ceillier A. Para-osteo-arthropathies des paraplegiques par lesion medullaire; etude clinique et radiographique. Ann Med 1918;5:497.

[2] Roberts P. Heterotopic ossification complicating paralysis of intracranial origin. J Bone Joint Surg Br 1968;50-B:70-7.

[3] Dai L. Heterotopic ossification of the hip after spinal cord injury. Chin Med J (Engl) 1998;111:1099-101.

[4] Lal S, Hamilton BB, Heinemann A, Betts HB. Risk factors for heterotopic ossification in spinal cord injury. Arch Phys Med Rehabil 1989;70:387-90.

[5] Stover SL, Niemann KM, Tulloss JR. Experience with surgical resection of heterotopic bone in spinal cord injury patients. Clin Orthop. 1991;263:71-7.

[6] Wittenberg RH, Peschke U, Bötel U. Heterotopic ossification after spinal cord injury: epidemiology and risk factors. J Bone Joint Surg (Br). 1992;74-B:215-8.

[7] Citta-Pietrolungo TJ, Alexander MA, Seg NL. Early detection of heterotopic ossification in young patients with traumatic brain injury. Arch Phys Med Rehabil 1992;73:258-62.

[8] Connor JM, Evan DA. Fibrodysplasia ossificans progressiva: the clinical features and natural history of 34 patients. J Bone Joint Surg Br 1982;64:76–83.

[9] Minare P. Neurologic injuries, paraosteoarthropathies and human leukocyte antigens. Arch Phys Med Rehabil. 1984;65:5531.

[10] Genet F, Jourdan C, Lautridou C, et al. The impact of preoperative hip heterotopic ossification extent on recurrence in patients with head and spinal cord injury: a case control study. PloS One 2011;6:23129.

[11] Garland DE. Clinical observations on fractures and heterotopic ossification in the spinal cord and traumatic brain injured populations. Clin Orthop 1988;233:86-101.

[12] Gennarelli TA. Heterotopic ossification. Brain Inj 1988;2:175-8.

[13] Flin C, Curalucci H, Duvovelle A, Viton JM. Heterotopic ossification and brain injury. Ann Readapt Med Phys 2002;45:517-20.

[14] Ebinger T, Roesch M, Kiefer H, Kinzl L, Schulte M. Influence of etiology in heterotopic bone formation of the hip. J Trauma 2000;48:1058-62.

[15] Mielants H, Vanhove E, de Neels J, Veys E. Clinical survey of and pathogenic approach to para-articular ossifications in long-term coma. Acta Orthop Scand 1975;46:190-8.

[16] van Kuijk AA, Geurts AC, van Kuppevelt HJ. Neurogenic heterotopic ossification in spinal cord injury. Spinal Cord 2002;40:313-26.

[17] Hannallah D, Peng H, Young B, Usas A, Gearhart B, Huard J. Retroviral delivery of Noggin inhibits the formation of heterotopic ossification induced by BMP-4, demineralized bone matrix, and trauma in an animal model. J Bone Joint Surg Am 2004;86-A:80-91.

[18] Ahrengart L, Lindgren U, Reinholt FP. Comparative study of the effects of radiation, indomethacin, prednisilone and ethane-1-hydroxy-1, 1-disphonate (EHDP) in the prevention of ectopic bone formation. Clin Orthop 1988;229:265-73.

[19] Urist MR, Nakagawa M, Nakata N, Nogami H. Experimental myositis ossificans: cartilage and bone formation in muscle in response to diffusible bone matrix derived morphogen. Arch Pathol Lab Med. 1978;102:312-6.

[20] Mahy PR, Urist MR. Experimental heterotopic bone formation induced by bone morphogenetic protein and recombinant human interleukin-1B. Clin Orthop 1988;237:236-44.

[21] Wildburger R, Zarkovic N, Egger G, et al. Comparison of the values of basic fibroblast growth factor determined by an immunoassay in the sera of patients with traumatic brain injury and enhanced osteogenesis and the effects of the same sera on the fibroblast growth in vitro. Eur J Clin Chem Biochem 1995;33:693-8.

[22] Cadosch D, Toffoli AM, Gautschi OP, et al. Serum after traumatic brain injury increases proliferation and supports expression of osteoblast markers in muscle cells. J Bone Joint Surg Am 2010;92-A:645-53.

[23] Bidner SM, Rubins IM, Desjardins JV, Zukor DJ, Goltzman D. Evidence for a humorol mechanism for enhanced osteogenesis after head injury. J Bone Joint Surg Am 1990;72-A:1144-9.

[24] Collett GDM, Canfield AE. Angiogenesis and pericytes in the initiation of ectopic calcification. Circ Res 2005;96:930-8.

[25] Wang L, Tang X, Zhang H, Yuan J, Ding H, Wei Y. Elevated leptin expression in rat model of traumatic spinal cord injury and femoral fracture. J Spinal Cord Med 2011;34:501-9.

[26] Hohmann EL, Elde RP, Rysavy JA, Einzig S, Gebhard RL. Innervation of periosteum and bone by sympathetic vasoactive intestinal peptide-containing nerve fibers. Science 1986;232:868-71.

[27] Jones KB, Mollano AV, Morcuende JA, Cooper RR, Saltzman CL. Bone and brain: a review of neural, hormonal, and musculoskeletal connections. Iowa Orthop J 2004;24:123-32.

[28] Jensen LL, Halar E, Little J, Brooke MM. Neurogenic heterotopic ossification. Am J Phys Med Rehabil 1987;66:351-63.

[29] Garland DE. A clinical perspective on common forms of acquired heterotopic ossification. Clin Orthop 1991;263:13-29.

[30] Garland DE, Blum CE, Waters RL. Periarticular heterotopic ossification in head-injured adults: incidence and location. J Bone Joint Surg Am 1980;62-A:1143-6.

[31] Cipriano CA, Pill SG, Keenan MA. Heterotopic ossification following traumatic brain injury and spinal cord injury. J Am Acad Orthop Surg 2009;17:689–97.

[32] Pape HC, Lehmann U, van Griensven M, Gänsslen A, von Glinski S, Krettek C. Heterotopic ossifications in patients after severe blunt trauma with and without head trauma: incidence and patterns of distribution. J Orthop Trauma 2001;15:229-37.

[33] Spencer RF. The effect of head injury on fracture healing: a quantitative assessment. J Bone Joint Surg Br 1987;69-B:525-8.

[34] Orzel JA, Rudd TG. Heterotopic bone formation: clinical, laboratory and imaging correlation. J Nucl Med 1985;26:125-32.

[35] van Kuijk AA, Geurts AC, van Kuppevelt HJ. Neurogenic heterotopic ossification in spinal cord injury. Spinal Cord 2002;40:313-26.

[36] Garland DE, Varpetian A. Heterotopic Ossification in Traumatic Brain Injury. In: Ashley MJ (ed.) Traumatic Brain Injury. Rehabilitation, Treatment, and Case Management. CRC Press; 2004:119-34

[37] Schurch B, Capaul M, Vallotton MB, Rossier AB. Prostaglandin E2 measurements: their value in the early diagnosis of heterotopic ossification in spinal cord injury patients. Arch Phys Med Rehabil. 1997;78:687-91.

[38] Ho SSW, Stern PJ, Bruno LP, et al. Pharmacological inhibition of prostaglandin E-2 in bone and its effect on pathological new bone formation in a rat brain model. Trans Orthop Res Soc. 1988;13:536.

[39] Shehab D, Elgazzar AH, Collier BD. Heterotopic ossification. J Nucl Med 2002;43:346-53.

[40] Mavrogenis AF, Guerra G, Staals EL, Bianchi G, Ruggieri P. A classification method for neurogenic heterotopic ossification of the hip. J Orthopaed Traumatol 2012 13:69-78.

[41] Falsetti P, Acciai C, Palilla R, Carpinteri F, Patrizio C, Lenzi L. Bedside ultrasound in early diagnosis of neurogenic heterotopic ossification in patients with acquired brain injury. Clin Neurol Neurosurg 2011; 113(1):22-7.

[42] Argyropoulou MI, Kostandi E, Kosta P, Zikou AK, Kastani D, Galiatsou E, Kitsakos A, Nakos G. Heterotopic ossification of the knee joint in intensive care unit patients: early diagnosis with magnetic resonance imaging. Crit Care 2006;10:R152.

[43] Carlier RY, Safa DM, Parva P, Mompoint D, Judet T, Denormandie P, Vallée CA. Ankylosing neurogenis myositis ossificans of the hip: an enhanced volumetric CT study. J Bone Joint Surg Br 2005;87-B:301-5.

[44] Kaplan FS, Glaser DL, Hebela N, Shore EM. Heterotopic ossification. J Am Acad Orthop Surg. 2004;12:116-25.

[45] Stover SL, Hataway CJ, Zeiger HE. Heterotopic ossification in spinal cord injured patients. Arch Phys Med Rehabil. 1975;56:199–204.

[46] Garland DE, Razza BE, Waters RL. Forceful joint manipulation in head-injured adults with heterotopic ossification. Clin Orthop 1982;169:133-8.

[47] Brissot R, Lassalle A, Vincendeau S, et al. Treatment of heterotopic ossification by extracorporeal shock wave: 26 patients. Ann Readapt Med Phys 2005;48:581-9.

[48] Reznik JE, Gordon SJ, Barker RN, Keren O, Arama Y, Galea MP. Extracorporeal shock wave therapy (ESWT) as a treatment for recurrent neurogenic heterotopic ossification (NHO). Brain Inj. 2013;27(2):242-7.

[49] Genet F, Marmorat JL, Lautridou C, Schnitzler A, Mailhan L, Denormandie P. Impact of late surgical intervention on heterotopic ossification of the hip after traumatic neurological injury. J Bone Joint Surg Br 2009;91-B:1493-8.

[50] Banovac K, Williams JM, Patrick LD, Haniff YM. Prevention of heterotopic ossification after spinal cord injury with indomethacin. Spinal Cord 2001;39:370-4.

[51] Banovac K, Williams JM, Patrick LD, Levi A. Prevention of heterotopic ossification after spinal cord injury with COX-2 selective inhibitor (rofecoxib). Spinal Cord 2004;42:707-10.

[52] Fransen M, Neal B. Non-steroidal anti-inflammatory drugs for preventing heterotopic bone formation after hip arthroplasty. Cochrane Database Syst Rev 2004, CD001160.

[53] Legenstein R, Bosch P, Ungersbock A. Indomethacin versus meloxicam for prevention of heterotopic ossification after total hip arthroplasty. Arch Orthop Trauma Surg 2003;123:91-4.

[54] Barthel T, Baumann B, Noth U, Eulert J. Prophylaxis of heterotopic ossification after total hip arthroplasty: a prospective randomized study comparing indemethacin and meloxicam. Acta Orthop Scand 2002;73:611-14.

[55] Banovac K, Gonzalez F, Wade N, Bowker JJ. Intravenous disodium etidronate therapy in spinal cord injury patients with heterotopic ossification. Paraplegia 1993;31:660–666.

[56] Banovac K. The effect of etidronate on late development of heterotopic ossification after spinal cord injury. J Spinal Cord Med 2000;23:40–44.

[57] Sullivan MP, Torres SJ, Mehta S, Ahn J. Heterotopic ossification after central nervous system trauma. A current review. Bone Joint Res 2013;2:51–7.

[58] Coventry MB, Scanlon PW. The use of radiation to discourage ectopic bone: a nine-year study in surgery about the hip. J Bone Joint Surg Am 1981;63-A:201-8.

[59] Knelles D, Barthel T, Karrer A, Eulert J, Kölbl O. Prevention of heterotopic ossification after total hip replacement: a prospective, randomised study using acetylsalicylic acid, indomethacin and fractional or single-dose irradiation. J Bone Joint Surg Br 1997;79-B:596-602.

[60] Lo TC. Radiation therapy for heterotopic ossification. Semin Radiat Oncol. 1999;9(2): 163-70.

[61] Sautter-Bihl ML, Hu●ltenschmidt B, Liebermeister E, Nanassy A. Fractionated and single-dose radiotherapy for heterotopic bone formation in patients with spinal cord injury: a phase-I/II study. Strahlenther Onkol 2001;177:200-5.

[62] Jang SH, Shin SW, Ahn SH, Cho IH, Kim SH. Radiation therapy for heterotopic ossification in a patient with traumatic brain injury. Yonsei Med J 2000;41:536-9.

[63] Hamid N, Ashraf N, Bosse MJ, Connor PM, Kellam JF, Sims SH, Stull DE, Jeray KJ, Hymes RA, Lowe TJ. Radiation therapy for heterotopic ossification prophylaxis acutely after elbow trauma: a prospective randomized study. J Bone Joint Surg Am 2010;92-A:2032-8.

[64] Pape HC, Marsch S, Morley JR, Krettek, Giannoudis PV. Current concepts in the development of heterotopic ossification. J Bone Joint Surg Br 2004;86-B:783-7.

[65] Garland DE, Hanscom DE, Keenan MA, Smith C, Moore T. Resection of heterotopic ossification in the adult with head trauma. J Bone Joint Surg Am 1985;67(8):1261-9.

[66] Ippolito E, Formisano R, Farsetti P, Caterini R, Penta F. Excision for the treatment of periarticular ossification of the knee in patients who have a traumatic brain injury. J Bone Joint Surg Am 1999;81-A:783-9.

[67] Freebourn TM, Barber DB, Able AC. The treatment of immature heterotopic ossification in spinal cord injury with combination surgery, radiation therapy and NSAID. Spinal Cord 1999;37:50–3.

[68] Gacon G, Deider Ch, Rhenter J-L, Minaire P. Ectopic bone formation in neurological lesions. Rev Chir Orthop Reparatrice Appar Mot 1978;64:375-90.

[69] Moreta-Suárez J, Sáez de Ugarte-Sobrón O, Martínez-de los Mozos JL. Osificaciones heterotópicas neurogénicas de cadera. A propósito de 2 casos. Rev esp cir ortop traumatol 2011;55:292-7.

4

The Non Invasive Brain Injury Evaluation, NIBIE – A New Image Technology for Studying the Mechanical Consequences of Traumatic Brain Injury

Hans von Holst and Svein Kleiven

1. Introduction

Traumatic brain injury (TBI) is an epidemiologically well-known disorder that ranges from minor to severe conditions (Kleiven, Peloso, von Holst, 2003). The aetiology of TBI is due to external violence and similar all over the world. About 80% is defined as mild and in this category, most patients recover completely after a certain time, ranging from days to months. Another 10% is defined as moderate with a prolonged recovery period, depending on a number of causes such as type and localisation of injury. The final 10% covers severe injuries, where the recovery period usually remains for life. In contrast to most other diseases, TBI has a sudden onset with a substantial impact on the patient´s close relatives, as complications are obviously not only of a physiologically handicapped nature but also psychological, due to the presence of personality changes. With an increase in worldwide social standard, TBI may unfortunately increase further. Thus, the World Health Organization has predicted TBI to surpass many diseases as one of the major causes of disability and death during the next decade unless external causes are reduced (World Health Organization, 2003).

As the external causes of TBI in most cases are known, the focus on primary prevention has already reduced the number of TBI successfully. One of the reasons for this reduction is due to the reconstruction of accidents by means of simulation. By using simulation methods and models, it is easier to discover innovations for prevention of the most severe accidents. The use of simulations will be of even greater importance in the future. Of equal importance is secondary prevention at the scene of the accident, in hospital care and the subsequent tertiary prevention during neurological rehabilitation. The overall mechanisms associated with TBI have been extensively investigated during the last decades by focusing on the biochemical and biomechanical consequences (Narayan, R.K, Wilberger, J.E, Povlischock, J.T, 1995). The introduction of new and advanced image technologies such as computerized tomography (CT) and magnetic resonance tomography (MRI) have, together with the introduction of neurological intensive care units, further improved the knowledge and consequences of TBI (von Holst, 2007). Today the recommended treatment is based on clinical practice and personal experience, with an increased interest in evidenced-based medicine an even more comprehensive and generally accepted treatment of TBI resulting in an expected improved outcome. Utilisation of simulation models and methods in clinical practice will further improve future intensive care treatment after TBI. The same scenario holds true also for tertiary prevention in neurological rehabilitation, as simulation methods and models will be introduced. Thus, the combined increased activities of primary prevention, pre-hospital care, neurosurgical interventions and neurological rehabilitation have certainly improved outcomes following TBI.

In this chapter we present the concept of a new image technology defined as non-invasive brain injury evaluation technology focusing on reconstructive potentials of TBI and how this can be implemented into clinical practice aimed at improvement of outcomes.

2. Biomechanics in TBI

Clinically, brain injuries can be classified into two broad categories: focal injuries and diffuse injuries. The focal brain injury is a lesion causing local damage, which can be seen by the naked eye. The diffuse brain injury is associated with global disruption of brain tissue and is usually invisible. Focal injuries consist of epidural haematomas (EDH), subdural haematomas (SDH), intracerebral haematomas (ICH) and contusions (coup and contrecoup). Diffuse injuries consist of brain swelling, concussion and diffuse axonal injury (DAI) (Melvin, 1993).

The human brain is sensitive to rotational motion (Holbourn, 1943; Gennarelli et al., 1987). In pioneering work, Holbourn (1943) observed shear strain patterns in 2D gel models and claimed that translation is not injurious; on the other hand, rotation could explain the majority of traumatic brain injuries due to the nearly incompressible properties of brain tissue. The bulk modulus of brain tissue is roughly five to six orders of magnitude larger than the shear modulus (McElhaney et al., 1976), so that for a given impact, it tends to deform only in shear. This gives significant sensitivity of the strain in the brain to rotational loading and small sensitivity to linear kinematics (Kleiven, 2006). Therefore, rotational kinematics should be a better indicator of traumatic brain injury risk than linear acceleration. Additionally, it has been shown that the most common severe injuries, such as subdural haemorrhage and diffuse axonal injury are more easily caused by rotational head motion (Gennarelli et al., 1972, 1987). Gurdjian and Gurdjian (1975) suggested that a combination of skull deformation, pressures and inertial brain lag could present a clearer picture of head injury (Gennarelli et al., 1982) stated that all types of brain injury can be produced by angular acceleration. According to Ommaya (1985), rotation can produce both focal and diffuse brain injuries, while translation is limited to focal effects.

2.1. Focal injuries

2.1.1. Epidural haematoma (EDH) and subdural haematoma (SDH)

Epidural haematoma is a relatively infrequently occurring sequel to head trauma (0.2-6%, Cooper, 1982). It occurs as a result of trauma to the skull and the underlying meningeal vessels and is not due to brain injury (Melvin et al., 1993). The mortality rate of SDH in most studies is greater than 30%. Acute subdural haematoma, together with diffuse axonal injury account for more head injury deaths than all other lesions combined (Gennarelli, 1981). SDH is the most common of the severe traumatic brain injuries, accounting for around 50% of the total number of injuries in this category in Sweden (Kleiven et al., 2003). The most common mechanism of subdural haematoma is tearing of the veins that bridge the subdural space as they go from the brain surface to the various dural sinuses (Gennarelli and Thibault, 1982). Based on previous primate experiments, Gennarelli (1983) suggested that SDH was produced by short duration and high amplitude of angular accelerations. Lee and Haut (1989) studied the effects of strain rate on tensile failure properties of human bridging veins and determined the ultimate strain to be about εf=0.5, which they found to be independent of the strain rate (=0.1-250 s-1). Earlier research done by Löwenhielm (1974) showed that the failure strain was markedly reduced from about 0.8 to 0.2 as the strain rate was increased. Lee et al. (1987) used a 2D sagittal model and Huang et al. (1999) used a 3D model (Shugar, 1977) to study the mechanisms of SDH. They found that the contribution of angular acceleration to tearing of bridging veins, measured as observed change in distance between a node in the interior of the skull and a node in the brain, was greater than the translational acceleration. Substantially larger relative motions between the skull and the brain, as well as higher strain in the bridging veins have been found when switching from a translational to a rotational mode of motion using a detailed 3D head model including 11 pairs of the largest bridging veins (Kleiven, 2003).

2.1.2. Contusion

Cerebral contusion is one of the most frequently found lesions following head injury. It consists of heterogeneous areas of necrosis, pulping, infarction, haemorrhage and oedema (Melvin et al., 1993). Contusions generally occur at the site of impact (coup contusions) and at remote sites from the impact defined as contrecoup contusions. Contrecoup lesions are more significant than coup lesions. Cerebral contusion at the site of impact in the presence of skull fracture is likely to be induced by the direct impression of the skull against the underlying brain tissue and therefore, in terms of skull fracture, caused by contact force and predicted by linear acceleration. In the absence of skull fracture,cerebral contusion is likely to be induced by shearing and scratching of the brain tissue against edges and sharper ridges in the dura/skull, and therefore caused by excessive head rotational loading (Löwenhielm, 1974). Moreover, Shreiber et al. (1997) derived a threshold of 0.19 in principal logarithmic strain in the cortex for a 50% risk of cerebral contusions. As previously mentioned, this strain is sensitive only to the rotational kinematics and not the translational motion (Ueno, Melvin, 1995; Kleiven, 2007).

2.1.3. Intracerebral haematomas (ICH)

Intracerebral haematomas are well defined homogeneous collections of blood within the cerebral parenchyma. They are most commonly caused by sudden acceleration/deceleration of the head. Other causes are penetrating wounds and blows to the head. Through reconstruction of a motocross accident, it was possible to re-create the injury pattern in the brain of the injured rider using the maximal principal strain (Kleiven, 2007b). The strain levels at maximum for two locations of intra-cerebral haematomas were around 0.4-0.5, which is close to known thresholds for rupture of cerebral veins and arteries (Monson, 2003; Löwenhielm, 1974; Lee, Haut, 1989), indicating that the risk of intra-cerebral haematomas can be predicted by the pattern and magnitude of maximum principal strain.

2.2. Diffuse Injuries

2.2.1. Concussion

The classical cerebral concussion involves immediate loss of consciousness following injury (Melvin et al., 1993). This is the most commonly occurring head injury, accounting for around 70% of total injuries, with more than 99% of patients leaving the hospital within 14 days (Kleiven et al., 2003). Studies on giant squid axons (Thibault, 1993) suggest a maximal principal strain of around 0.10 to cause reversible injury to the axons, which could be used as an approximate axonal strain threshold for concussion. During simulations of concussions in the National Football League (NFL), the strain magnitude in the brain was found to be sensitive to only rotational kinematics and not translational motion (Kleiven, 2007b).

2.2.2. Diffuse axonal injury (DAI)

Diffuse axonal injury is associated with mechanical disruption of many axons in the cerebral hemispheres and subcortical white matter (see Fig. 3). Microscopic examination of the brain discloses axonal tearing throughout the white matter of both cerebral hemispheres. It also involves degeneration of long white matter tracts extending into the brain stem. High-resolution CT scans may show small haemorrhages and axonal swelling (Fig. 3). DAI involves immediate loss of consciousness lasting for days to weeks. Severe memory and motor deficits are present and posttraumatic amnesia may last for weeks. At the end of one month, 55% of patients are likely to have died (Gennarelli, 1982).

The maximum strain that may cause damage to the axons has been estimated in previous publications. Studies have been performed with giant squid axons (Thibault et al., 1990) and a strain of 0.3 was suggested as threshold of diffuse axonal injury. Bain and Meaney (2000) proposed a threshold of 0.2 in maximal principal strain in the brain tissue for the onset of the malfunction of the neurons in the brain, which could be seen as a first stage of DAI. Maximum principal Green Lagrange strain of 0.2 has also been shown to correlate with cell death and neuronal dysfunction associated with DAI (Morrison et al., 2003). Gennarelli et al. (1972) subjected squirrel monkeys to controlled sagittal plane head motions. It was found that in the animals subjected to pure translation of the head, cerebral concussion was not obtainable. In contrast, the animals who were subjected to head rotations were all concussed. Visible brain lesions were noted in both translated and rotated groups but with a greater frequency and severity after rotation. Ueno and Melvin (1995) found, when applying kinematics to a 2D head model, that rotational acceleration has a dominant effect on shear deformation, while linear acceleration is related to pressure.

3. The concept of NIBIE

NIBIE, Non-Invasive Brain Injury Evaluation, is a technology for measuring and evaluating parameters such as intracranial pressure, strain and stress from CT, MRI and Positron Emission Tomography (PET) scans (Fig. 1). The primary purpose of NIBIE is as a diagnostic tool for screening of patients with TBI and observation of intensive care patients with neurosurgical disorders such as haematoma, oedema or tumours. In addition, stroke patients may benefit from the method. NIBIE was created as a result of an interdisciplinary collaborative research project between engineers at the Royal Institute of Technology and neurosurgeons at the Karolinska University Hospital in Stockholm, Sweden.

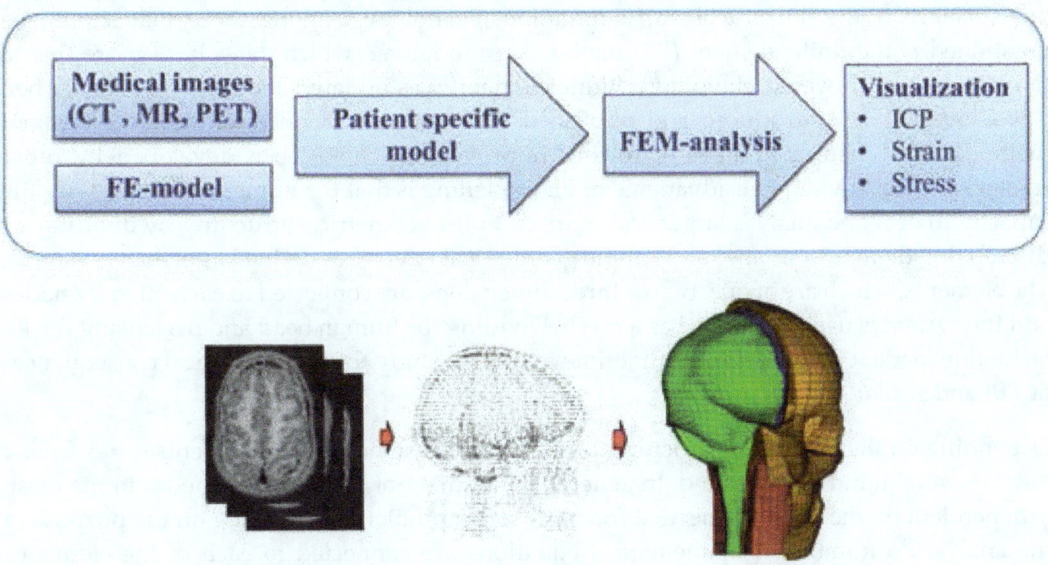

Figure 1. From medical image to FE modelling for visualization of ICP, strain and stress.

Research on numerical modelling of the head, which resulted in one of the most accurate finite-element models of the head available, made possible the use of the numerical model for medical applications in combination with existing medical diagnostic imaging data. The new image technology is well integrated with existing diagnostic tools and adjusted for each individual patient. NIBIE is unique in the sense that it can measure and define intracranial pressure without any neurosurgical procedure. It is the first non-invasive simulation method that is able to define biomechanic parameters in brain tissue on healthy and diseased people. Additionally, NIBIE has the capacity to define the strain level in the brain in order to evaluate the impact on the fibre tracts and classify what local and regional areas need to be focused on following TBI and stroke. Moreover, in neurosurgical procedures, NIBIE has proven to be safe for calculating the optimal neurosurgical approach into the brain with regard to the skull bone opening. Calculation of the most optimal head position with regard to gravitation is another possibility for reducing the pressure and strain level in the injured area. Further possibilities include the calculation of strain levels in fibre tracts following hydrocephalus and brain tumours to potentially explain gait apraxia, incontinence and cognitive dysfunctions. Thus, it is clear that the NIBIE software program is superior for the identification of biomechanical influence on brain tissue when compared to that found in CT, MRI and PET images.

4. Technology of NIBIE

The introduction of CT, MRI, PET and other images for medical use has substantially improved clinical knowledge and practice. Further improvement is to be expected parallel with developments in computer capacity. The next generation of innovative images supporting clinical neuroscience is the introduction of simulation technology. Among those that should be mentioned is the finite element (FE) method, or modelling, which dates back more than a hundred years. However, the phrase 'finite element' was initiated about 60 years ago when Ray Clough (1980) introduced and published what today is defined as the finite element method. Since then, a number of further improvements have been developed by other researchers worldwide. The advantage of FE modelling is that the numerical method has the capacity to deal and analyse larger and more complex geometrical structures by dividing, or discretizing them into smaller and simple geometrical structures defined as elements (Fig. 2). The elements, which are of one, two or three dimensions, are connected to each other by nodes and the system is usually defined as a mesh. Dividing the human head and neck using the FE technique made it possible for the first time to further study the biomechanical consequences of TBI and stroke.

Depending on the size of the structure to be analysed, the number of elements differ from a few to several hundred thousand. In general, the number of elements and nodes in the mesh is dependent on the accuracy needed for analysing a problem. Depending on the purpose of the analysis, a number of mathematical equations are connected to each of the elements, thereby giving the mesh a relationship between different mechanical loadings of, for instance, forces and displacements in the mesh. Parallel with the introduction of CT, MR and PET images, the FE method was further developed for engineering purposes such as simulations, of which the transportation industry should be mentioned in particular. Of special interest was the introduction of colour graphics in combination with powerful computers, which gave the FE method better understanding and capacity for clinical implementation.

In the last twenty years, an increased interest in the FE method has been highlighted in the health care sector mainly due to its capacity for performing reconstructive biomechanical

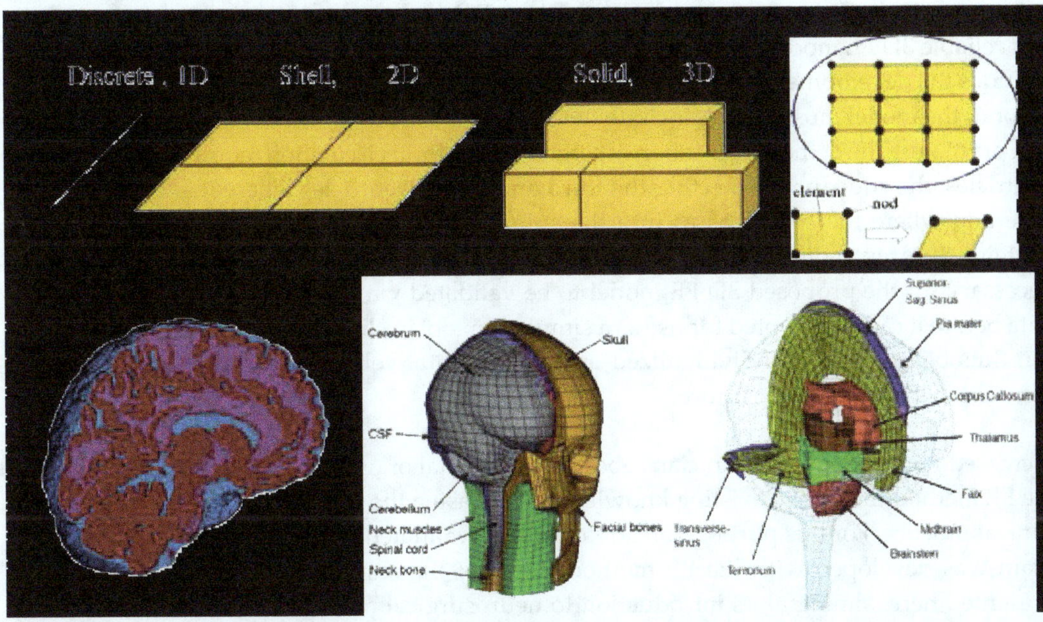

Figure 2. Schematic illustration of FE model development process from 1D, 2D and 3D elements to the construction of human head and neck models.

simulations of accidents (Kleiven, 2007). Although existing image technologies have substantially increased knowledge, there are still areas in need of new innovative image methods. This holds true especially in the field of clinical neuroscience. For instance, there is no image technology today that has the capacity to analyse a number of important biomechanical issues, which in turn will improve clinical assessment and clinical practice. Some of these problems include analysis of intracranial pressure in the brain tissue, the strain level in nerve fibres and stress in bone materials.

4.1. A computational 3D FE model

The development of advanced computational technology that started roughly three decades ago has increased interest in introducing human FE head models today (Ward and Thompson, 1975; Kumarezan, Radhakrishnan and Ganesan, 1995; Zhou, Khalif and King, 1995; Krabbel and Muller, 1996). With increased knowledge and interdisciplinary collaboration, more advanced 3D FE models have seen the light (Kleiven and von Holst, 2002; Johnson, 2008; Li, 2012). The technology has also become more accessible through easy-to-use interfaces, provided by most commercial FE-codes. The latest 3D versions include all anatomical structures of the human brain. As such, today a modern 3D FE head model includes the skin, all three bone layers, meninges, cerebrospinal fluid, brain tissue and aqueduct – including the foramina located in the skull base of the brain tissue. Depending on the purpose and need for analysis, the elements may consist of shell and solid tetrahedral or hexahedral configurations and can be used where they are most appropriate.

A prerequisite for using a modern FE method for TBI in clinical practice is access to a realistic and reliable 3D FE model of the human head. First, a FE model of the human head and brain includes the development of the outer and inner skull bone with the porous bone in between. Second, the model must further include the meninges including the dura, falx and tentorium and pia mater. Third, the construction of cerebrospinal fluid circulation requires the two lateral ventricles, the aqueduct connecting the third and fourth ventricles where it ends in the skull base and where the brain passes into the spinal cord. Fourth, the complete 3D FE model contains the grey and white matter of the brain tissue. Following complete development, it is necessary for the proposed 3D FE model to be validated via a significant amount of patient data before it can be accepted for use as a simulation tool in clinical practice. The 3D FE model can thus be extensively individualized and might tentatively have a substantial impact on clinical practice in the near future.

Increased knowledge from clinicians about the potential of using 3D FE modelling and what the FE method can add to existing knowledge will hasten the method to be implemented into clinical practice. For this purpose, an advanced and validated numerical model of the human brain was developed with the FE method; some of the results from such simulations are presented here, aiming at its introduction to neurosurgical practice of TBI and other neurological disorders. It can be tentatively suggested that the advanced FE model, including geometrically detailed descriptions, will predict injuries with good accuracy (Kumarezan, Radhakrishnan and Ganesan, 1995). It should be stressed that the FE method provides a means for studying how complex structures are affected by external loading and has long been used for applications in civil engineering and in the manufacturing industry. Thus, the method is well-suited for analysis of complex biological structures in the head and neck, as it will likely improve clinical practice in neurosurgery in the future.

5. Applied neuroscience

One of the most important neurological complications of moderate and severe traumatic brain injury (TBI) is the development of brain tissue oedema, which consists of an abnormal accumulation of fluid within the brain parenchyma. Oedema and its associated complications account for approximately 50% of deaths in patients with TBI (Marmarou, 2003). Raised intracranial pressure (ICP) is found in the majority of severe traumatic brain injuries caused by intracranial haematomas and brain swelling, and may be deleterious for the patient unless treated effectively (von Holst, 2007). Vasogenic and cytotoxic oedema are the two major types of oedema after TBI. Vasogenic oedema is due to blood-brain barrier disruption, resulting in increased extracellular water accumulation, while cytotoxic oedema is defined as increased intracellular water collection (Marmarou, 2003). As the aetiology of vasogenic oedema is relatively well understood, the treatment thereof is fairly effective. However, the mechanisms of cytotoxic brain oedema are still unclear, which renders a treatment of choice inadequate. Research has shown that the brain swelling observed in patients with TBI appears to be predominantly cellular, while vasogenic oedema is present at a minor degree (Marmarou,

Singoretti and Fatouros et al., 2006). This makes the clinical treatment of TBI oedema more complicated.

Although improvements in outcome have been made in recent decades, much remains to be done, especially since the recommended treatment is predominately based on clinical practice and personal experience. Clinically, local and minor oedema may be treated conservatively only by observation, while more extensive oedematous areas demand intensive care and where the treatment of choice usually follows evidence-based practice (Rabinstein, 2006; von Holst, 2007). Monitoring the ICP is an integral part of intensive care treatment following moderate and severe TBI. The longer the ICP exceeds 20–25 mm Hg, the poorer the outcome for the patient is expected (von Holst, 2007). On admittance to hospital, the patient with moderate and severe TBI is placed with the head at a 30-degree elevation aimed at optimizing the ICP, the cerebral perfusion pressure, the venous drainage from the head as well as the pulmonary function (Rabinstein, 2006; von Holst, 2007). Anatomically detailed FE models have been developed in an effort to simulate consequences of various impacts to the human head in the same group (Ho and Kleiven, 2009), which gives both researchers as well as clinicians a better understanding of TBI. Poroelasticity has been used to simulate hydrocephalus and brain oedema in early studies (Nagashima, Tamaki and Matsumotu et al., 1987). In more recent studies, simplified geometry, such as cylindrical or spherical geometry, has been adopted to investigate the mechanisms behind hydrocephalus (Kaczmarek, Subramaniam and Neff, 1997; Levine, 1999; Smille, Sobey and Molnar, 2005). Three dimensional (3D) FE models with anatomically detailed brain structures have also been used (Dutta-Roy, Wittek and Miller, 2008; Li, von Holst and Kleiven, 2009). Gravity has been shown to play an important role in brain shift during craniotomy in a series of studies using FE models (Coffey, Garg and Miga et al., 2010; Miga, Roberts and Kennedy et al., 2001). However, to date, there has been no experimental or clinical study evaluating the patient's head position with regard to oedema localization considering the gravity aspects, which could potentially alter both the clinical treatment as well as the outcome following TBI.

Formation of brain oedema involves fluid movement from the vasculature directly into the intracellular space (cytotoxic brain oedema) or extracellular space defined as the vasogenic oedema (Marmarou, 2003). The circulation of CSF tends to be disturbed for oedema patients with high ICP. However, the detailed mechanisms behind oedema and disturbed CSF circulation fall outside the range of this study. We used a fluid source added to the oedema to simulate extra fluid accumulation. In this model, we considered the influence of gravity on a patient with oedema at the posterior part of the brain for the supine and prone positions. The model was based on the normal CSF circulation model with the addition of a focal oedema at the posterior part of the brain. A higher localized interstitial fluid pressure (IFP) at the oedema zone due to extra oedema fluid accumulation is seen for both positions. The average IFP at the oedema zone decreased around 15%, from 3,331 Pa to 2,824 Pa when changing from the supine to prone position. For the supine position, the IFP decreased from the oedema zone the whole way to the frontal part of the brain. For the prone position, the IFP at tissue adjacent to the oedema showed a similar tendency to the supine position; however, IFP started to increase at a certain distance from the oedema zone due to hydrostatic pressure induced by gravity. The tissue pressure gradient drove the interstitial fluid away from the oedematous zone to other parts of the brain. When IFP increased, the brain tissue swelled due to the pressure gradient acting on the tissue skeleton. Since brain cells and CSF were nearly incompressible (Kaczmarek, Subramaniam and Neff, 1997), the enlarged volume was expected to be filled with extra fluid. The predicted water content increment was about 10% at the centre of the oedema and decreased towards other areas of the brain. The value of water content increment was nearly identical for both positions. This was to be expected, since the swelling of oedematous tissue was caused by the IFP gradient acting on the solid skeleton rather than the IFP. Both IFP and water content increment distribution in the brain was similar to those reported in experiments on cold-injured oedema in cats (Reulen and Kreysch, 1973).

5.1. Epidural, subdural haemorrhages and intracranial pressure

On arrival at the hospital from the scene of an accident it is not always easy to clinically judge the patient´s condition with regard to potential injuries in the brain tissue that might be in need of immediate handling by emergency staff. A better clinical evaluation can be done by performing a CT scan, which can be done within a short period of time. Among the most important injuries are the presence of epidural haematomas (EDH) and any signs of increased ICP. As shown in Fig. 3, the EDH is clearly visible. As this EDH will cause a substantial midline shift, the ultimate choice of treatment is an acute neurosurgical evacuation of the haemorrhage, which aims to reduce the expanding volume to avoid further secondary injuries. Additionally, as the ICP is probably increased in this patient, it is important to judge whether it should be monitored continuously or not. These two types of injuries are of great interest when it comes to the application of the NIBIE software image. The CT image is digitized over to NIBIE (Fig. 1) for the evaluation of secondary complications such as potential increased strain and ICP levels, two criteria which may have a dramatic effect on brain tissue with regard to secondary injuries.

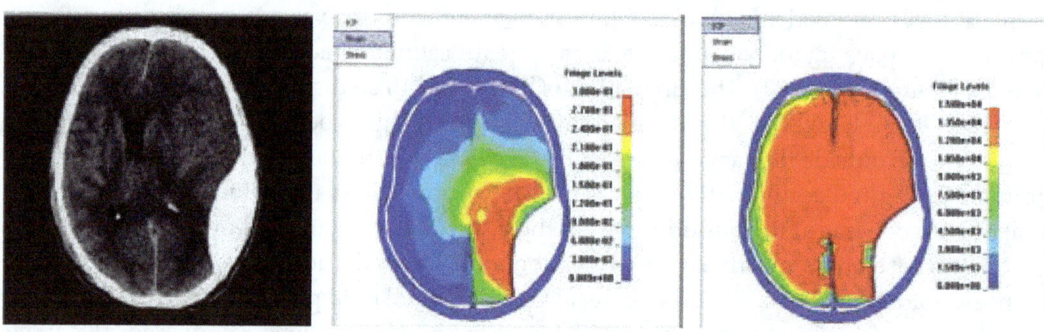

Figure 3. CT-verified epidural haematoma (left) analysed with NIBIE with regard to strain (middle) and ICP (right).

The increased strain level shown in Fig. 3 is highest in the nearest vicinity of the EDH and reduces with distance from the EDH. After the acute evacuation of the EDH, the strain level is simultaneously reduced, thereby preventing further secondary injuries. The strain level shown in Fig. 3 offers significant support to clinicians in neurological intensive care and for rehabilitation staff. Comparing the CT scan with the degree of strain level, NIBIE may also have the capacity to define the anatomical area of most importance for treatment and observation. This is also beneficial to the rehabilitation staff in terms of what region to focus on when the time is ready for more active neurological rehabilitation.

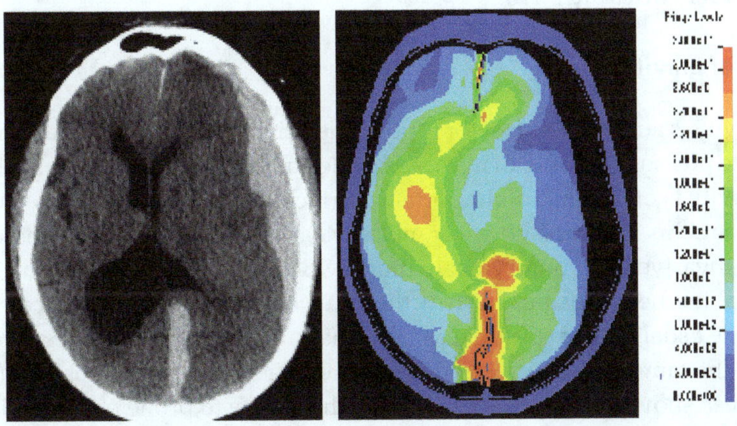

Figure 4. CT verified subdural haematoma (left) evaluated with NIBIE and strain level (right).

In contrast to the strain level, the FE model of NIBIE shows that the ICP is substantially increased throughout the brain. The evacuation of the EDH volume will not only reduce the increased strain level, but also the increased ICP. Usually, monitoring equipment is obligatory for a suspected increased ICP and is implanted right after the evacuation of the EDH during the same neurosurgical procedure. As NIBIE has proven reliable in defining normal or increased ICP levels, an implantation of monitoring equipment is not always necessary. In future, ICP can easily be defined by repeated CT and NIBIE evaluation during the neurological intensive care treatment period.

Not only patients suffering from EDH, but also those admitted with subdural haematomas may also benefit for the same reasons. While EDH is mostly acute and found in about two per cent of all types of injury, SDH is more frequent and divided into acute, sub-acute and chronic injury, depending on the age of the haematoma, which is not always easy to estimate. One possible and more precise age definition of the SDH could be the definition of strain level, which should be reduced when the haematoma has transferred from a clot to fluid (Fig. 4). In this case, NIBIE has the capacity to define the area of potential secondary injury and that may be found in nerve fibres showing an increased strain level.

With the introduction and use of NIBIE for clinical application, new injury criteria may be defined by focusing on strain and ICP levels. It is therefore quite possible that the new criteria will successively increase knowledge among health care staff. By using each slice from the CT and evaluating them in NIBIE, it is possible to gain a holistic view of the severity of the injury and hence better information on potential secondary injuries, and what clinicians should focus on when it comes to direct and more long term treatment. Of interest are patients with asymptomatic chronic SDH. Here, evaluation with NIBIE may give insight to whether the brain tissue shows any evidence of strain, which will be clinically helpful for clinicians in terms of their decisions for clinical treatment in some of the more questionable patients. This new insight will further encourage better clinical evaluation and treatment, resulting in better clinical outcomes for patients with EDH, SDH and increased ICP. This scenario also holds true for other cerebral injuries after TBI.

5.2. Influence of gravity

In general, gravity is an important factor for consideration in TBI, since it may have a dramatic influence on the pressure around an intracerebral lesion or haemorrhage. In the neurosurgical procedure, gravity is of paramount importance to facilitating an operation. When it comes to clinical treatment, this aspect is, however, not always considered in the intensive care phase. Here, the non-invasive brain injury evaluation, NIBIE, has proven promising in evaluating optimization of the head position. When the head of the patient with a cerebral lesion is positioned in the usual supine position, as is normally the case, the pressure is usually higher compared to if the same patient is instead considered for a more prone position (Fig. 5). Using NIBIE, it has been shown that by switching from the supine to prone position, the pressure in the injured area is reduced by about 15%, depending on the size and localization of the injury. Switching from a supine to a more prone position may thus cause a substantial reduction in secondary injury, thereby promoting shorter in-hospital treatment and a better outcome.

It has been shown that reducing an increased ICP after severe TBI can significantly reduce mortality rate. This is supported in clinical treatment where the patient's head is elevated to about 30 degrees to facilitate cerebral blood flow (Rabinstein, 2006). The pressure gradient in the central nervous system is not always equally distributed inside the cranium following TBI (Miindermann, 1999). Instead, it has been found that pressure gradients also exist between the two hemispheres or even between neighbouring areas of the same hemisphere, especially in the oedema zone, where local tissue pressure increases as a result of a pathological accumulation of extra fluid (Reulen and Kreysch, 1973). Additionally, it can be tentatively suggested that even a slightly increased interstitial fluid pressure IFP might trigger a series of pathological processes to the already injured and vulnerable tissue inside and surrounding the oedema zone (Li, von Holst and Kleiven, 2011). Following the biomechanical cascades of events in moderate and severe TBI, both necrosis and apoptosis was seen to be present, although they differed in some aspects. Necrosis was found as a response to tissue damage due to biomechanical or ischemic influences.

In contrast, neurons undergoing apoptosis are morphologically intact during the immediate post-traumatic period, with adequate biochemistry providing the existence of normal membrane potential (Werner and Engelhard, 2007). When the hydrostatic pressure reaches 30 mmHg the neurochemical cascade of events is initiated, thereby having the potential to trigger both neurodegenerative diseases and apoptosis in the brain tissue (Ju, Liu, Kim and Crowston et al., 2007). From a biomechanical point of view, the consequence of an increased interstitial fluid pressure may result in larger deformation of the cellular membranes, thus altering the

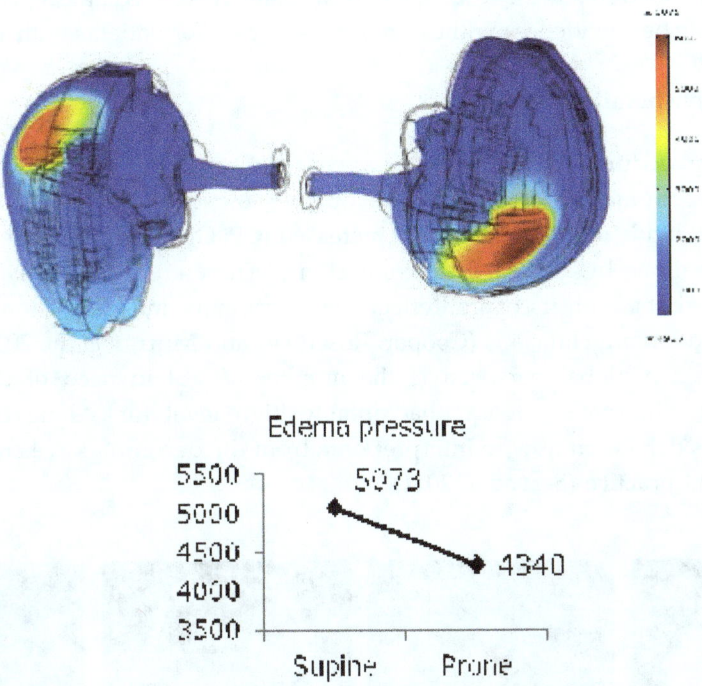

Figure 5. By changing the patient's head position from supine to a more prone position the pressure in the oedematous tissue is reduced by about 15 %.

pressure between the extracellular and intracellular environment. An elevated interstitial fluid pressure due to oedema compresses the vasculature, the consequence of which is reduced cerebral blood flow, potential ischemia and arteriolar dilatation. This makes the capillary pressure increase, which results in even more interstitial fluid accumulation (Werner and Engelhard, 2007).

Gravity causes a hydrostatic pressure gradient in compartments filled with fluid. The same pressure is present in the centre of gravity in the head and is thus set to zero. As is found in neurosurgical procedures, a postural change of the head position alters the distribution of hydrostatic pressure patterns according to the body's alignment to the gravity field (Hinghofer-Szalkay, 2011). However, at a certain location – referred to as hydrostatic indifferent point – the pressure remains constant during a given change of body position. When it comes to defining the most optimal head position in clinical practice between supine and prone positions, this remains to be evaluated when the indifferent point is presented. Thus, when positioning the TBI patient in the supine position as a routine, the treatment of choice is suboptimal, as it does not consider the anatomical localization of the injury. The potential verification of changing from supine to a more prone position has been shown by using an anatomically detailed 3D FE model in simulation research (Li, von Holst and Kleiven, 2011), where the effects of gravity on the oedema zone at the posterior part of the brain were investigated. It is hoped that these results may be implemented into clinical practice and may change the existing best evidence synthesis of intensive care for patients with TBI.

5.3. Decompressive hemicraniectomy

Decompressive procedures in neurosurgery are excellent methods for reducing the ICP in patients suffering from TBI or stroke. The number of such procedures has increased substantially worldwide with good effect on increased ICP. Of specific interest is decompression of the brain tissue by a larger hemicraniectomy. There are no real answers for these results. Thus, the debate on its overall effectiveness remains and complete consensus has not been achieved among clinicians (Cooper, Rosenfeld and Murray et al., 2011; Vashu and Sohail, 2011) From a global perspective, the number of TBI in need of decompressive hemicraniectomy will remain at an unacceptably high level for a long time to come. Presently, there is debate on how to interpret data from the decompressive craniotomy and apply it to clinical practice (Servadei, 2011).

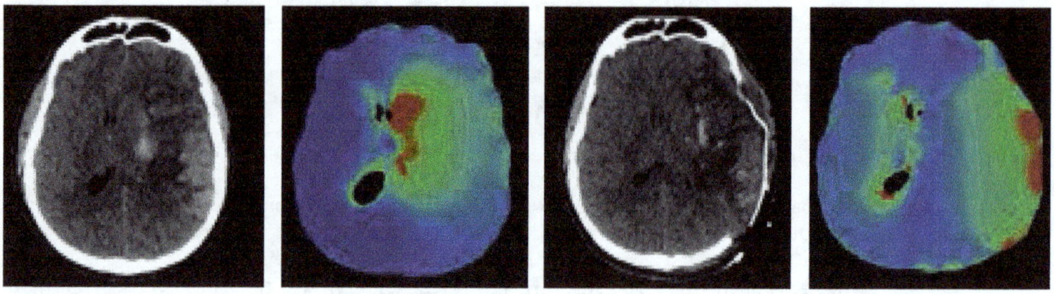

Figure 6. Evaluation of strain level in different anatomical areas in the brain tissue before (left black image with CT, left colour image with NIBIE) and after the decompressive hemicraniectomy (right black image with CT, right colour image with NIBIE).

The purpose of decompressive craniotomy is to reduce the ICP by allowing expansion of the brain tissue outside the skull bone. However, the treatment also results in stretching of the axonal fibres, which has been suggested to contribute to an unfavourable outcome for patients treated with decompressive craniotomy (Cooper, Rosenfeld and Murray et al., 2011; Stiver, 2009). Thus, there is a need for new clinical methods that may have the capacity to better consider the biomechanical consequences of swollen brain tissue after decompressive hemicraniectomy. With the new image technology of NIBIE, it is possible to evaluate the consequences by focusing on strain level before and after the neurosurgical procedure, which may have possibly improve our knowledge in this context. In fact, an increased strain may account for why we don´t see more significant improvement in these patients.

Prior to the neurosurgical procedure (Fig. 6, left), the CT showed increased strain levels of various degree in and around the injured brain tissue. When evaluating the consequences of decompressive hemicraniectomy, the strain level of the nervous tissue on the same side was also increased to over 60% and also more widespread (Fig. 6, right), and interfering with the remote hemisphere. Increased strain level can also be found when evaluating several slices from NIBIE, where the decompressive hemicraniectomy causes the injured brain tissue to expand beyond the skull bone. This results in strain levels well over 60% (Fig. 7).

- Strain level in %

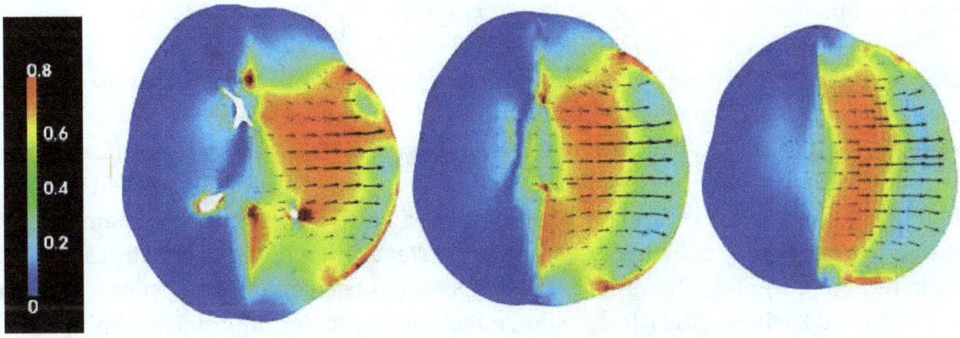

Figure 7. Three image sections from NIBIE showing increased strain levels of over 40% on the injured side (right hemisphere) after decompressive hemicraniectomy.

When biomechanical effects cause the nerve fibres to become stretched abnormally high during the neurosurgical procedure, the normal biochemical metabolism is also altered. Axons transfer electrical-chemical impulses between neurons, including their intact axons. These activities are critical for establishing normal clinical function in the nervous system. When parts of the axonal fibres are stretched, the capacity to transfer physiological impulses is altered and may even result in permanent loss of functional capability when stretched too much (Joseph, 1996). *In vitro* models for studying injury have shown that axonal stretch causes a number of neural derangements including neurofilament structure alterations (Chung, Staal and McCormack, 2005), immediate rise in intracellular calcium level after injury (Staal, Dickson and Gasperini, 2010), mechanical breaking of microtubules during stretch in axons (Tang-Schomer, M.D, Patel, A.R and Baas et al., 2010) and axonal swelling formation (Smith, Wolf and Lusardi et al., 1999).

An increase in strain levels as low as a 5% increase will alter neuronal function, while a strain level higher than 20% induces significant levels of cell injury in vitro (Morrison III, Cater, Wang et al., 2003). Bain et al. (2000) demonstrated that a strain level of approximately 21% will initiate electrophysiological changes, while a strain of approximately 34% results in morphological signs in the white matter. Combined, these studies have increased the knowledge in response to biomechanical stretch as found after the neurosurgical procedure. This may explain why decompressive craniotomy not only reduces ICP, but may also contribute to unfavourable outcomes for patients by increasing the strain level. Thus, with NIBIE, it is possible to quantify the axonal stretching to better understand the consequences of the neurosurgical procedure for many of the most severely injured patients, thereby having a better insight into the potential damages to the nervous tissue after TBI and stroke. In general, decompressive craniotomy results in complex axonal deformation; it is difficult to apply these cellular level thresholds to the tissue level, since the axons within the white matter do not necessarily lie in the same orientation as the stretching direction. Most of the previous axonal injury models use dynamic brain tissue during impact to study strain. This is different to the case of axonal stretch for the post-craniotomy stage, under which the axons are enduring slow dynamic events similar to a quasi-static stretching. The incorporation of fibre tracts in biomechanical simulation models is therefore necessary to obtain stretching along the axons, thus making it comparable with the threshold obtained from laboratory investigations.

The displacement and stretching of injured cerebral tissue after TBI and stroke is usually found for several days. This may further challenge the cerebral metabolism. Using a model of sciatic nerve stretch, it was reported that even minimal tension, if maintained for a significant amount of time, may result in loss of neuronal function (Fowler, Leonetti and Banich, 2001). Hence, it should be expected that the central nervous system will also sustain potential damage under long duration stretch, such as in the post-craniotomy stage, but with a different threshold level. The strain level representing the stretch of brain tissue has been quantified in a previous study (von Holst, Li and Kleiven, 2011). It was shown that following decompressive craniotomy, the strain level, as well as the water content in the brain tissue, was substantially increased. This may influence the axonal fibres in such a way that the neurochemical events are jeopardized. Axonal fibre tracts extracted from diffusion weighted (DW) images have been included in a biomechanical model simulating an impact event in order to study the axonal elongation occurring at the primary injury stage (Chatelin, Deck and Renard et al., 2011). Results from this study showed that stretching of axons correlates closely with diffuse axonal injury (DAI). However, axonal stretching during the post-craniotomy period, which may have prognostic value for the cognitive and neurological sequelae of patients treated with decompressive craniotomy, has not been previously studied.

6. Conclusion

Parallel with an increased theoretical knowledge of TBI, clinical neuroscience practice has witnessed a remarkable improvement with new technological equipment aimed at emergency care at the scene of accident, intensive care, as well as for neurosurgical procedures. Concurrently, the significant development of computer capacity during the last two decades has made it possible to implement various software programs having the capacity to better understand the mechanical consequences following an accident to the central nervous tissue. Thus, the integration of clinical practice with neuroengineering used for applied neurosurgery may further improve the future outcome of patients suffering from moderate and severe TBI. The integrated research between clinical neurosurgery and neuronic engineering has resulted in the development of a method for generating a numerical model based on 3D medical images, from either computer tomography (CT) or magnetic resonance imaging (MRI). We have found that simulation of TBI in numerical models can define the intracranial pressure without neurosurgical procedures. In addition, the strain level, which is related to the stretching of axons, can be used as a new predictive value in diagnoses, e.g., the effect of oedema and haemorrhage. Moreover, it is now possible to analyse the outcome of a treatment in, for instance, decompressive hemicraniectomy. By using numerical models of the human brain, it is possible to further optimize present treatments of TBI. Finally, using NIBIE in education of health care staff in all categories in the new field of neuroengineering is of significant importance in order to better understand the consequences of diseases in the central nervous system.

Acknowledgements

The present chapter was sponsored by Vinnova, Karolinska University Hospital and the Royal Institute of Technology, Stockholm, Sweden.

Author details

Hans von Holst[1,2] and Svein Kleiven[2]

1 Dept. of Neurosurgery, Karolinska University Hospital, Stockholm, Sweden

2 Division of Neuronic Engineering, Royal Institute of Technology, Stockholm, Sweden

References

[1] Bain, B.C. and Meaney, D.F, (2000) Tissue-Level Thresholds for Axonal Damage in an Experimental Model of Central Nervous System White Matter Injury. J. Biomech. Engng.16, pps 615-622.

[2] Chatelin, S, Deck, C, Renard, F, Kremer, F, Heinrich, C, Armspach, J.P, Willinger, R, (2011). Computation of axonal elongation in head trauma finite element simulation. Journal of the Mechanical Behavior of Biomedical Materials, 4(8):1905–1919.

[3] Chung, R.S, Staal, J.A, McCormack, G.H, Dickson, T.C, Cozens, M.A, Chuckowree, J.A, Quilty, M.C, Vickers, J.C, (2005) Mild axonal stretch injury in vitro induces a progressive series of neurofilament alterations ultimately leading to delayed axotomy. Journal of neurotrauma, 22(10):1081–1091.

[4] Clough, R. W., (1980). The finite element method after twenty-five years: A personal review. Computers and Structures, Vol 12 (4), 361-370.

[5] Coffey A.M, Garg I, Miga M.I, Thompson R.C (2010). An evaluative tool for preoperative planning of brain tumor resection. Proc SPIE 7625:762531. doi:10.1117/12.844477

[6] Cooper, D.J, Rosenfeld, J.V, Murray, L, Arabi, Y.M, Davies, A.R, D'Urso, P, Kossmann, T, Ponsford, J, Seppelt, I, Reilly, P, Wolfe, R (2011). Decompressive craniecto-

my in diffuse traumatic brain injury. New England Journal of Medicine, 364(16): 1493–1502.

[7] Cooper, P.R, (1982). Post-traumatic intracranial mass lesions, in: Head injury, Williams and Wilkins, Baltimore/London. pages 185-232.

[8] Dutta-Roy T, Wittek A, Miller K (2008) Biomechanical modeling of normal pressure hydrocephalus. J Biomech 41:2263–2271.

[9] Fowler, S.S, Leonetti, J.P, Banich, J.C, Lee, J.M. Wurster, R, Young, M.R.I, 2001) Duration of neuronal stretch correlates with functional loss. Otolaryngology-Head and Neck Surgery, 124(6):641–644.

[10] Gennarelli, T.A, et al., (1972). Pathophysiological Responses to Rotational and Translational Accelerations of the Head, SAE Paper No. 720970, in: 16th Stapp Car Crash Conf., Society of Automotive Engineers, pp. 296-308.

[11] Gennarelli, T.A, et al., (1982) Diffuse Axonal Injury and Traumatic Coma in the Primate. Ann. Neurol. 12, 564-574.

[12] Gennarell, T.A, (1983). Head injuries in man and animals: clinical aspects. Acta neurochir suppl. 32, 1-13.

[13] Genarelli T.A, et al., (1987) Directional dependence of axonal injury and traumatic coma in the primate. Ann. Neurol. 12, 564-574.

[14] Gurdjian E.S, Lissner, H.R, (1944) Mechanisms of head injury as studied by the cathode ray oscilloscope: preliminary report. J Neurol Neurosurg Psychiatry 1:393-399.

[15] Hinghofer-Szalkay H, (2011) Gravity, the hydrostatic indifference concept and the cardiovascular system. Eur J Appl Physiol 111:163–174.

[16] Ho, J, (2008) Generation of patient specific finite element head models. Doctoral thesis report:7 ISBN: 978-91-7415-191-6.

[17] Ho, J, von Holst, H, Kleiven, S, (2009) Automatic generation and validation of patient specific finite element head models suitable for crashworthiness analysis. International Journal of Crashworthiness, 14(6): p. 555-563.

[18] Ho J, Kleiven, S, (2009) Can sulci protect the brain from traumatic injury? J Biomech 42: 2074–2080.

[19] von Holst, H, (2007) Traumatic brain injury. In: Feigin VL, Bennett DA (eds) Handbook of clinical neuroepidemiology. Nova Science, New York, pp. 197–232.

[20] von Holst, H, Li, X.G, Kleiven, S, (2011) Increased strain levels and water content in brain tissue after decompressive craniotomy evaluated with numerical analysis.

[21] Holburn, A.H.S, (1943) Mechanics of head injury. Lancet 2. October 9, 438-441.

[22] Huang H.M, Lee, M.C, Chiu, W.T, Chen, C.T, Lee, S.Y, (1999) Three-dimensional finite element analysis of subdural hematoma. The Journal of Trauma, Injury, Infection and Critical Care. 47 (3) 538-544.

[23] Joseph, R, (1996) Neuropsychiatry, neuropsychology, and clinical neuroscience: emotion, evolution, cognition, language, memory, brain damage, and abnormal behavior. Williams & Wilkins.

[24] Ju, W.K, Liu, Q, Kim, K.Y, Crowston, J.G, Lindsey, J.D, Agarwal, N, Ellisman, M.H, Perkins, G.A, Weinreb, R.N, (2007) Elevated hydrostatic pressure triggers mitochondrial fission and decreases cellular ATP in differentiated RGC-5 cells. Invest Ophthalmol Vis Sci 48:2145–2151.

[25] Kaczmarek, M, Subramaniam, R.P, Neff, S.R, (1997) The hydromechanics of hydrocephalus: steady-state solutions for cylindrical geometry. Bull Math Biol 59:295–323.

[26] Kleiven, S, von Holst, H,(2002) Consequences of head size following trauma to the human head. Journal of Biomechanics 35, 153-160.

[27] Kleiven, S., Peloso, P.M. von Holst, H, (2003) The epidemiology of head injuries in Sweden from 1987 to 2000. Inj Control Saf Promot, 10(3): p. 173-80.

[28] Kleiven, S, (2006) Evaluation of head injury criteria using an FE model validated against experiments on localized brain motion, intra-cerebral acceleration, and intracranial pressure, International Journal of Crashworthiness 11 (1), 65-79.

[29] Kleiven, S, (2007) Predictors for traumatic brain injuries evaluated through accident reconstructions. Stapp Car Crash J. 51: p. 81-114.

[30] Kleiven, S, (2007) Predictors for traumatic brain injuries evaluated through accident reconstructions. Stapp Car Crash J 51:1–35.

[31] Kumarezan, S, Radhakrishnan, S, Ganesan, N, (1995) Generation of geometry of closed human head and discretization for finite element analysis. Med. Biol Eng Comput 33, 349-353.

[32] Krabbel, G, Muller, R, (1996) Development of a finite element model of the human head using the visible human database. Abstract of the visible human project conference, 71-72.

[33] Lee, M.C, Haut, R.C, (1989). Insensitivity of tensile failure properties of human bridging veins to strain rate: Implications in biomechanics of subdural hematoma. J. Biomech. 22 (6/7), 537-542.

[34] Levine, D.N, (1999) The pathogenesis of normal pressure hydrocephalus: a theoretical analysis. Bull Math Biol 61:875–916.

[35] Li, X.G, (2012) Finite element and neuroimaging techniques to improve decision making in clinical neuroscience. Doctoral thesis report 2012:1 ISBN: 978-91-7501-240-7.

[36] Li, X.G, von Holst, H, Ho, J, Kleiven, S, (2009) Three dimensional poroelastic simulation of brain edema: initial studies on intracranial pressure. Proceedings of World Congress on Medical Physics and Biomedical Engineering, September 7–12, Munich. Springer, Heidelberg, pp. 1478–1481.

[37] Li, X, von Holst, H, Kleiven, S, (2011) Influence of gravity for optimal head positions in the treatment of head injury patients. Acta Neurochirurgica, 153(10): p. 2057-2064.

[38] Lövenhjelm, P, (1974) Dynamic Properties of the Parasagittal Bridging Veins. Z. Rechtsmedizin 74, pages 55-62.

[39] Marmarou, A, (2003) Pathophysiology of traumatic brain edema: current concepts. Acta Neurochir Suppl 86:7–10.

[40] Marmarou, A, Signoretti, S, Fatouros, P.P, Portella, G, Aygok, G.A, Bullock, M.R, (2006) Predominance of cellular edema in traumatic brain swelling in patients with severe head injuries. J Neurosurg 104:720–730.

[41] McElhaney, J, Roberts, V, Hilyard, J, (1976) Handbook of human tolerance, Japan Automobile Research Institute Inc., Tokyo, p. 143.

[42] Melwin, J.W, (1995). Injury assessment reference values for the CRABI 6-Month Infant Dummy in a Rear-Facing Infant Restraint with Air Bag Deployment. in: SAE International Congress and Exposition. , SAE Paper No. 950872, Society of Automotive Engineers.

[43] Miga, M.I, Roberts, D.W, Kennedy, F.E, Platenik, L.A, Hartov, A, Lunn, K.E, Paulsen, K.D, (2001) Modeling of retraction and resection for intraoperative updating of images. Neurosurgery 49:75–85.

[44] Morrison III, B.C, Cater, H.L, Wang, C.C-B, Thomas, F.C, Hung, C.T, Ateshian, G.A, Sundström, L.E, (2003) A tissue level tolerance criterion for living brain developed with an in vitro model of traumatic mechanical loading. 47TH Stapp Car Crash Conference Journal.

[45] Nagashima, T, Shirakuni, T, Rapoport, S.I, (1990) A two dimensional, finite element analysis of vasogenic brain edema. Neurol Med Chir 30:1–9.

[46] Narayab, R.K, Wilberger, J.E, Povlischock, J.T, (Editors) (1995) Neurotrauma. McGraw-Hill. ISBN 0-07-045662-3.

[47] Ommaya, A.K, Hirsch, A.E, (1971) Tolerances for Cerebral Concussion from Head Impact and Whiplash in Primates. J. Biomech, 4, 13-21.

[48] Rabinstein, A.A, (2006) Treatment of cerebral edema. Neurologist 12:59–73.

[49] Reulen, H.J, Kreysch, H.G, (1973) Measurement of brain tissue pressure in cold induced cerebral oedema. Acta Neurochir (Wein) 29:29–40.

[50] Schugar, T.A, (1977) A finite element head model Vol I: Theory, development and results. U.S. Depat. of Transportation Report No. DOT-HS-289-3-550-IA.

[51] Servadei, F, (2011) Clinical value of decompressive craniectomy. New England Journal of Medicine, 364(16):1558–1559.

[52] Shreiber, D.I, Bain, A.C, Meaney, D.F, Schreiber, D.I, Bain, A.C, (1997) In vivo thresholds for mechanical injury to the blood-brain barrier. 41st Stapp Car Crash Conf.

[53] Tang-Schomer, M.D, Patel, A.R, Baas, P.W, Smith, D.H, 2010 Mechanical breaking of microtubules in axons during dynamic stretch injury underlies delayed elasticity, microtubule disassembly, and axon degeneration. The FASEB Journal, 24(5):1401–1410.

[54] Thibault, L.E, (1993) Brain injury from the macro to the micro level and back again: What have we learned to date? in: IRCOBI Conf. 3-25.

[55] Smillie, A, Sobey, I, Molnar, Z, (2005) A hydroelastic model of hydrocephalus. J Fluid Mech 539:417–443.

[56] Smith, D.H, Wolf, J.A, Lusardi, T.A, Virginia, M.Y.L, Meaney, D.F, (1999) High tolerance and delayed elastic response of cultured axons to dynamic stretch injury. The Journal of neuroscience, 19(11):4263–4269.

[57] Staal, J.A, Dickson, T.C, Gasperini, R, Liu, Y, Foa, L, Vickers, J.C, (2010) Initial calcium release from intracellular stores followed by calcium dysregulation is linked to secondary axotomy following transient axonal stretch injury. Journal of neurochemistry, 112(5):1147–1155.

[58] Stiver, S.I, (2009) Complications of decompressive craniectomy for traumatic brain injury. Neurosurgical focus, 26(6):E7.

[59] Ueno, K, Melvin J.W,(1995) Finite element model study of head impact based on Hybrid III head acceleration; The effect of rotational and translational acceleration. Journal of Biomechanical Engineering. 117(3) 319-328.

[60] Vashu, R, Sohail, A, (2011) Decompressive craniectomy is indispensable in the management of severe traumatic brain injury. Acta neurochirurgica, 10:2065–2066.

[61] Ward, C.C, Thompson, R. B, (1975) The development of a detailed finite element brain model. SAE Paper No. 751163.

[62] Werner, C, Engelhard, K, (2007) Pathophysiology of traumatic brain injury. Br J Anaesth 99:4-9.

[63] World Health Organization (2003) World Health Report 2003: A vision for global health. Shaping the future. World Health Organization.

[64] Zhou, C., Khalif, T.B, King, A.I, (1995) New model comparing impact responses of the homogenous and inhomogeneous human brain. Stapp Car Crash Conference Proceedings, 121-137.

5

Understanding, Assessing and Treating Prospective Memory Dysfunctions in Traumatic Brain Injury Patients

Giovanna Mioni, Shawn M. McClintock and Franca Stablum

1. Introduction

Our capacity to shape and direct our future behaviour is of fundamental importance in the development, pursuit, and maintenance of independence and autonomy from early childhood to late adulthood. A cognitive ability required for those functions is prospective memory (PM), which is the ability to form and remember to prospectively perform the intended action [1, 2]. Researchers have extensively focused on PM impairment in patients with traumatic brain injury (TBI) [3]. However, there has been limited research into the assessment and treatment of PM impairment in TBI patients. Reliable and valid tests with normative data are necessary for health professionals working with people with PM impairments. This chapter reviews the principal findings on PM impairment in TBI patients, and the main procedures used to assess and rehabilitate PM.

2. Prospective Memory

Prospective Memory (PM) refers to the cognitive ability to form and remember to perform an intended action at a specific moment in the future [1, 2]. That cognitive ability is essential for many daily activities, such as remembering to pick up something at the market after work, send a gift for a birthday, or call a friend at a specific time. Although past researchers tended to characterize PM as a unitary process, it is very complex and comprised of various components [4]. For example, consider the situation in which a principal asks a teacher to relay a message to a student. The teacher has committed him/herself to two memory tasks: one is to remember the content of the message, and the second is to deliver it as soon as he/she sees the student. Remembering the content of a PM task is essential to perform the PM task, which researchers refer to as the *content* of a PM task (*retrospective component*). However, remembering only the content of the PM task will not produce successful performance. The action must also be performed at the appropriate moment in the future. This is referred to as the *prospective component* of PM tasks. Thus, a critical aspect to success on PM tasks is not only recalling the content of the intended action, but also performing the action at the appropriate moment in the future [4].

A four stages model has been proposed to explain the functioning of PM [1, 4-6]:

1. *Intention formation* - the first phase consists on the formation of the delayed intention, which often involves forming a plan. Different degrees of motivation may influence the strength of encoding the delayed intention. In fact, the strength of an intention may reflect not only the personal importance, but also the potential benefits and costs of realizing the delayed intention.
2. *Intention retention* - the retention intervals describe the delay between the formation of and execution of the intended action. The retention interval, most of the time, is filled with an "ongoing task" [7]. Some authors found lower performance after a long relative to a short delay [8], though others failed to find an association between delay length and decline [9, 10] or improvement in performance [11]. In addition to the length of the delay interval, the cognitive load added during the delay interval (filled or un-filled intervals) may influence performance [7, 9].
3. *Intention initiation* - the point in time at which execution of the intention is (or should be) initiated. Successful performance on PM tasks, not only required to accurately encode the intended action and maintain the intended action active during the interval delay, but also to recognize the cue, retrieve the action associated with that intention, and perform the action. People may fail on their performance not only because they fail to recall the intended action when the target occurs, but also because their cognitive resources were captured by the demands of the ongoing task.
4. *Intention execution* - where and when the intended action is executed. This may be considered the final stage with the execution of the delayed intention. However, successfully completing all previous phases, errors can occur and the delayed intention may not be performed. Distractions or failure to complete the task due to external circumstances may compromise performance. For example, the intention to phone a friend may fail because of interruption by the doorbell or the friend was not at home. When the delayed intention is not executed, it is necessary to re-establish the intended action and re-form the plan [1].

A fifth phase, *Evaluation of outcome* was proposed and is concerned with monitoring the output of the execution of the intended action. The evaluation of outcome describes the process by which a person checks if the intended action has been accurately performed [1].

According to Einstein and McDaniel's model [12], there are two types of PM targets, event-based and time-based tasks[1], that trigger the execution of our delayed intention. In conditions that require event-based PM, a person performs an action when a specific event occurs (i.e.

passing a message when a friend calls); while in situations that require time-based PM, the action has to be performed at a specific time in the future (i.e. remembering the appointment with a friend at 4:00 p.m.) [12]. Event-based PM tasks are considered to be less cognitively demanding than time-based PM tasks because they require less self-initiated retrieval and external cue(s) are available to help recall the task [13, 14].

2.1. Prospective memory in traumatic brain injury patients

It has been suggested that the prefrontal cortex predominantly mediates executive control mechanisms [15], which are required to successfully initiate and execute the intended action [5, 13, 14, 16]. Because of this link between executive functions and the prefrontal cortex, and because prefrontal areas are commonly damaged after a TBI, it is not surprising that individuals with TBI are often impaired on PM tasks [3]. For individuals with TBI, frequent PM failures (e.g., forgetting to repay a loan to a friend, maintain an appointment, take medication, turn off the stove) can be frustrating, embarrassing and in some cases, life threatening. These failures have the potential to limit the independence of these individuals, causing them to rely on a carer for prompting and completion of activities and instrumental activities of daily living. Moreover, these failures may affect their opportunity to return to work or start a new vocation [3, 17, 18].

Impairment of PM in TBI patients would differ according to the complexity and requirement of the tasks [7, 19]; moreover, when tested both on event- and time-based tasks, TBI patients are particularly impaired on time-based tasks consistent with the idea that those tasks require more self-initiation. Dysfunctions on time-based tasks may also be due to less strategic monitoring behaviour engaged by TBI patients [1, 4, 16].

The earliest studies that examined the effect of TBI on PM performance used self-rating scales [20] or few PM items [21, 22]. In those studies, the Prospective Memory Questionnaire (PMQ) was tested along with attentional and memory tasks [20]. Adults with TBI and older adults performed more poorly than younger adults on short-term PM tasks, and TBI patients rated themselves more poorly than younger adults. Two PM tasks were used to assess PM performance [22]: the first task involved telling the participants about a self-report memory questionnaire at the beginning of an assessment session and instructing them to ask for the questionnaire at the end of the session (even-based task). The second task involved asking the participants to return (by mail) an evaluation form with the date written in the top corner (time-based task). Because of the small number of items used and the correct/incorrect nature of these items, the PM scores obtained with these tasks were limited in range and thus were unreliable [23].

To assess PM more reliably and accurately, it is necessary to increase either the number of items used or the number of responses required for each item. Recent studies considered these limitations and developed more appropriated tasks to investigate the effects of TBI on event- and time-based PM performance (Table 1).

---

1 A third prospective remembering task, called, activity-based [1]. An activity-based prospective memory task required to carry out an intended action at the end of an activity (i.e., torn off the oven when you have finished cooking).

			TBI characteristics			Type of prospective memory tasks	
Study[1]	**Year**	**Sample**	**GCS**	**Time since injury (months)**	**NPS assessment**[2, 3]	**Event-based**	**Time-based**
[25]	1999	12 TBI and 12 controls	8 or less	24.58 (15.58)	-	Response to questions and the target word	Press a key every 5 min and monitor the time
[26]	2001	13 TBI and 13 controls	6.6 (3.3)	1.8 (0.7)	WCST, COWAT and DASS	Deliver a message (unfilled and filled conditions)	Stop the timer after 5 min (unfilled and filled conditions)
[28]	2003	14 TBI and 14 controls	3 to 15	9.71 (7.5)	TOL, COWAT and LNST	Response to a cue (low and high cognitive demand)	-
[11]	2004	16 TBI and 16 controls	8 or less	108	-	Perform actions when the target appeared (related-unrelated cues) (10 vs. 45 min delay)	Perform actions after the interval (related-unrelated cues) (10 vs. 45 min delay)
[19]	2004	7 TBI, 21 older and 19 younger controls	severe	41.71 (11.79)	Verbal intelligence and WCST	Complex tasks following the multiprocess model	-
[29]	2004	24 TBI and 24 controls	8 or less	25.75 (21.63)	Digit span forward and backward, TMT, LM Visual recognition, COWAT, Stroop, WCST	Press a designed key on focal cue or peripheral cue	-
[27]	2005	25 TBI and 25 controls	8 or less	7	Visual (Story sub-test, RAVLT) and verbal (Pictures, Faces and Routes sub-tests of RBMT) declarative memory, digit span, TMT, COWAT and WCST	RBMT	Stop a timer and send the envelop
[7]	2007	17 TBI and 16 controls	11.67 (3.50)	41.28 (32.52)	-	Response to a cue (one or four cue targets)	-
[18]	2008	44 TBI but no controls	7.08 (3.89)	-	TMT, COWAT and metacognitive variables	CAMPROMPT	CAMPROMPT

			TBI characteristics			Type of prospective memory tasks	
Study[1]	Year	Sample	GCS	Time since injury (months)	NPS assessment[2, 3]	Event-based	Time-based
[24]	2010	31 TBI and 31 controls	13-15	0.89 (0.22)	-	MIST	MIST
[16]	2012	18 TBI and 18 controls	6.77 (2.13)	24.50 (19.67)	Stroop and N-Back	-	Press a key every 5 min and monitor the time

1 Studies included here have been conducted with behavioral measures.

2 References of neuropsychological tests are not reported because the authors referred to different versions. Please refer to the specific articles for the appropriate references.

3 Appendix A reports the full name of neuropsychological tasks employed in the studies with a brief description.

Table 1. Studies that used behavioural tasks to investigate PM performance on TBI patients. GCS = Glasgow Coma Scale (Scores < 8 = severe; scores 9-12 = moderate; scores 13-15 = mild); Time refers to the time post injury (months); NPS assessment refers to the neuropsychological tasks included in the studies; WCST = Wisconsin Card Sorting Test; COWAT = Controlled Oral Word Association Test; DASS = Depression, Anxiety, Stress Scale; TOL = Tower of London; LNST = Letter-Number Sequencing Test; TMT = Trial Making Test; RBMT = Rivermead Behavioural Memory Test; CAMPROMPT = Cambridge Behavioural Prospective Memory Test; MIST = Memory for Intention Screening Test.

Among the studies identified[2], only one included patients with mild TBI [24]. Most studies included have evaluated event-based PM performance, 6 examined both event- and time-based performance, and one only analyzed time-based PM performance. When both event- and time-based tasks were included in the studies, TBI patients obtained lower performance on time-based PM tasks [11, 25-27], which substantiated that time-based tasks are more difficult to execute probably due to more self-initiated retrieval impairment [12]. Generally, TBI patients showed PM dysfunctions compared to healthy controls, but the degree of impairment varied according to the characteristics of the employed tasks. By varying the cognitive demand on the ongoing task TBI patients performed more poorly than controls on the high, but not low demand condition [28]. Some authors also manipulated the salience of the event cue in PM performance [29]. The cue was either integrated (focal cue) or peripheral (no-focal cue) to the ongoing working memory task. TBI patients and controls showed no differences on the ongoing task, but PM performance was poorer in TBI patients in both focal and peripheral cue conditions. That finding suggested that even with highly salient cues, TBI patients exhibit PM failures. Moreover, both TBI and controls self-reported that greater monitoring effort was required for the peripheral, rather than for the focal-cue condition. Instead, when the cue is maintained in a focal condition, but is varied the number of distractions during the ongoing task, TBI patients performed more poorly both on one and four target conditions [7]. Finally, some authors have varied the delay between encoding and task performance (10 vs 45 min) expecting lower performance in the longer delay condition. Researchers have also manipulated the functional link (semantic inter-item associative link) between intended actions with the expectation that

2 Studies were included if conducted with TBI patients and match controls. Research was conducted on Psychinfo and PubMed with key words: "Prospective Memory", "Traumatic brain injury", "Event-based" and "Time-based".

performance would improve. Patients with TBI performed significantly lower than controls; however, there were no significant effects of delay interval or functional link of the intended actions [11].

A subset of studies included executive functions tasks to determine whether impairment on PM was associated with executive dysfunctions. The available evidences were mixed regarding the relationship between PM and executive functions, as some studies found significant [16, 22, 28] and others no [27] association between those two constructs. For example, we found [16] that working memory significantly correlated with PM accuracy only in TBI patients, while inhibition was involved in controls. Also, working memory significantly correlated with PM performance in the low cognitive demand condition in both TBI and controls [28]. These results suggested that for the employed dual-task event-based paradigm, participants had to actively maintain in memory the requirement while undertaking the ongoing task [16, 28]. Spontaneous flexibility assessed through the Controlled Oral Word Association Test (COWAT) [30] significantly correlated with event-based PM performance in the high-demand condition in TBI patients. TBI event-based PM performance significantly correlated with attention/speed processing tasks, which added further support to the notion of a strong relationship between attention and PM performance [29, 31]. In particular, the authors pointed out that those PM dysfunctions may be due to momentary lapses of attention to task details rather than to complete forgetting of the task instructions. Retrospective memory also accounted for a significant amount of variance in PM tasks of TBI patients independent of executive functions [25]. In particular, it was found that executive functions were involved both on time- and event-based PM performance, but it particularly influenced time-based PM performance, whereas retrospective memory contributed most to event-based performance. Finally, a complex PM paradigm was adopted [19, 32] to investigate which of the four phases of PM were affected in TBI patients. Impairment of PM was found on intention formation, intention re-instantiation, and intention execution. That finding confirmed that executive functions are involved on these three phases rather than only on intention retention. Only one study investigated the involvement of temporal abilities in time-based PM performance and found that adequate temporal abilities were involved in monitoring behavior rather than PM [16].

In addition, two studies have investigated PM performance according to demographic, clinical and metacognitive variables [18, 25]. Depressive symptoms were found to adversely affect successful performance on the timing component of the time-based task [20], while anxiety symptoms adversely affected performance on event-based tasks [25]. In a more recent study, the localization of the damage (mainly frontal) significantly correlated with event-based Cambridge Test of Prospective Memory (CAMPROMPT) scores, whereas duration of post-traumatic amnesia (PTA) and metacognitive variables significantly correlated with both time- and event-based scores [18].

2.2. Virtual tasks to investigate prospective memory in TBI patients

For adequate clinical assessment and rehabilitation programs, neuropsychologists need information about how a patient functions in routine daily activities, and laboratory-based tasks may be unable to always provide such information [33]. Chaytor and Schmitter-Edgecombe (2003) found that the relationship between neuropsychological tests and measures of outcome is often limited. Recently, it was concluded that most PM tasks lack adequate reliability [23]. As a consequence, it is often impossible to translate test scores into either goals for rehabilitation or conclusions about the level of impairment; that is, many conventional tests of memory-related abilities lack ecological validity [23, 33, 34]. To solve this important discrepancy between performance on neuropsychological tests and performance in everyday life, researchers, following the evolution of computer programs, have developed tasks that can bridge conventional neuropsychological tests with behavioral observations. Virtual tasks, in fact, can simulate the activity of everyday life in a controlled setting [33].

Study	Year	Sample	GCS	Time since injury (months)	NPS assessment[1]	PM Tasks
[38]	2005	25 TBI and 20 controls	-	113.76 (75.13)	NART, WCST, LM, COWAT and TMT	Videotape: Performing activities when the cue appeared on the screen by saying to the experimenter the activities required
[37]	2005	2 brain injury patients[2] and 3 controls	Patients SR GCS = 3 and Patients TJ GCS = 4	Patients SR 6 months; Patients TJ 3.5 months	Word list from WMS, Digit span, Stroop, WCST and NART	Virtual Street: Imagine walking on a street and performing 3 activities. The list of activities was either visible or hidden after instruction
[39]	2006	20 TBI and 20 controls	-	160.2 (91.66)	DEX, Logical memory from WMS and Ruff 2&7 selective attention test	Virtual Street: Imagine being a street inspector and performing 3 activities under low and high distraction. Moreover performing 10 errands
[40]	2009	16 TBI and 16 controls	8 or less	at least 3 month	HVLT, TMT and Digit span	The supermarket shopping trip: "buy" 8 items while watching a 8-min DVD of a supermarket trip
[44]	2013	18 TBI and 18 controls	4.54 (1.37)	66.94 (95.22)	Phonemic and Semantic fluency; TMT; WCST	Virtual Week

1 References of neuropsychological tasks are not reported because the authors referred to different version of the tasks. Please refer to the specific articles for the appropriate references.

2 The study includes 3 patients with brain injury: SR suffered a severe TBI as a result of assault, TJ suffered a TBI as a result of motor vehicle accident and RW suffered cerebellar and sub-arachnoid haemorrhages. Only information on patients SR and TJ were included because TBI patients.

Table 2. Studies that used ecological tasks to investigate PM performance on TBI patients. GCS = Glasgow Coma Scale; NPS assessment refers to the neuropsychological tasks included in the studies; NART = National Adults Reading Test; WCST = Wisconsin Card Sorting Test; LM = Logic Memory; COWAT = Controlled Oral Word Association Test; TMT = Trial Making Test; WMS = Wechsler Memory Scale; DEX = questionnaire from the Behavioural Assessment of Dyexecutive Syndrome; HVLT = Hopkins Verbal Learning Test.

In Table 2 are revised studies that were conducted with virtual tasks. This literature is presented separately from other studies on PM because it is more representative of everyday PM performance, and focused on filling the gap between performance on laboratory tasks and PM performance in real life.

The Prospective Remembering Video Procedure (PRVP) was designed to test PM abilities in virtual street simulation [35]. The task involves remembering to carry out a set of activities while watching a videotape filmed by a person walking slowly through a shopping complex. Participants virtually visited a shopping centre, with a set of event-based activities, each of which involved an action (`buy a record') and a cue (`from the record stand'). As each cue comes into view, the associated action must be recalled. The view that was presented focused mostly on the shop-front, although the footage also included views of passengers crossing the street. Studies conducted with health students and mix-brain injury patients demonstrated that the PRVP procedure was reliable and easier to complete when the video was set in a familiar location. Moreover, it was found that the video-based task was correlated with performance on an equivalent real life memory task, and provided evidence for criterion validity [35, 36, 37]. Twenty severe TBI patients and 20 matched controls were also tested with PRVP and completed the ongoing and PM tasks while "walking" along the street. Severe TBI patients showed poorer performance and were more affected by distractions on the PM tasks compared to controls [38]. Previous findings were confirmed and extended with a Virtual Street task [37, 38, 39]. Results showed that TBI patients performed more poorly than the control group on the PM tasks, but had similar performance on the Wechsler Memory Scale (3rd Edition) Logical Memory subtest. The authors discussed this result in favor of sensitivity of the Virtual Street task to measure PM performance. These results also suggested that TBI patients may show normal performance on memory tests, particularly in a controlled and quiet setting, but when memory performance is tested in a less controlled setting with distractors and tasks that require more strategic processes (like in real life conditions), real TBI dysfunctions may emerge [39].

Interesting, following the idea to create tasks more representative to real life situations, other authors have investigated the "generation effect", which refers to the effect of people demonstrating better memory for self-generated material than for experimenter-generated materials [40, 41, 42]. Considering the instructions often presented in PM setting to perform the action at a specific time or when a specific cue occurs, these instructions may allow control over the tasks, but they are unable to produce the same level of motivation in participants compared to self-generated activities [42]. Some authors reasoned whether people with TBI were more likely to remember a PM task if it is self-generated as opposed to experimenter-generated [40]. TBI patients were less accurate than controls, but the source of the to-be-remembered item exerted minimal influence on PM performance in both TBI patients and controls. Additional analyses were conducted to further investigate the source of errors, and it was found that both groups were able to recognize at post-test the shopping item they had intended to buy, but TBI patients failed to activate their intention to buy the intended item at the appropriate time. Moreover, significant correlations were found between working memory, attention-set shifting and PM performance, which provided further support to the notion that higher order cognitive functions are necessary in PM [19, 40, 42].

Although they showed a high level of correspondence with real-life situations, the PRVP and the Virtual Street required participants to perform only event-based tasks. This was a limitation as PM performance should be investigated both with event- and time-based tasks. To resolve these limitations, the Virtual Week task was developed [42]. This task simulates daily life activities in a board game, where participants move around the board with the roll of a dice. Each circuit around the board represents one virtual day. Participants are required to perform 10 PM activities each virtual day (5 virtual days from Monday to Friday; additional information about the task procedures are presented in the section "Behavioral measures"). We found that people with TBI had significant difficulties executing PM tasks, which were more pronounced for time-based than event-based tasks [44]. These data suggested a relatively global PM deficit in people with TBI. Of particular interest was the finding that the magnitude of TBI impairment was consistent across regular and irregular tasks. Because the key distinction between regular and irregular tasks was that they place low and high demands on retrospective memory, respectively, these data suggested that failures of retrospective memory were not the major cause of TBI-related impairment in PM [44].

Taken together, TBI patients showed PM impairment when measured with laboratory based PM tasks. Some studies have reported that TBI patients were particularly impaired when they performed time-based tasks [11, 25-27] consistent with the view that time-based tasks are demanding and require more self-initiated processes [12]. However, other studies found a more generalized PM impairment in TBI patients [3, 44]. General agreement was observed between authors concerning the involvement of executive functions in PM performance; participants with lower executive functions would also present lower PM performance [16, 22, 25, 26, 28, 29, 31, 44]. The degree of the involvement of executive functions in PM performance varies according to the task employed and cognitive load. It is important to note that some authors have observed lower correspondence between PM performance obtained with laboratory-based tasks and real life situations [23, 33, 34, 45, 46]. Studies conducted with virtual reality tasks are trying to fill this gap, but further research is required to provide reliable and valid scores, and to develop tasks that can be used in clinical settings to screen for PM performance.

3. Assessment of prospective memory dysfunctions in clinical settings

Reliable and valid PM tools with normative data are necessary for health professionals working with people with any type of neurological disorder to acquire reliable information regarding PM performance. Such psychometrically sound tools are important not only to evaluate the degree of PM impairment, but also to provide useful information to inform the appropriate rehabilitation program. This section provides the most commonly used tools to investigate PM in clinical settings.

3.1. Self-report questionnaires

Self-report questionnaires are the most commonly employed tools to assess PM in real life situations. They assess PM dysfunctions by asking participants to rate their memory abilities by answering questions regarding their frequency of forgetting or remembering. They are particularly useful in clinical settings and in the rehabilitation process, because they can provide information about the patients' PM dysfunctions. However, it is very important to consider that a common problem after TBI is an inability to recognize impairments or disabilities that resulted from injury. This phenomenon has been termed "lack of insight" [22] or impaired "self-awareness" [47]. Self-report questionnaires have been recognized for their value in contributing to the understanding of patients' everyday PM dysfunctions; however, when used with TBI patients, impaired self-awareness may compromise the validity of self-report measures. Useful information can be acquired from relatives or caregivers. Questionnaires completed by significant others of the patients' general PM function have been found to correlate with objective PM test scores, and reliably address the patients' PM dysfunction in daily life [17, 18, 45].

The first developed questionnaires investigated general memory dysfunction in daily life with no specific distinction between retrospective or PM dysfunctions. These questionnaires included the Memory Functioning Questionnaire [48], Inventory of Everyday Memory Functioning [49], Cognitive Failure Questionnaire [50], Everyday Memory Questionnaire [51] and the Subjective Memory Questionnaire [52].

The Prospective Memory Questionnaire (PMQ) is a 52-item questionnaire that includes four PM subscales: 1) the *long-term episodic subscale* is related to memory for irregularly scheduled tasks, which require completion some hours or days after a cue to perform it (i.e. "I forgot to return books to the library by the due date"), 2) the *short-term habitual subscale* addresses memory for tasks to be completed shortly after the relevant cue that occur on regular basis (i.e. "I forgot to put a stamp on a letter before mailing it"), 3) the *internally cued subscale* addresses memory for tasks that do not have a clear external cue (i.e. "I was driving and temporarily forgot where I was going"), and 4) the *techniques to remember subscale* measures the use of strategies to aid prospective memory (i.e. "I rehearse things in my mind so I will not forget to do them") [20]. The PMQ questionnaire was administrated to 114 younger adults, 27 older adults and 15 patients with TBI [20]. Coefficient alpha was.92 for the PMQ total score, and ranged from.78 to.90 for the subscales. Factor analysis confirmed the 4-subscale structure. Test-retest reliability was found to be high, r =.88for the PMQ total and ranged from.64 to.88 for the subscales. Overall, the results found that the ratings of TBI patients were significantly different from those of controls on one of the short-term habitual subscales of the PMQ, however, very few studies have used the PMQ with TBI patients [53].

The Comprehensive Assessment of Prospective Memory (CAPM) measure was developed to evaluate the frequency of PM failure, and to evaluate the perceived amount of concern about these memory lapses and the reasons why people are successful or unsuccessful in performing PM tasks [54]. The items include both basic and instrumental activities of everyday life and are divided into three sections. Section A analyses frequency of failure (39 items; i.e. "Forgetting an appointment with your doctor or therapist", "not locking the door when leaving home"), and is considered to be the best section to evaluate PM dysfunction and outcome after rehabilitation [55]. Section B analyses the amount of concern about these failures (39 items; the same items used in the first session), and Section C analyses the reasons associated with the success or failures of PM tasks (15 items; "I rely to other people to remind me when I have to remember to do things"). Section A was used with 33 severe TBI patients (GCS = 5.1; PTA = 6.66 days), 33 relatives and 29 healthy controls to investigate frequency of PM failure [54]. Analyses were conducted on self-rating and informant-rating, and the difference between these two indices provided a measure of self-awareness on PM dysfunction. The results showed no significant differences between the TBI and controls' self-ratings of the frequency of PM failure. However, a significant difference was found between the informant-ratings, which suggested that relatives and/or caregivers reported higher levels of PM failure. These findings are likely to be due to the commonly found self-awareness difficulties in patients with TBI [47, 54]. The section C was used to investigate how TBI patients perceived and self-rated the reasons for PM failure [56]. Relatives and caregivers were also asked to rate TBI patients' PM failures. One-hundred thirty-six participants were included in the study and divided into four groups: 38 severe TBI (GCS = 5.1, PTA = 62.6 days), 34 significant others of TBI patients, 34 controls, and 30 significant others of controls. Results showed that patients with TBI were more likely to forget planned activities; moreover, TBI patients forgot to do things when they focused on other tasks or if they considered other activities unimportant. Patients with TBI seemed also to rely more on relatives to remind them to do things. However, no significant differences were found between TBI patients and controls on reporting reason of remembering or forgetting, and indicated that TBI patients tended to overestimate their PM abilities [54, 56]. It is important to note that authors reported that some TBI patients included in the study indicated that they have difficulty understanding some questions included in section C and suggested to further investigate the internal consistency of the section C [56]. The validity of CAMP (section A) was investigated in a study conducted with 45 patients with moderate and severe TBI (age M=30.02 years; GCS = 7.08; PTA = 47.89) and their relatives [45]. Participants also performed two tests of PM, the CAMPROMPT [57] and the Memory Intentions Screening Test (MIST) [58]. Concurrent validity was investigated by the comparison of scores on the CAPM with scores on the CAMPROMPT and MIST. Results showed that self-report CAPM scores did not significantly correlate with scores on the CAMPROMPT or MIST. TBI patients reported very few PM failures on the CAPM, but demonstrated impairments on neuropsychological testing. Interestingly, results showed that the responses provided by the relatives on CAPM correlated with CAMPROMPT and MIST performance. These findings suggested that the relative version of the CAPM has some concurrent validity when compared with performance on neuropsychological assessments, and that the relative version of the CAPM is an objective and valid measure of PM failure in TBI patients [17, 45]. To our knowledge, no studies have been conducted with TBI on section B of CAMP.

Finally, the Prospective and Retrospective Memory Questionnaire (PRMQ) was developed to investigate the rate of frequency with which patients make particular types of memory errors [59]. The PRMQ consists of 16 items that are divided into 8 categories (two items in each category) that tap different aspects of memory failure: prospective short-term self-cued, prospective short-term environmentally-cued, prospective long-term self-cued, prospective long-term environmentally cued, retrospective short-term self-cued, retrospective short-term environmentally-cued, retrospective long-term self-cued, and retrospective long-term environmentally-cued [59]. Different forms of the PRMQ are available for patients and caregivers. In addition to the 16 items included in the patient form, caregivers are asked to respond to four additional questions. Two of the questions concern the caregivers' frustration and two ask the caregivers to rate the patients' frustration. The PRMQ has never been used with TBI patients, but was tested with 242 healthy older adults (age M = 72.74 years) and 155 patients with Alzheimer disease (AD; age M = 73.95 years). One-hundred fifty-five caregivers of AD patients (age M= 56.85) and younger participants (age M = 44.19) were also included in the study. The split half reliability of the PRMQ conducted in younger and older adults (n = 406) compared the two items within each category was found to be.84. Results showed that memory dysfunction was highest for AD patients and lowest for caregivers, with younger and older adults in between. Moreover, caregivers rated PM dysfunctions of AD patients more frustrating than patients did, and PM errors were rated as significantly more frustrating than retrospective memory errors. The authors concluded that the PRMQ might be a potentially useful tool for investigating differences in frequency of prospective and retrospective memory failure in non-patient samples, but that the questionnaire needed to be adapted to increase its sensitivity to allow for more extensive clinical use [59]. These results were extended through the testing of 87 younger adults (age M = 44.11 years) with PRMQ and with a standard laboratory procedure of PM [60]. The reliability of PRMQ was.86 (Cronbach's alpha) for the total scale,.72 for the PM scale, and.72 for the retrospective memory scale. Participants reported higher scores (higher memory failure) for the PM than retrospective memory scale. To examine whether the PRMQ scores may predict actual performance in the laboratory PM tasks, correlation analyses were conducted and showed that only the PM scale was a significant predictor for the standard laboratory PM performance. In sum, the study extended initial findings and added additional support for the validity of the PRMQ. In addition, it provided the first evidence for the utility of the PRMQ subscales in differentiating between prospective and retrospective memory task performance [59, 60].

To our knowledge, no other studies appear to have examined the relationships between PM performance and measures of self-awareness in TBI patients. This may reflect the unreliability of self-rated PM measures [47]. Despite previous studies that have provided good validity and reliability of questionnaires, the results are mixed when self-rated scores were compared with laboratory-based measures of PM performance [3, 56, 60, 61]. There are two important caveats to the questionnaires. First, it is important to consider that some authors have reported lower correspondence between the PM tasks used in the examination condition, and PM activities in the everyday situation. Indeed, in real word situations, people required higher levels of executive functioning to perform multiple tasks than in a controlled experimental standardized setting. Therefore, some authors have found that TBI patients showed unimpaired performance on neuropsychological PM tests, but reported impaired PM performance in real life [45, 46]. Second, it is important to consider the self-awareness dysfunction often observed in TBI patients that might compromise the validity of TBI participants' self-report measures [22, 47].

3.2. Behavioral measures

In 2002, Shum et al. [61] published the first review about PM dysfunctions in TBI patients. The authors identified three neuropsychological tests that provided objective scores of PM, and that were used in clinical settings. These tests included the Rivermead Behavioural Memory Test (RBMT) [62], Cambridge Behavioural Prospective Memory Test (CBPMT) [63], and Memory Intentions Screening Test (MIST) [58]. More recently, a second review about PM dysfunctions in TBI patients was published [3]; despite the increasing number of studies conducted, very few studies were dedicated to the development of valid and reliable measures to investigate PM failure in clinical settings. We briefly present the main tools that were highlighted in the prior reviews [3, 61] and a newly developed task.

The RBMT was the first widely used task in clinical practice that explicitly tests PM performance. It includes three PM tasks: (1) remembering where a belonging is hidden and asking for it to be returned, (2) asking for the next appointment time when an alarm sounds, and (3) delivering a message. Six neurologically impaired adults (age M = 42 years) with a length of stay in the post acute rehabilitation program that ranged from 22 to 101 days (M = 66.2 days) were tested with the RBMT [64]. Participants were required to perform RBMT and some real-life activities every morning with or without verbal or visual cues. Low or no significant correlations were found between the number of activities correctly performed and RBMT score, which indicated that the RBMT was an invalid predictor of PM performance. Different results were obtained in a study with a larger sample size [65]. One-hundred-nineteen participants were divided into four groups: 20 severe TBI, 29 moderate TBI, 39 mild TBI, and 31 controls. Participants performed the RBMT together with other clinical memory measures (Wechsler Memory Scale-Revised and Luria Nebraska Neuropsychological Battery). The authors found the RBMT to be an accurate and valid measure to test PM memory failure in everyday life. However, RMBT had ceiling effects when used with 25 TBI patients (10 moderate and 15 severe; age = 28.6 years) and 25 controls [27]. In addition, the authors found that only one of the three RBMT PM items (RBMT delayed message) successfully differentiated between TBI patients and controls. Although the RBMT was widely used in clinical settings and in several neuropsychological studies, it provided only a limited range of scores and is unlikely to be sensitive to deficits in non-severe patients [27, 61, 64]. Importantly, the test does not assess time-based PM performance [62]. A new version of the RBMT, The Rivermead Behavioural Memory Test Extended Version (RBMT-E) was created by combining two parallel forms of the RBMT [66]. The idea was to develop a more demanding test that eliminated the ceiling effects and thus would be more sensitive to minor PM impairments. The RBMT-E includes 8 subtests: (1) First and second names: remembering the names of three people; (2) Appointment and belongings: retrieving to ask for two belongings previously hidden; (3) Picture recognition: recognizing 20 previously-seen pictures and distinguishing them from distractors; (4) Face recognition: recognizing 15 previously-seen faces and distinguishing them from distractors; (5) Story: recalling a story immediately and after a delay; (6) Route: remembering 7 routes immediately and after a delay; (7) Message: remembering to pick up and deliver to the correct location a message immediately and after a delay and (8) Orientation and date: answering 12 orientation questions and giving the correct date. The RBMT-E was tested with 16 TBI patients (age M = 40.5 years; time since injury M = 47.5 months, range 8-92 months) and 16 controls [67]. Patients included in the study were all previously evaluated with RBMT and all scored in the normal range (screening score between 9-12), but all lamented PM dysfunctions in daily life. The authors intended to compare the performances obtained with RBMT and the RBMT-E. The results, however, were mixed and inconclusive. In fact, when patients were retested with the RBMT, some participants scored outside the normal range, which indicated poor test-retest reliability. Moreover, when the analyses of RBMT-E performance were conducted on those patients who scored in the normal range at test and retest (data collected with RBMT) and compared with controls, no differences were found between groups [16].

The CBPMT includes four time-based and four event-based tasks and requires approximately 40 minutes to be completed [63]. Participants were allowed to use any strategy to remember the tasks. The time-based tasks included (1) remembering the experimenter to not forget the keys after 15 minutes; (2) requesting the tester for a newspaper after 20 minutes; (3) switching task after working for 20 minute and (4) stop working on the booklet after 3 minutes. The event-based tasks included (1) reminding the tester about five hidden objects; (2) when the alarm rings, putting a briefcase under the desk; (3) Changing pens after having completed seven filler assignments and (4) give the envelope with the message. The CBPMT was used with 36 people with mixed brain injury (age M = 35.61 years; time since injury 75.56 months) and 28 control participants [63]. Participants also performed the EMQ along with general intelligence, attention, working memory, executive functions and retrospective memory tasks. Results showed good correlation between the CBPMT and measures of working memory and executive functions. No correlations were found between the CBPMT and EMQ in brain injury patients, but significant correlations were found with controls. Subsequently, the CBPMT was used to create the CAMPROMPT [47], which included three time-based and three-event based tasks to be completed in 25 minutes. PM tasks are executed while performing a filler activity, and participants are allowed to spontaneously use strategies (i.e. take notes). The time-based tasks included: (1) remembering his/her belongings when there were 7 minutes left to the end of the session; (2) when the timer shows 16 minutes, the participants had to remember to stop the task in 7 minutes time and (3) at 10:11 and 5 minute after the end of the session, remembering to call the reception. For the event-based tasks participants were asked (1) to return a book to the examiner when he/she came to a question about the television program 'EastEnders'; (2) to return an envelope with "MESSAGE" written on it and (3) to remind the examiner to pick up five objects that had been hidden when the session is over. The CAMPROMPT was used with 44 moderate and severe TBI patients (age M = 29.64; GCS = 7.08) [18]. Participants also completed executive functions tasks and the CAMP section A. Results showed that PTA was a good predictor of PM performance, and patients with lower executive functioning showed lower PM performance with a higher degree of impairment on the time-based tasks. Overall, the CAMPROMPT showed very high reliability (Pearson r = .99) and high internal consistency (Cronbach's alpha = .75), but moderate test–retest reliability (Kendall's Tau-b = of .64) [57, 68].

The MIST includes four event-based and four time-based tasks to be performed in 30 minute sessions while playing a word-search puzzle that serves as a distractor [58]. The 8 PM activities are balanced in terms of delay interval (2 or 5 minutes delay), cue (time-based or event-based), and response modality (verbal or a physical response). The MIST also includes an 8-item multiple-choice recognition test and a more naturalistic task that has to be performed in a 24-hour delay (calling the examiner the next day and report how many hours of sleep the night before). The MIST test has been widely used with healthy older adults and various clinical populations [58]. No significant correlation was found between the MIST score and CAMP in 45 moderate and severe TBI patients (age M = 30.02 years; GCS = 7.08; PTA = 47.89) and their relatives, but TBI patients showed lower performance on the time-based tasks [45]. The MIST task was used with 38 mild TBI (mTBI) patients (age M = 40.6 years, GCS range 13-15, no PTA, loss of consciousness < 20 minutes) and matched controls were included in the study [24]. Patients were tested within a month of injury (M = 26.6 days) and 3 months post-injury. Mild TBI (mTBI) patients performed more poorly than controls on the MIST task within the first month following injury, which indicated that PM impairment is part of the acute cognitive dysfunction profile of mTBI. PM dysfunctions were also observed after 3 months post-injury, suggesting that PM may be a sensitive indicator of cerebral compromise in mTBI patients. Taken together, these studies conducted with mild and severe TBI patients [24, 45, 58, 69] showed a consistent deficit on the MIST summary score and total number of errors. Both TBI patients and controls demonstrated higher performance when they executed activities after a short time delay. Better performance was obtained with event-based than with time-based tasks in both TBI patients and controls. The controls demonstrated higher performance for action responses compared to verbal responses, though no effect of response type was observed in TBI patients. Overall, the MIST demonstrated good validity and test-retest reliability when performed across a two-week interval [70]. The split half reliability was .70 (Spearman-Brown coefficient), internal reliability (Cronbach's alpha = 0.89) of the six subscales was high, but the internal reliability (Cronbach's alpha = .47) for each trial was poor.

The Royal Prince Alfred Prospective Memory Test (RPA-ProMem) includes three alternative forms, each of which has two time-based (i.e., "in 15 minutes time I would like you to tell me it's time for a coffee break") and two event-based tasks (i.e., "At the end of our session today, I would like you to ask me for an information sheet on note-taking strategies") that have to be performed within the session (short-term: "In 15 minute interval I would like you to remind me to move my cat so I don't get the ticket") or at a later moment (long-term: "When you arrive home today, I want you to phone and leave a message on my voice mail, telling me your mother's name") [69]. External aids are permitted during the testing session. The RPA-ProMem was used with 20 patients with brain lesions (stroke n = 7, epilepsy n = 5, tumour/cyst n = 2, TBI n = 2, arteriovenus malformation removal n = 2, encephalitis n = 1 and systemic lupus erythematosus n = 1) and 20 controls [69]. Participants also performed the MIST, CAMP section A, and EMQ. Patients with brain lesions showed lower performance on the RPA-ProMem compared to controls, even when they rated their own PM performance in daily life as normal. No differences were found between the scores of the three parallel form of RPA-ProMem, and they showed good alternate form reliability (Spearmen-Brown coefficient = .71). These finding are consistent with those obtained from studies with self-report questionnaires [3, 61] and support the use of RPA-ProMem as an objective clinical measure of PM performance.

Finally, Virtual Week was developed as a laboratory PM task that would more closely represent PM activities in everyday life [43]. Two clocks are placed above and below the dice. The clock above the dice is a chronometer that starts at the beginning of each virtual day and the clock below is a virtual clock that moves when participants roll the dice and indicates the virtual time of the day (the clock moves 15 minute every two squares). Participants are required to perform 10 activities every virtual day. The original version [43] included 7 virtual days, but the later versions include 3 or 5 days and maintained task validity [71]. A training day is included at the beginning of the task to familiarize patients with task procedures. Interestingly, Virtual Week also includes regular and irregular tasks. Every virtual day, participants are required to perform 4 regular tasks that simulate regular activities that occur as one undertakes normal health care duties every day (i.e. "take medications every day at breakfast"), and 4 irregular tasks that simulate the kinds of occasional activities that are new (i.e., Monday: pick up the laundry when shopping). Within the regular and irregular tasks, two are time-based (i.e., "call the plumber at 3pm") and two are event-based (i.e., "return the book to Philip when you see him").. We tested 18 TBI patients (age M = 31.72 years; GCS M = 4.54, time since injury M = 66.94 months) and 18 controls with Virtual Week and other neuropsychological tasks [44]. Results showed a generalized PM impairment in TBI patients, and significant correlations were found between PM performance, indices of cognitive recovery (Level of Cognitive Functioning and Functional Independence Measure/Functional Assessment Measure), and semantic fluency. These results indicated that participants with better cognitive recovery obtained better PM performance. Since the first publication [43], Virtual Week has been widely used with healthy and clinical populations [71], with corresponding evidence indicated good psychometric properties [71, 72]. The reliability of Virtual Week was investigated in a study that involved younger and older adults [72]. Across the entire sample, reliability estimates ranged from .84 to .94 for the regular, irregular, and time-check tasks. In another study, the split-half reliability for the overall Virtual Week measure was estimated to be: 74 in a clinical group with schizophrenia [73]. In a recent study, test-retest reliability was investigated in older adults by use of the same (Study 1) or parallel (Study 2) versions across two testing time points separate by 1 month [74]. Preliminary results in Study 1 showed good internal consistency (Cronbach's alpha) of .64 at the initial and .83 at the retest session. In Study 2, for version A, internal consistency was .70 at the initial test and .89 at the retest session, and for Version B was .82 at the initial test and .65 at the retest session.

4. Prospective memory trainings

Traditionally, the rehabilitation of memory impairment in TBI patients has focused on retrospective memory. Only recently has the importance of PM impairments following TBI been recognized and resulted in the development of specific training programs [17, 18]. Considering that PM is not a unitary process, it is difficult to address the optimal rehabilitation paradigm that can be solely focused on treating PM as a unitary system, or can focus on treating specific PM components. In this section, we review the main rehabilitation approaches (Remedial vs. Compensatory) used in the treatment of PM impairment.

4.1. Remedial/Restorative approaches

Cognitive interventions have been developed to restore "the underlying defective cognitive functions usually via repetitive drills or training activities designed to stimulate damaged neural networks or establish new networks" [61, pp 9]. The first studies investigated the effect of repeating PM tasks after different retention intervals on PM performance. The Spaced Retrieval Technique (SRT) required participants to remember a task over an interval of time. If the task was recalled correctly, the retention interval was an increase. The SRT was tested with two TBI patients over 4.5 and 3.5 months of training. Results showed positive effects on PM performance, in fact, TBI patients increased their performance from being unable to complete a PM task following a 60 seconds delay to being able to complete a PM task following 8 minute delay, for patients 1; and an increment from 4 to 8 minutes delay was observed in patients 2 [75]. Based on these encouraging results, the authors further investigated the generalization effects of SRT with one TBI patient [76]. The training paradigm consisted of repetitive administration of PM tasks, with systematic lengthening of the delay period between task administration and task execution. Probes were taken that evaluated generalization to performance on naturalistic PM and retrospective memory tasks. Results confirmed previous findings and showed that patients were able to increment of temporal interval between task administration and task execution an maintain good PM performance. However, the results were less encouraging as tasks showed poor ecological validity [76]. Moreover, two TBI patients were tested with SRT training and retrospective memory drills [77]. The first patient increased the delay interval from 1 to 5 minutes, while the second patient increased the delay interval from 2 to 10 minutes. Results were consistent across the two TBI patients who showed improvement on PM task performance at the delayed target time in both experimental and real-life settings. A more ecologically valid training program called the Prospective Memory Re-training Package (PMRP) was developed [78]. Six TBI patients were first tested with the Prospective Memory Screening test (PROMS) [75] and then were trained on the PMRP. The training required the patients to perform real-life activities (i.e., putting a stamp on an envelope) at specified target times, with a maximum delay of 6 minutes. The delay between task administration and task execution increased depending on correct or incorrect responses. Results showed better PM performance after 2 months of training [78]. In addition, positive effects were found when space retrieval was combined with Error Learning (EL) technique, which was achieved by the discouragement of participants from guessing if they were uncertain of a response [79].

The effects of cognitive strategies on PM performance were also investigated [80]. Some authors showed that participants had better performance on PM tasks when they had previously made a strong and explicit association between PM cue and intended action through imagining themselves performing that PM action. By reinforcing the cue-action association during the encoding phase, future intentions are more likely to be supported by automatic cognitive processes according to the McDaniel & Einstein's Multiprocess Model [4]. The authors [4] showed that less attentional resources and executive processes are required to perform the PM action because the intended action is spontaneously retrieved when the prospective cued is encountered. Following this finding, a training program was developed with visual imagery technique [81]. The training included three successive phases. The first phase evaluated the individual visual imagery capacity, the second focused on acquisition of visual imagery skills using spaced retrieval techniques, and the third focused on visual imagery techniques that are progressively applied to real-life situations in order to promote learning transfer. During the third phase, participants are encouraged to identify challenging daily-life situations and to develop more appropriate visual imagery strategies to successfully complete the real-life activities. Twenty-one patients with various brain injuries were included in the study: 12 participants were included in the control group (age M = 36.6 years; time since injury = 60 months) and 9 were included in the experimental group using visual imaginary technique (age M = 41.9 years; time since injury = 65 months). Participant included in the control group performed different memory trainings respective with the training used in their centre. The trainings were different for each patient, but intensity and frequency of training were the same in both groups. Results showed that visual imagery training significantly improved delayed recall of everyday verbal information (i.e., stories, appointments). Relatives also reported a reduction in PM problems and the effects were stable after a 3-month follow-up. Successive, visual imagery technique was used with 30 severe TBI patients [82]; 10 of who were assigned to the experimental condition using visual imaginary technique (age M = 35.00 years; PTA = 30.60 days; time since injury = 43.40 months) and 20 to the control condition (age M = 30.90 years; PTA = 29.20 days; time since injury = 34.00 months). The program required the patients to learn flexible cognitive strategies by creating gradually more complex and ecological associations between cue and intended action that could be used in real life situations. Participants who took part in the rehabilitation program improved their PM performance (measured by Test écologique de mémoire prospective; TEMP [83]), and also reported the use of imagery techniques in everyday life situations with corresponding improvement in PM function. Relatives also confirmed this improved performance [82].

The positive results obtained with visual imagery techniques seem to rely on the strong cue-action association and engagement required by the training. Repeated imagination of the retrieval situation and increased cue-action association might increase the detection of retrieval cues with the occurrence of the situation. This technique seems to be particularly effective for event-based PM tasks in which the PM cue is available. For time-based actions, maybe additional effort is needed and patients should try to associate a visual cue even if the action is time-based. For example, if the action is to make a call at 3 pm, participants should look at the phone and remember to make the phone call. Thus, imagination may help to translate a time-based into an event-based task. However, such a transference of time to an event based task presumably will only be possible in patients with mild impairment.

Some studies have attempted to resolve PM dysfunction with a different approach. Considering that PM is not a unitary system [4], one line of rehabilitation might be to restore the components of PM. These approaches followed the idea that retrospective memory and/or executive dysfunction may underlie PM impairment [16, 25, 27], and that improvement of these cognitive components should result in better PM performance [84]. Hypothetically, training programs devoted to improve attention, working memory, and executive functions could have positive effects on PM performance [3, 61, 84]. In general, approaches to the rehabilitation of executive deficits have focused on training patients to follow step-by-step problem solving strategies (i.e., define the problem and generate potential solutions) [85]. Positive effects were found when retrospective memory dysfunctions were rehabilitated [86, 87]; however, the value of such an approach for PM improvement remains to be investigated. Other studies have found that structured group experience facilitate the PM rehabilitation. Participants who enrolled in Goal Management Training (GMT) were encouraged to highlight common executive difficulties and discover which were the best strategies (i.e., breaking down goals into sub-goals, using mental imagery) [88]. Attempts to promote generalization included homework exercises and recording of everyday errors [85, 89]. Despite efforts to foster generalization and maintenance, the everyday benefits of such training still largely depend on strategies that spontaneously "come to mind" in everyday life [90]. Remedial strategies seem to work on the mental organization and encoding of prospective actions that should help recall. However, PM not only involves encoding and storing the content of PM action, but also recalling the intended action at the appropriate moment in the future. The remedial strategies previously presented may have more application to the rehabilitation of PM by enhancing recall of the content (the retrospective component) than enhancement of the intention. These techniques have demonstrated good effects on PM performance but need to be further developed in line with PM models and real life situations [1, 4, 5, 91]. For example, training paradigms need to include both event- and time-based tasks, with the knowledge that routine tasks (i.e., daily regular tasks [43]) can be better encoded, remembered, and performed. Novel activities can be difficult to remember, but in such cases researchers and clinicians can manipulate the salience of the PM cue [4, 72]. Preliminary data suggested that PM training based on remedial strategies can improve individual's PM performance, but further research is needed to investigate the generalizability to real-life situations.

4.2. Adaptive/Compensatory approaches

In contrast to the remedial approaches that are aimed to restore the impaired PM function, adaptive/compensatory strategies are aimed to compensate the PM dysfunction. These techniques are widely used in clinical practices and patients often spontaneously report the use of compensatory strategies such as a timer or diary. Memory aids are widely available, can be inexpensive, and have the potential to be highly effective in compensating for PM problems in mild to moderately impaired patients. Although patients can find it difficult to learn and remember to use such aids, it is possible to implement an effective system, even in patients with profound amnesia [61].

There is a substantial body of evidence supporting the use of external memory devices [90, 92], which can be categorized into non-electronic and electronic external memory devices. *Non-electronic memory devices* include a diary, calendar, and to-do lists. These are easily available, but are only beneficial if patients make the effort to use them at the appropriate time [92]. Despite the fact that patients often spontaneously report to take notes on calendar and use a pin-board, very few studies have investigated the effectiveness of non-electronic memory devices on PM rehabilitation. Of the few conducted. one study used a memory book in training with TBI patients with amnesic disorders [93]. Patients were first introduced to the different functions and learned how to use the memory book. Then, patients used the memory book in a controlled laboratory environment followed by use in everyday life. Patients had to demonstrate mastery of criteria before they moved to the next step (use the memory book in real-life condition). For severe patients, the training lasted 6 months. Memory improvement was observed and effects were stable over a long time period. Previous results were extended to evaluate the effectiveness of the memory book in comparison to a more social therapy in which patients were trained with problem-solving strategies [94]. Eight TBI patients were randomly assigned to one of the two experimental conditions: memory book (mean age = 29.9 years; days of coma = 39.7; time since injury = 77.7 months) and supportive therapy (mean age = 26.8 years; days of coma = 37.5; time since injury = 86.8 months). After the training, the authors reported reductions in the number of errors in everyday life in patients who used the memory book. However, 6-months later, there were no longer differences between the two groups. This may raise the problem of generalization and long-term use of learned memory strategies. Some authors have noted that many patients quickly abandon diary use once they are discharged [95]. To overcome such problems, several formal training approaches worked also on self-awareness of PM deficits in order to minimize patients' resistance to use memory aids when back in their home environment. In fact, some studies showed the importance of involving family and friends in the training and the need to have practice sessions in community-based settings [96]. Taken together, these results are encouraging regarding the utility of non-electronic memory aids; also, a later study showed that participants who spontaneously took notes (13 out of 36 people with brain injury and 14 out of 28 controls) performed significantly better on a PM test than those who did not take notes [63]. Results lead to the conclusion that note-taking significantly benefits PM performance. The suggestion is therefore to integrate non-electronic memory aids in other memory training programs such as group or remedial therapies [3, 92, 97].

Considering the increasing use of electronic devices in everyday life, it has been observed a consequent increase of electronic memory devices in clinical training and PM rehabilitation. *Electronic memory devices* have the clear benefit of not merely telling the patients what he/she is intended to do, but also drawing the patient's attention to this information at the appropriate time. A brief summary of electronic memory aids in PM training for TBI patients is provided in Table 3.

Probably the most used and commercialized electronic memory device used to compensate for PM deficits is the NeuroPage system [98, 99, 100], which enables an individual to receive timed reminders or cues that appear on a portable pager carried by the person. The aim is to help individuals maintain independence by reminding them to carry out everyday tasks. Messages appear on a big screen and the user can control the system with a single large button, which makes the NeuroPage suitable for patients with motor difficulties. Messages have to be confirmed by the patients by calling the central system, in the case of no answer, the message is displayed again. All messages are also stored in the central system. The authors also

Memory Aids	References	Advantages	Disadvantages
NeuroPage	[98, 99, 100]	Very small and little learning is required. The system can ring or vibrate and a text message appeared on the screen.	The appointments are changed through a paging company and user cannot change them.
Mobile Extensible Memory and Orientation Sustem (MEMOS)	[102, 103, 104]	Therapists and caregivers can access to the system from any computer with internet and modify to encode data.	Problem with connection between server and devices.
Memojog	[105, 106]	Users, therapists and caregivers can access to the system. Possibility to add others information beside PM tasks (i.e. birthdays, addresses).	Problem with connection between server and devices. Difficulties with touch screen system.
Voice Organizer	[107, 108]	User can autonomously record new messages.	Patients with speech and motor impairments might have difficulties in using the system.
Palmtop	[109]	User can autonomously add new messages.	Too difficult to use for patients with severe impairments

Table 3. Overview of electronic memory devices.

presented the results of a large study conducted with 143 patients aged between 8 and 83 years [98]. All patients had brain damage (mainly TBI or stroke) and memory, attentional, and planning deficits. Results showed that patients generally benefitted from the use of NeuroPage with improvement in everyday goals by an average of 30% when the pager was used relative to baseline performance. Importantly, in the same patients, there was evidence that the benefits persisted when the system was no longer used, except in those with more pronounced executive impairment [84; 98, 99, 101]. Many patients suggested the pager served as a training function (i.e., consolidating intentions into a everyday life).

The Mobile Extensible Memory and Orientation System (MEMOS) [102, 103, 104] is a system specially designed for patients with brain injuries. The system includes a central server to communicate with a personal memory assistant over a wireless cellular phone. Similar to the NeuroPage, MEMOS includes a large screen with few buttons to accommodate patients with cognitive and motor impairments. Of interest, the device allows patients to leave messages for future appointments that are transferred to the central system where the caregiver can input them. The system sends reminders for PM tasks with feedback and step-by-step guidance. Important tasks, as taking medication, can be set as "critical tasks" for which the caregivers can be advised if the patient executed them.. The effectiveness of MEMOS was compared with a Palm organiser in 13 patients with brain injury [104]. Patients reported positive effects from both devices, but during the interview after the training, patients reported that the MEMOS was more helpful in the execution of PM tasks and desired to continue using it. The long-term use of MEMOS was evaluated with 3 TBI patients [103]. The authors reported that the MEMOS alone was unable to compensate for memory deficits in patients with severe TBI. For those patients, additional support for relatives is necessary [103].

Another interesting memory aid is Memojog [105, 106], which is similar to the MEMOS device [102]. Memojog is a remote and interactive communication system that provides prompting for people with memory impairments. A central system is used to deliver text prompts to a mobile device that are announced by an alarm. Interestingly, both the user and the caregivers can add new information into the devices from any internet station. Also, new tasks can be phoned in by others to add them into the system. The reminders are then wirelessly transmitted at the appropriate times and users have to respond to them. As for MEMOS, "crucial tasks" can be monitored with particular attention. Moreover, the system can record other information such as birthdays, addresses, contact information, pictures, and details of any appointments. Limitations of the system are the connectivity problems, thus authors and caregivers are unsure if the patients are doing something wrong or if the system is malfunctioning. Besides that, users (both older adults and patients with brain injury) are motivated by the system and haven shown improvement in memory performance with Memojog [106].

Also commercialised are systems in which it is possible to record messages that are played back at the appropriate time. One of them, Voice Organiser is a phone-type device that requires no input messages trough the central system, but the user can autonomously add new task and reminders [107]. Five TBI patients (mean age = 42.6 years; time since injury = 38.6 months) were trained in an A-B-A experimental design and performance was monitored for 9 weeks. Results showed that all but one patient improved in PM performance. The improvement was evident immediately at the beginning of the training. A limitation of the Voice Organiser device is that patients with significant speech disorders or poor motor ability might have difficulties in using it. In such conditions, relatives can program the system [107]. More recently, 8 patients with brain damage (mean age 46.25 years) and PM impairments were trained with an IC Recorder for a maximum of 3 months [108]. The names of the experimenter and patients were said before the alarm to attract attention and motivate the user. Soon after, the recorded message was said, indicating the task to be performed. Results showed that tasks prompted by the IC Recorder were better remembered and executed for five of the eight patients. The study added further support to the high quality of memory aids and suggested that the IC Recorder has great potential as a voice memory aid to assist patients with PM impairments [108].

Finally, microcomputers can be used to facilitate everyday PM performance. They have the advantage to be hand-held computers that can be easily carried around. Moreover, they provide visual as well as auditory messages to prompt the PM actions. Twelve patients (11 TBI patients and 1 with cerebrovascular accident; mean age = 49.6 years) were trained with a palmtop organiser and evaluated at follow-up between 2 months and 4 years after initial training [109]. Participants were asked about prior experiences with computer devices, then whether the device was useful, and if and how often they still used it. Nine out of 12 patients reported that the palmtop computer was very useful during the training, and they were still using it. Of the remaining three patients, 1 never learned how to use it and 2 found no appropriate situation in their daily life where use it. Later PM performance was investigated in 12 patients (mean age = 4 years; time since injury = 49.5 months) using Palm organiser or mobile phone. The authors were not only interested in training PM performance, but also in training patients to enter appointments into the devices. The study showed that only patients with mild impairment were able to correctly enter the appointments [110].

The electronic market moves very quickly and memory devices need to be updated accordingly. We would like to report two interesting devices tested with older adults, but that can be extremely promising with patients with brain injuries: Autominder [111] and Coach [112]. Autominder is a mobile robot platform with an integrated screen display and portable mobile device designed to assist older adults in their home. As with the other memory systems, Autominder transmits reminders for PM activities, but interestingly has the ability to adapt to the user's schedule depending on the behaviour detected by sensors installed throughout the home. Coach consists of a video camera installed in the home and provides support for both prospective and retrospective memory deficits. In fact, Coach provides cues to initiate future actions and helps users to execute the action by suggesting the procedure step-by step. Interestingly, Coach is requires no learning on its use and thus has limited demands of the patient in terms interfacing with the device. The system verbally communicates the reminders so no reading is required. The advantages from using these systems are clear and users showed improvement in their PM performance. However, for some older adults, technology is still intimidating and work with it may generate apprehension. Future generations would benefit more from high quality technology [3, 84, 92, 113].

5. General conclusion and future directions

This chapter reviewed the literature regarding assessment and treatment of PM impairment in TBI patients. Dysfunctions in PM are often observed in TBI patients, they can be very frustrating and limit the independence of TBI patients, causing them to rely on caregivers for prompting. Moreover, these failures may affect their chance to return to work or start new activities after injury [2, 17, 18]. The PM impairment in TBI patients may be due to underling dysfunctions in working memory, inhibition, and executive functions [16, 22, 25, 28, 29].

Evaluation of PM performance in clinical setting was initially assessed with questionnaires, the most known are the PMQ [20], CAPM [54] and PRMQ [59]. Questionnaires have the advantage to be easly administrated, but they are unreliable and non-objective measures of PM dysfunction [47]. Despite some previous studies that have provided good reliability and validity of questionnaires [3, 56, 60, 61], the results are mixed when self-rated scores are compared with laboratory-based measures on PM performance. The main issue concerning the employment of questionnaires to evaluate PM performance is the impairment in self-awareness that is often observed in TBI patients [22, 47] that might compromise the validity their responses to the questions.

Laboratory based tests to investigate PM performance have also been developed. The most popular are the RBMT [62], CAMPROMPT [45], and MIST [58]. More recently, to overcome the limitation of a few numbers of trials observed in the previous tests, two new testes have been developed: Virtual Week [71] and RPA-ProMem [69]. These tasks have the advantage of assessing PM performance under more controlled conditions. Nevertheless, they often lack ecological validity. More studies should be dedicated to develop reliable and ecologically valid measures to assess PM performance in clinical settings. The evolution of new technologies might help in this direction (i.e., virtual reality) to bridge the gap between performance in experimental controlled settings and real life situations. Researchers also need to develop PM test according to PM models [4, 32, 91] and ensure measurement of both event-based and time-based activities.

In terms of PM rehabilitation, two main approaches can be followed: remedial and compensatory. Remedial strategies are dedicated to restore the underlying cognitive functions with the intent to restore the damage neural networks or to create new networks. Compensatory strategies are implemented to modify the environment to overcome patients' limitations [3, 84, 92]. Most patients report the use of calendars and diaries to keep track of their duties, but these tools are limited as they require the patient to initiate using them. Electronic memory devices have the advantage to attract attention and display messages that indicate the action that has to be conducted. The most popular and commercialized electronic memory devices are the NeuroPage [98] and MEMOS [102], but many more devices are available, and some have the option to record messages as Voice organizer, [108] and add birthdays, addresses, or photos [105, 106, 109]. However, the problem with electronic devices may be that most patients are unable to learn how to properly operate them. This may be of less relevance in upcoming years when there are more individuals who are familiar with the use of such technological devices.

Aside from technology, however, the most relevant aspect seems to be whether or not patients are aware of their deficits, and therefore willing to use any kind of compensatory strategy. In any case, training with memory aid needs to be integrated into a more general neuropsychological treatment. Before administering any kind of treatment, the therapist needs to analyze what the patient is capable of accomplishing in everyday life. Therapy has to reflect the fact that acceptance of any device is highly related to awareness and acceptance of impairment.. In addition, external memory aids may be combined with other compensatory strategies such as changes in work behaviors and management of work breaks. Finally, caregivers need to work together with patients and and the treatment team to identify the more suitable memory aids and training.

Appendix A

Description of neuropsychological tests and questionnaires included in the studies.

	Full name	Characteristics
NEUROPSYCHOLOGICAL TESTS		
Executive functions		

WCST	Wisconsin Card Sorting Test	The materials included four stimulus cards and two identical decks of 64 fixed sequence response cards. Participants were required to place the card according to a criterion and they were notified only whether the responses were right or wrong. Once 10 consecutive correct matches are made, the sorting criterion is changed, without warning.
COWAT	The Controlled Oral Word Association Test	It is measures rapid strategy formation, organization, cognitive flexibility and generation of words given a phonetic (letter) cue (C, F, L or F, A, S, depending on the study).
VERBAL FLUENCY		The test includes phonemic and semantic sub-tests. In the phonemic sub-test participants are required to produce word starting with a certain letter (as in the COWAT). In the semantic sub-test participants are required to produce word part of a category (animal, cities and color).
TOL	Tower of London	Participants are presented with a standard array of four colored disks (white, yellow, blue and black) on three pegs of varying lengths and asked to achieve a given arrangement in a stated number of moves by shifting the disks one at a time from one peg to another.
Attention		
TMT (Part A and B)	Trail Making Test	Required participants to rapidly draw lines between 25 consecutively numbered circles or between alternating numbers and letters.
Stroop		Participants were instructed to identify the color of the central word. Two possible conditions (congruent and incongruent) are included. In the congruent condition, the color of the central word corresponded with the written word; whereas, in the incongruent condition, the written word appeared in a different font color.
RUFF 2 & 7		Participants are asked to cross out the digits 2 and 7 in two conditions. In one condition, the 2s and 7s are randomly interspersed among other digits, and in the second condition the distractors are made up of alphabetical letters.
Memory		
LNST	Letter-Number Sequencing Test	It involves the auditory presentation of lists of letters and numbers. Participants are then required to repeat the numbers first in ascending order, and then the letters in alphabetical order.
Digit Span	Digit Span (Backward and forward from Wechsler Memory Scale)	Participants were required to immediately recall strings of numbers that increased in length (maximum score 16).

Word List	Word Lists sub-tests from the Wechsler Memory Scale	
LM	Logical Memory sub-test from Wechsler Memory Scale	The task includes immediate (LM-I) and 30-min delayed (LM-II) prose recall.
N-Back		Common bi-syllabic word stimuli are presented sequentially. Participants were instructed to press a designed keys to indicate when they recognized a word that was the same as one of the N words back.
HVLT	*The Hopkins Verbal Learning Test*	The test includes three learning trials of 12 orally presented words. A yes/no recognition task was administered immediately following learning trial.
Verbal declarative memory		
Story sub-test of RBMT		Recall a short passage, both immediately and after a delay of approximately 15 minutes.
RAVLT	Rey Auditory Verbal Learning Test	Learning and recalling lists of words both immediately and after a delay.
Visual declarative memory		
Pictures, faces and routes sub-tests of RBMT		Participants have to remember a series of 10 line drawings of common objects and to identify them from a larger group of 20 drawings; remember five photographs, which they had to identify from a set of 10 photographs, finally, retracing a five-part pathway around the room.
QUESTIONNAIRES		
DASS	The Depression, Anxiety, Stress Scales	Three self-report scales designed to measure the negative emotional states of depression, anxiety and stress.
DEX	The Dysexecutive Questionnaire from Behavioral assessment of the dysexecutive syndrome (BADS)	20-item questionnaire focusing on the symptoms of dysexecutive syndrome.
BDI	Beck Depression Inventory	Self-report questionnaire in which each item consists of four statements indicating different levels of severity of a particular symptom experienced over the past week. Scores for all items are summed to yield a single depression score.
PREMORBID INTELLIGENCE		

NART	National Adult Reading Test	The test requires subjects to read out loud a set of 50 words which are irregular in terms of their grapheme–phoneme correspondences. The responses are individually scored as correct or incorrect, according to their pronunciation. This score can then be used to derive a premorbid IQ estimate.

Author details

Giovanna Mioni[1,2*], Shawn M. McClintock[3] and Franca Stablum[2]

*Address all correspondence to: mioni.giovanna@gmail.com

1 École de Psychologie, Université Laval, QC, Canada

2 Department of General Psychology, Padova, Italy

3 Neurocognitive Research Laboratory, Division of Brain Stimulation and Neurophysiology, Department of Psychiatry and Behavioral Sciences, Duke University School of Medicine, Department of Psychiatry, UT Southwestern Medical Center, USA

References

[1] Ellis JA. Prospective Memory or the Realization of Delayed Intentions: A Conceptual Framework for Research. In: Brandimonte M, Einstein GO, McDaniel MA (eds.) Prospective memory: Theory and Applications. Mahwah, NJ: Lawrence Erlbaum; 1996. p1–22.

[2] Kliegel M, McDaniel MA, Einstein GO. (eds). Prospective Memory: Cognitive, Neuroscience, Developmental, and Applied Perspective. Mahwah, NJ: Lawrence Erlbaum; 2008.

[3] Shum D, Levin H, Chan RCK. Prospective Memory in Patients with Closed Head Injury: A Review. Neuropsychologia 2011; 49 2156-2165.

[4] McDaniel MA, Einstein GO. Strategic and Automatic Processes in Prospective Memory Retrieval: A Multiprocess Framework. Applied Cognitive Psychology 2000; 14 127-144.

[5] Kliegel M, Martin M, McDaniel MA, Einstein GO. Complex Prospective Memory and Executive Control of Working Memory: A Process Model. Psychologische Beiträge 2002; 44 303–318.

[6] Ellis JA, Freeman JE. Ten Years of Realizing Delayed Intentions. In: Kliegel M, McDaniel MA, Einstein GO. (eds.) Prospective Memory: Cognitive, Neuroscience, Developmental, and Applied Perspective. Mahwah, NJ: Lawrence Erlbaum; 2008. p1-22.

[7] Henry JD, Phillips LH, Crawford JR, Kliegel M, Theodorou G, Summers, F. Traumatic Brain Injury and Prospective Memory: Influence of Task Complexity. Journal of Clinical and Experimental Neuropsychology 2007; 1 1-10.

[8] Meacham JA, Leiman B. Remembering to Perform Future Actions. In Neisser U. (ed.) Memory Observed: Remembering in Natural Contexts. San Francisco: W. H. Freeman; 1982. p327-336.

[9] Einstein GO, Holland LJ, McDaniel MA, Guynn MJ. Age-Related Deficits in Prospective Memory: The Influence of Task Complexity. Psychology and Aging 1992; 7 471-478.

[10] Guynn MJ, McDaniel MA, Einstein GO. Prospective Memory: When Memories Fail. Memory and Cognition 1998; 26 287-298.

[11] Carlesimo GA, Formisano R, Bivona U, Barba L, Caltagirone C. Prospective Memory in Patients with Severe Closed-Head Injury: Role of Concurrent Activity and Encoding Instructions. Behavioural Neurology 2004; 22 101-110.

[12] Einstein GO, McDaniel MA. Normal Aging and Prospective Memory. Journal of Experimental Psychology: Learning, Memory and Cognition 1990; 16 717-726.

[13] McDaniel MA, Guynn MJ, Glisky EL, Rubin SR, Routhieaux BC. Prospective Memory: A Neuropsychological Study. Neuropsychology 1999; 13 103-110.

[14] McFarland CP, Glisky EI. Frontal Lobe Involvement in a Task of Time-based Prospective Memory. Neuropsychologia 2009; 47 1660-1669.

[15] Stuss DT. Traumatic Brain Injury: Relation to Executive Dysfunction and the Frontal Lobes. Current Opinion in Neurology 2011; 24, 584–589.

[16] Mioni G, Stablum F, McClintock SM, Cantagallo A. Time-based Prospective Memory in Severe Traumatic Brain Injury Patients: The Involvement of Executive Functions and Time Perception. Journal of the International Neuropsychological Society 2012; 18, 697–705.

[17] Fleming JM, Shum D, Strong J, Lighthouse S. Prospective Memory Rehabilitation for Adults with Traumatic Brain Injury: A Compensatory Training Program. Brain Injury 2005; 19 1-13.

[18] Fleming JM, Riley L, Gill H, Gullo MJ, Strong J, Shum D. Predictors of Prospective Memory in Adults with Traumatic Brain Injury. Journal of the International Neuropsychological Society 2008; 14 823-831.

[19] Kliegel M, Eschen A, Thöne-Otto AIT. Planning and Realization of Complex Intentions in Traumatic Brain Injury and Normal Aging. Brain and Cognition 2004; 56 43–54.

[20] Hannon R, Adams P, Harrington S, Fries-Dias C, Gibson MT. Effects of Brain Injury and Age on Prospective Memory Self-rating and Performance. Rehabilitation Psychology 1995; 40 289-297.

[21] Bisiacchi PS. The Neuropsychological Approach in the Study of Prospective Memory. In: Brandimonte M, Einstein GO, McDaniel MA. (eds.) Prospective Memory: Theory and Applications. Mahwah, NJ: Lawrence Erlbaum; 1996. p297–317.

[22] Kinsella GJ, Murtagh D, Landry A, Homfray K, Hammond M, O'Beirne L, Dwyer L, Lamont M, Ponsford, J. Everyday Memory Following Traumatic Brain Injury. Brain Injury 1996; 10 499-507.

[23] McDaniel MA, Einstein GO. Prospective Memory: An Overview and Synthesis of an Emerging Field. Thousand Oaks, CA: Sage; 2007.

[24] Tay SY, Ang BT, Lau XY, Meyyappan A, Collinson SL. Chronic Impairment of Prospective Memory After Mild Traumatic Brain Injury. Journal of Head Trauma 2010; 27 77–83.

[25] Shum D, Valentine M, Cutmore T. Performance of Individuals with Severe Long-term Traumatic Brain Injury on Time-, Event-, and Activity-based Prospective Memory Tasks. Journal of Clinical and Experimental Neuropsychology 1999; 21 49-58.

[26] Kinch J, McDonald S. Traumatic Brain Injury and Prospective Memory: An Examination of the Influence of Executive Functioning and Retrospective Memory. Brain Impairment 2001; 2 119-130.

[27] Mathias JL, Mansfield KM. Prospective and Declarative Memory Problems Following Moderate and Severe Traumatic Brain Injury. Brain Injury 2005; 4, 271–282.

[28] Maujean A, Shum D, McQueen R. Effect of Cognitive Demand on Prospective Memory in Individuals with Traumatic Brain Injury. Brain Impairment 2003; 4 135-145.

[29] Schmitter-Edgecombe M, Wright MJ. Event-based Prospective Memory Following Severe Closed-head Injury. Neuropsychology 2004; 18 353–361.

[30] Spreen O, Strauss E. A Compendium of Neuropsychological Tests (2nd ed.). New York: Oxford University Press; 1998.

[31] Maater CA, Sohlberg MM, Crinean J. Focus on Clinical Research: Perceptions of Memory Function in Individuals with Closed-head Injury. Journal of Head Trauma Rehabilitation 1987; 2 74-84.

[32] Kliegel M, McDaniel MA, Einstein GO. Plan Formation, Retention, and Execution in Prospective Memory: A New Approach and Age-related Effects. Memory and Cognition 2000; 28 1041-1049.

[33] Knight RG, Titov N. Use of Virtual Reality Tasks to Assess Prospective Memory: Applicability and Evidence. Brain Impairment 2009; 10 3–13.

[34] Burgess PW, Alderman N, Forbes C, Costello A, Coates LM, Dawson DR, Anderson ND, Gilbert SJ, Dumotheil I, Channon, S. The Case for the Development and Use of 'Ecologically Valid' Measures of Executive Function in Experimental and Clinical Neuropsychology. Journal of the International Neuropsychological Society 2006; 12 194–209.

[35] Titov N, Knight RG. A Video-based Procedure for the Assessment of Prospective Memory. Applied Cognitive Psychology 2001; 15 61-83.

[36] Titov N, Knight RG. A Procedure for Testing Prospective Remembering in Persons with Neurological Impairment. Brain Injury 2000; 14 877-886.

[37] Titov N, Knight RG. A Computer-based Procedure for Assessing Functional Cognitive Skills in Patients with Neurological Injury: The Virtual Street. Brain Injury 2005; 19 315-322.

[38] Knight RG, Harnett M, Titov N. The Effects of Traumatic Brain Injury on the Predicted and Actual Performance of a Test of Prospective Remembering. Brain Injury 2005; 19 27–38.

[39] Knight RG, Titov N, Crawford M. The Effects of Distraction on Prospective Memory Remembering Following Traumatic Brain Injury Assessed in a Simulated Naturalistic Environment. Journal of the International Neuropsychology Society 2006; 12 8-16.

[40] Kinsella GJ, Ong B, Tucker J. Traumatic Brain Injury and Prospective Memory in a Virtual Shopping Trip Task: Does it Matter who Generates the Prospective Memory Target? Brain Impairment 2009; 10 45–51.

[41] Ellis JA, & Kvavilashvili, L. Prospective memory in 2000: Past, Present and Future Directions. Applied Cognitive Psychology 2001; 14 1-9.

[42] Bertsch S, Pesta BJ, Wiscott R, McDaniel MA. The Generation Effect: A Meta-analytic Review. Memory & Cognition 2007; 35 201-210.

[43] Rendell PG, Craik FIM. Virtual and Actual week: Age-related Differences in Prospective Memory. Applied Cognitive Psychology. Special Issue: New Perspective in Prospective Memory 2000; 14 S43-S62.

[44] Mioni G, Rendell PG, Henry JD, Cantagallo A, Stablum F. An Investigation of Prospective Memory Functions in People with Traumatic Brain Injury Using Virtual Week. Journal of Clinical and Experimental Neuropsychology (in press).

[45] Fleming JM, Kennedy S, Fisher R, Gill H, Gullo M, Shum D. Validity of the Comprehensive Assessment of Prospective Memory (CAPM) for Use with Adults with Traumatic Brain Injury. Brain Impairment 2009; 1, 34-44.

[46] Fleming JM, Doig E, Katz N. Beyond Dressing and Driving: Using Occupation to Facilitate Community Integration in Neurorehabilitation. Brain Impairment 2000; 1 141-150.

[47] Fleming JM, Strong J, Ashton R. Self-awareness of Deficits in Adults with Traumatic Brain Injury: How to Best Measure? Brain Injury 1996; 10 1-15.

[48] Gilewski MJ, Zelinski EM. Memory Functioning Questionnaire. Psychopharmacology Bulletin 1988; 24 665-670.

[49] Hermann DJ, Neisser U. An Inventory of Everyday Memory Experience. In: Gruneberg MM, Morris PE, Sykes NR (eds.) Practical Aspects of Memory. New York: Academic Press; 1978.

[50] Broadbent DE, Cooper PF, FitzGerald P, Parkes KR. The Cognitive Failures Questionnaire and its Correlates. British Journal of Clinical Psychology 1982; 21 1-16.

[51] Sunderland A, Harris JE, Gleave J. Memory Failures in Everyday Life Following Severe Head Injury. Journal of Clinical Neuropsychology 1984; 6 127-142.

[52] Bennett-Levy J, Powell GE. The Subjective Memory Questionnaire: An Investigation into the Self-reporting of 'Real Life' Memory Skills. British Journal of Social and Clinical Psychology 1980; 19 177-188.

[53] Buchnan T, Ali T, Hefferman TM, Ling J, Parrott AC, Rodgers J, Scoley AB. Nonequivalence of On-line and Paper and-pencil Psychological Tests: The Case of the Prospective Memory Questionnaire. Behavior Research Methods 2005; 37 148-154.

[54] Roche NL, Fleming JM, Shum D. Self-awareness of Prospective Memory Failure in Adults with Traumatic Brain Injury. Brain Injury 2002; 16 931-945.

[55] Chau L, Lee J, Fleming J, Roche N, & Shum D. Reliability and Normative Data for the Comprehensive Assessment of Prospective Memory (CAPM). Neuropsychological Rehabilitation 2007; 17 707-722.

[56] Roche NL, Moody A, Szabo K, Fleming JM, Shum D. Prospective Memory in Adults with Traumatic Brain Injury: An Analysis of Perceived Reasons for Remembering and Forgetting. Neuropsychological rehabilitation 2007; 17 314-334.

[57] Wilson BA, Emslie H, Foley J, Shiel A, Watson P, Hawkins K, Groot Y, Evans J. The Cambridge Prospective Memory Test, London: Harcourt; 2005.

[58] Raskin SA. Memory for Intentions Screening Test: Psychometric Properties and Clinical Evidence. Brain Impairment 2009; 1 23-33.

[59] Smith G, Della Sala S, Logie RH, Maylor EA. Prospective and Retrospective Memory in Normal Ageing and Dementia: A Questionnaire Study. Memory 2000; 8 311–321.

[60] Kliegel M, Jäger T. Can the Prospective and Retrospective Memory Questionnaire (PRMQ) Predict Actual Prospective Memory Performance? Current Psychology: Developmental, Learning, Personality and Social Fall 2006; 25 182-191.

[61] Shum D, Fleming J, Neulinger K. Prospective Memory and Traumatic Brain Injury: A Review. Brain Impairment 2002; 3 1-16.

[62] Wilson BA, Cockburn JM, Baddeley AD. The Rivermead Behavioural Memory Test. Bury St Edmunds: Thames Valley Test Co; 1985.

[63] Groot YCT, Wilson BA, Evans J, Watson P. Prospective Memory Functioning in People with and without Brain Injury. Journal of the International Neuropsychological Society 2002; 8 645–654.

[64] Mills V, Kixmiller JS, Gillespie A, Allard J, Flynn E, Bowman A, Brawn CM. The Correspondence between the Rivermead Behavioural Memory Test and Ecological Prospective Memory. Brain and Cognition 1997; 35 322-325.

[65] Makatura TJ, Lam C, Leahy BJ, Castillo M, Kalpakjian C. Standardized Memory Tests and the Appraisal of Everyday Memory. Brain Injury 1999; 13 355-367.

[66] Wilson BA, Clare L, Baddeley AD, Cockburn J, Watson P, Tate R. The Rivermead Behavioural Memory Test Extended Version (RBMT-E). Bury St Edmunds: Thames Valley Test Company; 1999.

[67] Wills P, Clare L, Shiel A, Wilson BA. Assessing Subtle Memory Impairments in the Everyday Memory Performance of Brain Injured People: Exploring the Potential of the Extended Rivermead Behavioural Memory Test. Brain Injury 2000; 14 693-704.

[68] Delprado J, Kinsella G, Ong B, Pike K, Ames D, Storey E, Saling M, Clare L, Mullaly E, Rand E. Clinical Measures of Prospective Memory in Amnesic Mild Cognitive Impairment. Journal of the International Neuropsychological Society; 2012; 18 295-304.

[69] Radford KA, Lah S, Say M, & Miller LA. Validation of a New Measure of Prospective Memory: The Royal Prince Alfred Prospective Memory Test. The Clinical Neuropsychology 2011; 25 127-140.

[70] Woods SP, Moran LM, Dawson MS, Carey CL, Grant I, The HIV Neurobehavioral Research Center (HNRC) Group. Psychometric characteristics of The Memory for Intentions Screening Test. Clinical Neuropsychology 2008; 22 864-878.

[71] Rendell PG, Henry JD. A Review of Virtual Week for Prospective Memory Assessment: Clinical Implications. Brain Impairment 2009; 10 14-22.

[72] Rose NS, Rendell PG, McDaniel MA, Abele I, Kliegel M. Age and Individual Differences in Prospective Memory During a "Virtual Week": The Role of Working Memory, Task Regularity and Cue Focality. Psychology and Aging 2010; 25 595-605.

[73] Henry JD, Rendell PG, Kliegel M, Altgassen M. Prospective Memory in Schizophrenia: Primary or Secondary Impairment? Schizophrenia Research 2007; 95 179–185.

[74] Mioni G, Stablum F, Rendell PG, Gamberini L, Bisiacchi PS. Test-retest Reliability of Virtual Week: A Task to Investigate Prospective Memory (in preparation).

[75] Sohlberg MM, White O, Evans E, Mateer C. Background and Initial Case Studies into the Effects of Prospective Memory Training. Brain Injury 1992a; 6 129-138.

[76] Sohlberg MM, White O, Evans E, Mateer C. An Investigation of the Effects of Prospective Memory Training. Brain Injury 1992; 6 139-154.

[77] Raskin SA, Sohlberg MM. The Efficacy of Prospective Memory Training in Two Adults with Brain Injury. Journal of Head Trauma Rehabilitation 1996; 11 32-51.

[78] Hannon R, Feliciano L, Messner A. Prospective Memory Retraining in Adults with Traumatic Brain Injury. Archives of Clinical Neuropsychology (abstract).

[79] Kixmiller JS. Evaluation of Prospective Memory Training for Individuals with Mild Alzheimer's Disease. Brain and Cognition 2002; 49 237–241.

[80] Chasteen AL, Park DC, Schwarz N. Implementation Intentions and Facilitation of Prospective Memory. Psychological Science 2001, 12, 457–461.

[81] Kaschel R, Della Salla S, Cantagallo A., Fahlböck A, Laaksonen R, Kazen M. Imagery Mnemonics for the Rehabilitation of Memory: A Randomised Group Controlled Trial. Neuropsychological Rehabilitation 2002; 12 127-153.

[82] Potvin MJ, Rouleau I, Sénéchal G, Giguère JF. Prospective Memory Rehabilitation Based on Visual Imagery Techniques. Neuropsychological Rehabilitation 2011; 21 899-924.

[83] Potvin MJ, Rouleau I, Audy J, Charbonneau S, Giguère, JF. Ecological Prospective Memory Assessment in Patients with Traumatic Brain Injury. Brain Injury 2011; 25 192-205.

[84] Fish J, Wilson BA, Manly T. The Assessment and Rehabilitation of Prospective Memory Problems in People with Neurological Disorders: A review. Neuropsychological rehabilitation 2010; 20 161-179.

[85] von Cramon, DY, Matthes-von Cramon GM, Mai N. Problem-solving Deficits in Brain Injured Patients: A Therapeutic Approach. Neuropsychological Rehabilitation 1991; 1 45-64.

[86] Hutchinson J, Marquardt TP. Functional Treatment Approaches to Memory Impairment Following Brain Injury. Topics in Language Disorders 1997; 18 45-57.

[87] Raymond MJ, Malia KB, Bewick KC, Bennett TL. A Comprehensive Approach to Memory Rehabilitation Following Brain Injury. The Journal of Cognitive Rehabilitation 1996; 14 18-23.

[88] Levine B, Robertson IH, Clare L, Carter G, Hong J, Wilson BA, et al. Rehabilitation of Executive Functioning: An Experimental Clinical Validation of Goal Management Training. Journal of the International Neuropsychological Society 2000; 6 299-312.

[89] Levine B, Schweizer T, O'Connor C, Turner G, Gillingham S, Stuss DT, Manly T, Robertson IH. Rehabilitation of Executive Functioning in Patients with Frontal Lobe Damage with Goal Management Training. Frontiers in Human Neuroscience 2011; 5-9.

[90] Bellezza FS. Mnemonic Devices: Classification, Characteristics, and Criteria. Review of Educational Research Summer 1981; 51 247-275.

[91] Smith RE, Persyn D, Butler P. Prospective Memory, Personality, and Working Memory: A Formal Modeling Approach. Zeischrift fur Psychologie 2011; 219 108-116.

[92] Thöne-Otto AIT, Walther K. Assessment and Treatment of Prospective Memory Disorders in Clinical Practice. In: Kliegel M, McDaniel MA, Einstein GO. (eds.) Prospective Memory: Cognitive, Neuroscience, Developmental, and Applied Perspective. Mahwah, NJ: Lawrence Erlbaum; 2008. p321-345.

[93] Sohlberg MM, Mateer CA. Training Use of Compensatory Memory Books: A Three Stage Behavioural Approach. Journal of Clinical and Experimental Neuropsychology 1989; 11 871–91.

[94] Schmitter-Edgecombe M, Fahy JF, Whelan JP, Long CJ. Memory Remediation After Severe Closed Head Injury: Notebook Training Versus Supportive Therapy. Journal of Consulting Clinical Psychology 1995; 484-489.

[95] Lynch WJ. You must Remember this: Assistive Devices for Memory Impairment. Journal of Head Trauma Rehabilitation 1995; 10 94–97.

[96] Burke JM. Danick JA, Bemis B, Durgin CJ. A Process Approach to Memory Book Training for Neurological Patients. Brain Injury 1994; 8 71-81.

[97] Ownsworth TL. McFarland K. Memory Remediation in Long-term Acquired Brain Injury: Two Approaches in Diary Training. Brain Injury 1999; 13 605–626.

[98] Wilson BA, Evans JJ., Emslie H et al. Evaluation of NeuroPage: A New Memory Aid. Journal of Neurology, Neurosurgery and Psychiatry 1997; 113-115.

[99] Wilson BA, Emslie HC, Quirk K, Evans JJ. Reducing Everyday Memory and Planning Problems by Means of a Paging System: A Randomised Control Crossover Study. Journal of Neurology, Neurosurgery, and Psychiatry 2001; 70 477-482.

[100] Evans JJ, Emslie H, Wilson BA. External Cueing System in the Rehabilitation of Executive Impairments of Action. Journal of the International Neuropsychology Society 1998; 4 399-408.

[101] Fish J, Manly T, Emslie H, Evans JJ, Wilson BA. Compensatory Strategies for Acquired Disorders of Memory and Planning: Differential Effects of a Paging System

for Patients with Brain Injury of Traumatic versus Cerebrovascular Aetiology. Journal of Neurology, Neurosurgery, and Psychiatry 2008; 79 930-935.

[102] Walther K, Schulze H, Thöne-Otto A. An Interactive Memory Aid Designed for Patients with Head Injury: Comparing MEMOS with Two Commercially Available Electronic Memory Aids. Poster at First Congress of the European Neuropsychological Societies in Modena, Italy, April 2004.

[103] Walther K, Thöne-Otto AIT. Long-term Usage of the Interactive Memory Aid System MEMOS. Poster presented at the Second International Conference on Prospective Memory, Zurich, Switzerland. Retrieved August 23, 2005.

[104] Thöne-Otto AIT, Walther K. Evaluation of MEMOS, an Interactive Memory Aid System for Brain Injured Patients: Personal Memory Assistant vs. Palm Organizer. Poster presented at the Second International Conference on Prospective Memory, Zurich, Switzerland. Retrieved August 23, 2005.

[105] Morrison K, Szymkowiak A, Gregor P. "Memojog–An Interactive Memory Aid Incorporating Mobile Based Technologies." Mobile Human-Computer Interaction-MobileHCI 2004. Springer Berlin Heidelberg, 2004. 481-485.

[106] Szymkowiak A, Morrison K, Gregor P, Shah P, Evans JJ, Wilson BA. A Memory Aid with Remote Communication Using Distributed Technology. Personal and Ubiquitous Computing 2005; 9 1-5.

[107] van den Broek MD, Downes J, Jhonson Z, Dayus B, Hilton N. Evaluation of an Electronic Memory Aid in the Neuropsychological Rehabilitation of Prospective Memory Deficits. Brain Injury 2000; 14 455-462.

[108] Yasuda K, Misu T, Beckman B, Watanabe O, Ozawa Y, Nakamura T. Use of an IC Recorder as a Voice Output Memory Aid for Patients with Prospective Memory Impairment. Neuropsychological Rehabilitation 2002; 12 155-166.

[109] Kim HJ, Burke DT, Dowds MM, Boone KA, Park GJ. Electronic Memory Aids for Outpatient Brain Injury. Brain Injury 2000; 14 187-196.

[110] Thöne-Otto AIT, Walther K. How to Design an Electronic Memory Aid for Brain Injured Patients: Considerations on the Basis of a Model of Prospective Memory. International Journal of Psychology 2003; 38 236-244.

[111] Pollack ME, Brown L, Colbry D, McCarthy CE, Orosz C, Peintner B, Ramakrishnan S, Tsamardinos I. Autominder: An Intelligent Cognitive Orthotic System for People with Memory Impairment. Robotics and Autonomous Systems 2003; 44 273-282.

[112] Mihailidis A, Fernie GR, Claghorn WL. The Development of a Computerized Cueing Device to Help People with Dementia to be More Independent. Technology and Disability 2000; 13 23-40.

[113] Caprani N, Greaney J, Porter N. A Review of Memory Aid Devices for an Ageing Population. PsychNology Journal 2006; 4 205-243.

[114] Shum D, Sweeper S, Murray R. Performance on Verbal Implicit and Explicit Memory Tasks Following Traumatic Brain Injury. The Journal of Head Trauma Rehabilitation 1996; 11 43-53.

6

Traumatic Brain Injury Rehabilitation

Wafa Al Yazeedi, Loganathan Venkatachalam,
Somaya Al Molawi and Fatma Al Kuwari

1. Introduction

Traumatic brain injury (TBI) is a leading cause of seizure, disorders, disability and death worldwide; regrettably, facilities for rehabilitation remain insufficient. One million Americans are treated and released from hospital emergency departments because of TBI [1]. The range of severity of TBI is broad, from concussion through to persistent vegetative states and categories are mild, moderate and severe (Box 1). In the European Union, brain injury accounts for one million hospital admissions per year. Many published studies support the notion that males are far more likely to incur a TBI than females. The highest rate of injury occurs between the ages of 15-24 years. Persons under the age of five or over the age of 75 are also at higher risk. Brain injury can cause many physical, cognitive and behavioural/emotional impairments, as well as common lifestyle consequences that may be either temporary or permanent (Box No 2). Brain injury may also result in seizure disorders. Brain injury is a public health concern that demands ongoing epidemiological study, increased efforts in the prevention of injuries occurring and research to advance medical options and therapeutic interventions.

Box No 1

Injury severity category	Initial Glasgow Coma Scale	Duration of post-traumatic amnesia
Mild	12-15	Less than 24 hours
Moderate	9-11	1-7 days
Severe	3-8	1-4 weeks

Box No 2
Consequences of traumatic brain injury

Neurological impairment (motor, sensory and autonomic)

- Motor function impairment – coordination, balance, walking, hand function, speech
- Sensory loss – taste, touch, hearing, vision, smell
- Sleep disturbance – insomnia, fatigue
- Medical complications – spasticity, post-traumatic epilepsy, hydrocephalus, heterotopic ossification
- Sexual dysfunction

Cognitive impairment

- Memory impairment, difficulty with new learning, attention and concentration; reduced speed and flexibility of thought processing; impaired problem-solving skills
- Problems in planning, organizing, and making decisions
- Language problems – dysphasia, problems finding words and impaired reading and writing skills
- Impaired judgment and safety awareness

Personality and behavioural changes

- Impaired social and coping skills, reduced self-esteem
- Altered emotional control; poor frustration tolerance and anger management; denial, and self-centeredness
- Reduced insight, disinhibition, impulsivity
- Psychiatric disorders – anxiety, depression, post-traumatic stress disorder, psychosis
- Apathy, a motivational state

Common lifestyle consequences

- Unemployment and financial hardship
- Inadequate academic achievement
- Lack of transportation alternatives
- Inadequate recreational opportunities
- Difficulties in maintaining interpersonal relationships, marital breakdown
- Loss of pre-injury roles; loss of independence

2. Body

The recovery process following TBI is a slow process that might take months or years, rather than weeks. Six months following an injury yields a clearer picture of what effect the injury has had, but waiting roughly a year after the accident before making any important decisions regarding the future is considered advisable. Physical recovery will take approximately a year, but psychological recovery might take considerably longer. Factors that may affect the rate of a person's recovery include injury type, severity, location of the individual's brain injury, age (younger patients tend to have better outcomes), pre-injury health, pre-injury personality, intelligence and lifestyle, social support from family and friends and other factors like alcohol or drug abuse. Depending on the individual's physical abilities and potential, a rehabilitation programme will be initiated accordingly.

The effectiveness of a comprehensive multidisciplinary rehabilitation team (Box No.3) is increased when compared to natural recovery following brain injury. The importance of recognizing the vegetative state and its management is emphasized. Finally, the important, but often neglected area of employment rehabilitation is covered. We plan to explain the rehabilitation process starting from the day of the accident with the aim of recovering from the posttraumatic brain injury sequlae and achieving reintegration into the community.

Box No 3 Rehabilitation team

- Patient and patient's family
- Rehabilitation medicine physician
- Rehabilitation nurse
- Allied health professionals: physiotherapist, occupational therapist, speech pathologist, social worker and orthotics
- Neuropsychologist, clinical psychologist
- Vocational rehabilitation services and counsellors
- Other medical specialties: neurosurgery, orthopaedic surgery and urologist

The iterative process of consultation yielded consensus definitions for each component of the rehabilitation service pathway for head-injured adults (Table 1). This chapter describes not only brain injury due to road traffic accident or fall from a great height but also brain injury in war victims. Modern rehabilitation practices are based around the concepts of impairment, disability and handicap, as outlined by the World Health Organization (WHO) in 1980. Recently, however, the WHO has redefined these concepts.

The modern terminology that will be introduced in the near future still encompasses the term 'impairment', but now replaces 'disability' with 'activity' and 'handicap' with 'participation'. This is not simply a sign of political correctness, but serves to emphasize the positive aspects of disability rather than its negative connotations. The rehabilitation approaches consist of three basic types; 1) reducing the disability; 2) acquiring new skills and their application for reducing the impact of disability; 3) alteration of the environment in physical and social contexts, so that existing disability will carry as little participation as possible. For example, a young male individual had a traumatic brain injury and recovery with residual hemiplegia with spasticity and urinary incontinence. A specific programme tailored to this individual's needs was offered during brain injury rehabilitation management process. (Box No. 4).

Title and description	Sites	Description of rehabilitation input
Minor HI: education – medically stable, requiring 24-48 hrs. observation prior to community rehabilitation, with low probability of acute neurological deterioration	Acute A&E observation ward	Assessment and observation – education, emotional and social support. Planned discharge home or moves to code 30 at 48 h
Supportive rehab – medically unstable, requiring neurosurgical or clinical care	Acute hospital	Identifying and addressing early rehab goals before medically stable and transfer of care to rehab team.
Supportive rehab – medically unstable, not requiring neurosurgical or critical care	Acute hospital	Identifying and addressing early rehab goals before medically stable and transfer of care to rehab team.
Rapid access rehab – medically stable, not (necessarily) able to actively participate due to amnesia, confusion, rejection, low response or awareness	Acute hospital	Needs inpatient care due to physical dependency and requires continuous clinical assessment to facilitate optimal timing for rehab input and detect clinical deterioration. Immediate early rehab delivered and judgment made on timing/ appropriateness of referral to next rehab sector.
Active participation inpatient rehab – medically stable, able to actively participate with and benefit from therapy	Acute or community hospital	Needs inpatient care due to physical dependency, or need for specialist therapy equipment, safe environment, supervision or intensity of therapy, which cannot be provided in community
Behavioural rehab – medically stable, but with prolonged confusion, amnesia or behavioural difficulties, requiring specialist behavioural management, intensive supervision and secure environment	Specialist inpatient unit	Specialist behavioural management, including high staff/patient ratio to ensure intensive supervision and secure environment; access to neuropsychology and neuropsychiatry.
Slow-stream rehab – medically stable, but with low awareness or response persisting beyond, e.g., three weeks after sedation; withdrawn and medically stable. Able to benefit from medical and physical therapy to prevent complications and support recovery	Community hospital or specialist inpatient unit	Assessment/active rehabilitation phase, which needs to be distinguished from long-term care, although planning of care an increasingly important aim after, e.g., six months. Patients may go to active participation unit if sufficient improvement occurs.

Title and description	Sites	Description of rehabilitation input
Community rehab – medically stable, able to actively participate with and benefit from, therapy. Will include spectrum of initial severity of injury with a small minority derived from code 05 category.	Domiciliary or day hospital	Interdisciplinary coordinated management therapy aimed at community reintegration/inclusion by enhancing independence and assisting return to work/education. In collaboration with social services, voluntary and statutory services. Includes treatment of patients in residential care or with live-in carers.
Intensive cognitive rehab – medically stable, independently mobile, primarily cognitive impairments likely to benefit from intensive neuropsychological therapy.	Domiciliary or day hospital	Aiming to return to work, studies or independent community life.
Specialist vocational rehab – medically stable, living in community, aiming to enter/ return to employment.	Domiciliary or residential	Aiming for return to work, where this is influenced by physical or cognitive problems, or needs residential placement.
Maintenance – medically stable but permanently disabled.	Domiciliary, residential or nursing home, respite unit	Prevent deterioration of physical, emotional and behavioural conditions, and long-term management of seating, pressure, spasticity, etc.
Social, patient and carer support – carer support for initial injury, patient support when able to communicate.	All sites	Developing social skills, stamina, confidence, attention and leisure pursuits, sorting out benefits, day supervision and respite care. Specific attention paid to: community involvement and integration (further education, etc.); personal social development; structured daytime activity; family support and outreach.

HI = head injury; rehab = rehabilitation;
A&E = accident and emergency

Table 1. Classification of head injury recovery and actual/potential rehabilitation services (adult).

Box No 4 Specific programme offered during brain injury rehabilitation

Post-traumatic amnesia assessment
Management of post-traumatic agitation
Neuropharmacological management
Cognitive rehabilitation therapy
Coma emergence and rehabilitation of minimally responsive states
Spasticity management including motor point/nerve blocks and Botulinum toxin therapy
Casting, splinting, orthotics, contracture management
Pain management services for cervicogenic headaches, trigger point injections
Balance and vestibular assessment and rehabilitation
Cognitive and behavioural assessment and remediation
Comprehensive dysphagia and speech therapy services
Assistive technology using augmentative and alternative communication
Rehabilitation nursing education
Intrathecal Baclofen pump therapy
Brain injury discharge advice and family education
Social support: discharge planning, caregiver training

Brain injury rehabilitation occurs in the following settings:

- **Inpatient rehabilitation:** This involves intensive specialist rehabilitation for people who are not yet ready to return home after discharge from hospital. Neurological rehabilitation centres provide an ideal setting for further treatment, where a structured rehabilitation programme is in place throughout the day.
- **Outpatient rehabilitation:** Some people may be well enough to return home and receive further treatment as an outpatient, either at a local hospital or at a separate rehabilitation centre.
- **Community rehabilitation:** Following an inpatient rehabilitation stay, some people may be transferred to a residential transitional living unit. Here people can develop their independent living skills so that they may be able to live in a place of their own. Others will go straight back to their homes, with a community rehabilitation team or outreach team helping them to make further progress; this may involve therapists working with the person in their home or community environment [2].

The main basic approach to treatment in the above example was to reduce disability through appropriate medication with which to control spasticity and for applying new skills of physiotherapy and occupational therapy to improve the individual's functional activity of gait training. This was done through means of ambulation in an indoor environment, with physical aid and wheelchair aid for long distances and, by using an adaptive device to facilitate feeding and other self-care activities. Additionally, adapted fittings to bathrooms and kitchens can be installed. Liaising with the injured individual's employer and having a dialogue for initiating his return to work in a part-time capacity or having downtime between working hours to reduce fatigue can also be instigated. The involvement of his family is also important to make them more accepting of his condition and for effecting the necessary adjustments to their own lifestyles.

The basic nature of rehabilitation is to work with the disabled person and family in partnership. The interdisciplinary rehabilitation team should provide accurate information and advice, explain the prognosis and natural history and work with the individual to establish realistic goals within an appropriate social environment. Whatever approaches implemented, setting a realistic goal is key to a good quality rehabilitation programme. For example, the long-term goal of independent walking requires a number of short stages to be implemented, such as sitting, balance training without support, standing balance without support, walking in parallel bar, walking with a person's assistance, walking with aids and lastly independent walking.

The rehabilitation team and disabled person should know what the goal is and when this goal has been achieved. Thus, valid and reliable outcome measures are very important for supporting the rehabilitation process. The most common measures used in the UK is the Barthel Index, but functional independence measures are also very common worldwide. Physiotherapy and occupational therapy using a 10-meter walking test for improvement of walking and a nine hole pick peg test for improvement of hand function, respectively, are also used. There are many other tools for measuring variable functional independence measure (FIM) cognitive and motor functions, the Glasgow coma scale (GCS), Rancho Los Amigos levels of cognitive functioning scale (RLA), disability rating scale and the Coma Recovery Scale-(Revised). It is important to highlight that the use of valid and reliable outcome measures is important in order to observe goals, assess progress and adjust the rehabilitation programme. The author has published articles related to the above-mentioned variables influencing and predicting functional outcomes after TBI [3].

For example, in her study [3], she pointed out that there was positive correlation of functional independence measure on discharge (FIMd) and RLA (Figure1). The researcher postulated GCS as a predictor of functional outcome and showed in her result positive correlation of GCS and FIM cognitive. Rehabilitation should begin as early as possible (even at the level of acute care) (Figure 3) [4]. It is common for individuals to ultimately be transferred to a rehabilitation unit when avoidable complications are already present. Unfortunately, muscle contractures, pressure sores and unnecessary aggressive behaviour are atypical during stay in rehabilitation unit . If the rehabilitation team can be involved in the early stage of acute care setting, perhaps even on the intensive care unit, it is more likely that such complications can be avoided. Studies provide evidence that undertaking rehabilitation within the first days of evolution improved cognition, perception and motor recovery of brain-damaged patients, and led to shorter lengths of stay (LOS) in rehabilitation units [5,6,8].

An early intervention rehabilitation team (EIRT) has been initiated by the author at the level of trauma or surgical intensive care units in Hamad General Hospital (HGH), Qatar. A rehabilitation programme focusing on cognitive stimulation and prevention of musculoskeletal complications of contractures has been offered. Pressure ulcers and aggressive behaviour has been limited by providing appropriate orthoses, frequent positioning, psychotropic

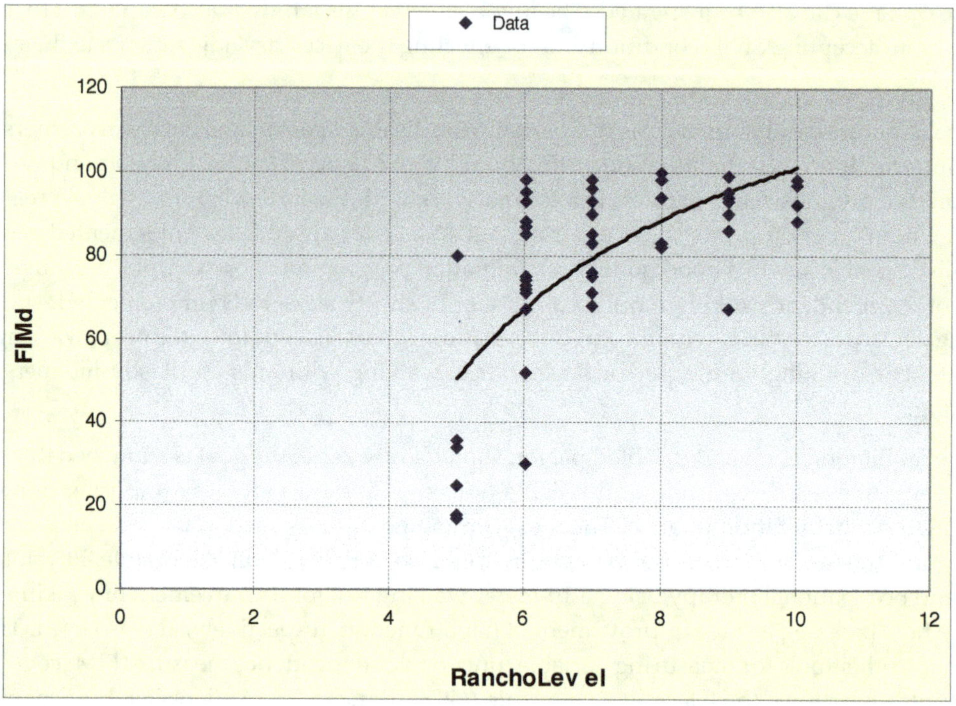

Figure 1. Correlation of FIM d and Rancho

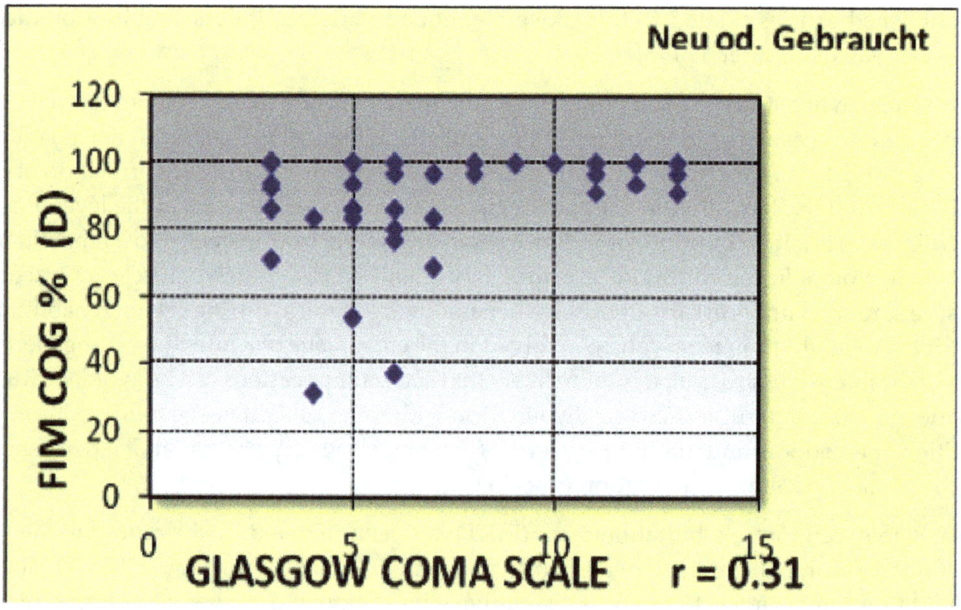

Figure 2. Correlation of FIIM cog D and GCS

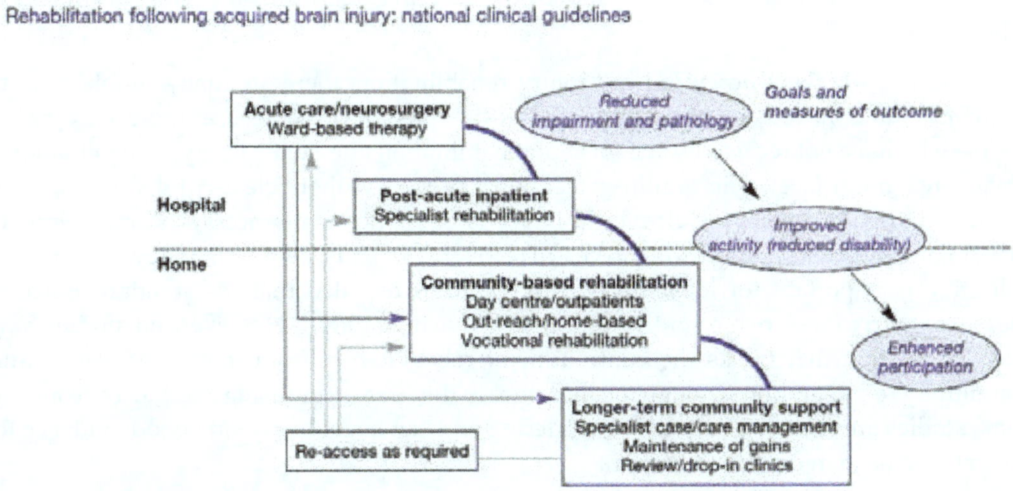

Figure 3. Rehabilitation following brain injury

medication or psychiatric consultation, while transfer to rehabilitation units as early as possible have resulted in shorter LOS in acute care units in HGH and have shown improvement in physical and mental impediments. This chapter will classify and promptly summarize the rehabilitation process of the slow stream rehabilitation programme, the active participation programme and long-term rehabilitation programme, the community based rehabilitation programme and returning to the community or work.

Most rehabilitation units will admit individuals a week or so after injury once they are medically stable. Generally, individuals have an average stay of about three months. However, longer-term rehabilitation is important if short-term gains are not to be lost. Outpatient rehabilitation should continue at least until physical recovery has plateaued. Recovery of cognitive and intellectual problems can take longer than physical problems and it is often such psychological difficulties that cause most handicaps and distress to the injured individual's family. This problem must be compensated by establishing a long-term facility that must be allowed to give the injured individual rehabilitation and medical service for at least one year. Following on, another important step in the rehabilitation setting is that the rehabilitation team will need to clearly establish links with social services as well as other relevant professionals, such as employment rehabilitation experts.

The rehabilitation team recommends developing close links with the established community rehabilitation centre (CRC) in the state or province, with CRC in turn having links with the regional rehabilitation unit or rehabilitation hospital. Most post-acute rehabilitation is conducted in the hospital setting or at the regional rehabilitation unit, before individuals are discharged back into the community. At this point, the community team becomes involved and is able to deliver ongoing physical and psychological rehabilitation through a multidisciplinary team, based in a peripheral hospital, as well as being able to deliver services within the home. The author is working on establishing CRC in Qatar under the national strategy of rehabilitation.

When addressing the efficacy of head injury rehabilitation, there are many problems to be overcome. Randomized and blind study is almost impossible to achieve, as there are very few people who have not received some form of rehabilitation after acute injury. Rehabilitation is obviously a multi-faceted and multi-professional process without clear-cut definitions. M.P. Barnes reported rehabilitation after head injury to be a long-term process with much impairment taking two years or more to achieve full recovery [5]. Thus, long-term follow-up and data collection is important for ideal study. More studies revealed that the standard outcome measures help to improve cognitive and motor functional level. However, no studies have been found that that tracks the continuum of rehabilitation from intensive care to final community re-integration. Though the literature in this area is confusing and hard to come by, some studies are nonetheless worth considering and can begin to provide good evidence for the value of head injury rehabilitation.

McKay and colleagues [6] compared matched groups of severe head injury individuals who did or did not receive formal rehabilitation during their acute trauma centre admission. All TBI rehabilitation individuals received physical, occupational or speech therapy, whereas in the non-rehabilitation group, only a very small minority did. In the rehabilitation group, therapy was also initiated quickly, whereas in the other group, therapy started about three weeks after the acute episode. Overall coma length, rehabilitation stay and cognitive functioning showed a significant benefit in the rehabilitation group. An interesting study by Blackerby [7] demonstrated that an increase in intensity of rehabilitation for five to eight hours a day produced a reduction in the average length of stay.

An important study by Cope and Hall [8] compared 34 head injured people who had either been referred 'early' or 'late' to a comprehensive inpatient rehabilitation programme. The early group had significant reduction in length of stay both in the acute care unit and in the rehabilitation unit. Many studies indicate better functional outcomes following a formal rehabilitation programme. For example, Aronow [9] produced one of the very few case controlled studies, where patients from an inpatient head injury programme were matched with similar patients in a neuro-trauma programme who received no formal rehabilitation. On the outcome scale used (not widely published in terms of validity and reliability), the rehabilitation group had a significantly better outcome than the non-rehabilitation group. Some published studies are supportive of the view that comprehensive TBI rehabilitation programmes produce benefits over and above standard care and spontaneous recovery.

Barnes [5] indicated in his study that early intervention by a specialist head injury service significantly reduced social morbidity and severity of post-concussion symptoms at six months. On referral to this study and her own experience, the author introduced an Early Intervention Rehabilitation Team at the level of intensive care and acute care units in Hamad General Hospital, Qatar, which resulted in reducing the length of stay in acute settings and preventing complications. It is clear that much work still needs to be done in this field. Nonetheless, valuable studies strongly support a comprehensive TBI rehabilitation programme, which produced worthwhile benefits over and above standard care and spontaneous recovery. The rehabilitation team of rehabilitation unit's focus is on a comprehensive assessment for TBI-related neurological and functional impairments and the development of an individualized specific programme based on functional goals and serial monitoring of outcomes (Box No. 4).

What follows will describe the process of a specialized rehabilitation programme for specific rehabilitation problems after traumatic brain injury. Physical disability is divided into three types – mild, moderate and severe. The severe type of disability consists of the following factors of muscle contracture: spasticity, heterotopic ossification and communication problems; these will be discussed in detail.

Severe physical disability. This occurred after severe head injury; relatively few people have had severe physical disability in the long-term. The longer-term problems of traumatic brain injury tend to include cognitive, intellectual, behavioural and emotional difficulties rather than physical problems. This has been confirmed by a number of studies [10, 11]. Spasticity can be particularly problematic after TBI and if not treated persistently, can often lead to muscle contracture and a functionally useless limb. Passive stretching in the acute phase is important, as may be the use of orthoses or even serial splinting and casts in order to prevent such contracture. Whilst there are a number of modern oral anti-spastic agents (e.g., Baclofen, Dantrium and Tizandine), troublesome spasticity tends to be focal and thus better treated by a local modality. Botulinum toxin has recently been introduced as a potent muscle relaxant and a number of studies have now demonstrated efficacy in the management of spasticity [12, 13]. Fortunately, the effects of Botolinium toxin wore off after three months and did not impair long-term recovery, which used to be the case in other focal techniques such as phenol and alcohol nerve blocks.

Heterotopic ossification. Neurogenic heterotopic ossification (HO) is characterized by the formation of bone in soft tissues following traumatic injury to the central nervous system, especially around large joints (CNS). The hip is the most commonly involved joint, but elbow and knee is also common in both spinal cord injury and traumatic brain injury (Figure 4]. HO was first described in 1883 by Reidel and in 1918, Dejerne and Ceillier reported that HO frequently occurred among soldiers who had experienced spinal cord trauma as combatants in World War I [14]. The development of HO is extra-articular and occurs outside the joint capsule. Bone forms in the connective tissue between the muscle planes and not within the muscle itself. The new bone can be contiguous with the skeleton but generally does not involve the periosteum. Mature HO shows cancellous bone and mature lamellar bone blood vessels and bone marrow with a minor amount of haematopoiesis.

Alkaline phosphatase has been recommended as a useful screening tool for HO [15]. Alkaline phosphatase levels become abnormal approximately two weeks after injury. In the typical case of HO, the alkaline phosphatase levels reached approximately 3.5 times the normal value 10 weeks after the inciting trauma, before returning to normal at approximately 18 weeks. The literature suggests reasonably good results for primary and secondary prevention with Non-Steroidal Anti Inflammatory Drugs, bisphosphonates and radiation. Surgical excision and joint release can provide improvements for many patients, but have varied results and often depend

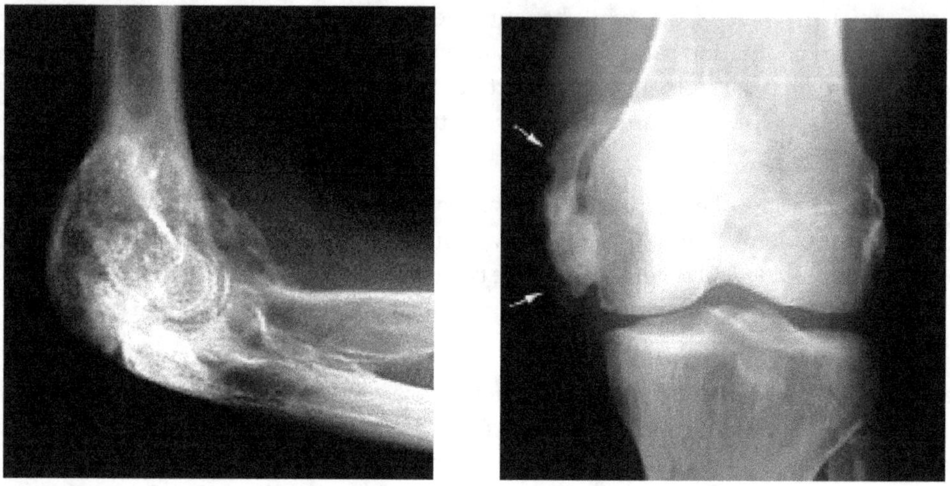

Lateral radiograph demonstrate the anterior and posterior ossification.

Anteroposterior radiograph of the left knee in a traumatic brain injury. Mature heterotopic ossification surrounds the medial femoral condyle, with a solid Peripheral cortex (arrows).

Figure 4. X Ray of heterotrophic ossification

on the degree of CNS injury. The role of physical therapy in patients with HO is somewhat controversial. There are those who believe that aggressive ROM may lead to increase bone formation. Most, however, agree that physical therapy preserves movement, leading to better function and prevention of ankylosis. Physiotherapy typically involves active and passive ROM, gentle terminal stretching and resisted ROM exercise [16].

Nutrition is a particular problem. The reasons are two-fold – an increased catabolic rate immediately after brain trauma compounded by the common occurrence of swallowing difficulties. If maintenance of good nutritional status is difficult, a judgment that should preferably be made only after adequate dietary advice, then nasogastric feeding can be used in the very short-term. However, if adequate nutrition cannot be maintained within a few days following iTBI, then a fine bore percutaneous endoscopic gastrostomy (PEG) tube should be inserted. This is a relatively simple and straightforward procedure with few complications. If nutrition is not maintained, it can have serious consequences for wound healing and an increased risk of pressure sores.

Pressure sores remained, unfortunately; they are rather common and are nearly always avoidable. Rigid adherence to regular turning regimens, as well as the use of appropriate pressure relieving mattresses and appropriate lifting and handling techniques should help to limit the occurrence of pressure sores. However, risks could be increased by poor nutrition as well as by other factors such as urinary or faecal incontinence. Regrettably, once sores are present, they can be extremely time consuming in terms of healing and often require surgical intervention to excise the ulcer, bony prominence or affected bone and to resurface the defect by skin grafting or other techniques such as a myocutaneous flap [17].

Urinary continence can also be problematic after head injury. Whilst in the short-term, indwelling catheterization can be used, in the long-term this is a most undesirable solution. Urodynamic study regarding the exact nature of the underlying detrusor and/or sphincter problem, combined with appropriate pharmacology, often relieves the situation. However, if impairment of bladder emptying remains, the technique of clean and intermittent self-catheterization can be invaluable - performed either by the patient or sometimes by an appropriate carer [18].

Communication problems can be troublesome after brain injury. Thus, an assessment by a speech therapist is important and various speech and language interventions can obviously be of benefit, particularly for dysarthria and dysphagia. However, those with very severe disablement are often unable to communicate orally and need to revert to an appropriate communication aid. These can vary from simple pointing boards to more complex pre-programmed artificial voice communicators. There are a number of Communication Aid centres who have particular expertise in this field and in the forms of assistive technology, which is becoming increasingly important in reducing disability and participation in those with severe physical problems.

Medical rehabilitation Problems. Urinary tract infections, pulmonary complications and derangement in electrolytes and liver function are common in 60% to 70% of acute TBI cases and may prolong acute hospital stay. Seizures may be reported in 20% of those with a severe TBI. Common neuroendocrine disorders include growth hormone deficiency, syndrome of inappropriate secretion of antidiuretic hormone, diabetes insipidus, secondary amenorrhoea, galactorrhoea and gynaecomastia. The common hormonal insufficiencies were found to be from the pituitary (hypothalamus) region. (Figure 5).In hypo pituitarism, the anterior pituitary insufficiency had higher incidence [19] rather than the posterior. There is an increasing amount of evidence that suggest that post TBI hormonal deficiency syndrome affects many people who have sustained TBI and mild TBI, and research is now beginning to show that replacement of deficient hormones can lead to significant improvements.

To evaluate patients, a full hormonal assessment via a spot or 24-hour urine should be performed to test for hormones and their metabolites (serum testing). It is also important to test for neuroendocrine markers. This can be done with either spot or 24-hour urine testing. It is important to use a laboratory with neurotransmitter capability. To treat hormonal insufficiencies after TBI, early hormonal supplementation should be considered to minimize the physical and psychological sequelae. Hormonal assessments can be done at three-month intervals from the date of injury, or more frequently, based on treatment [20].

Cranial nerve injury in TBI. TBI-complicated cranial nerve injury is subject to a high incidence rate, a high mortality rate and a high disability rate. One study explained that the extent of

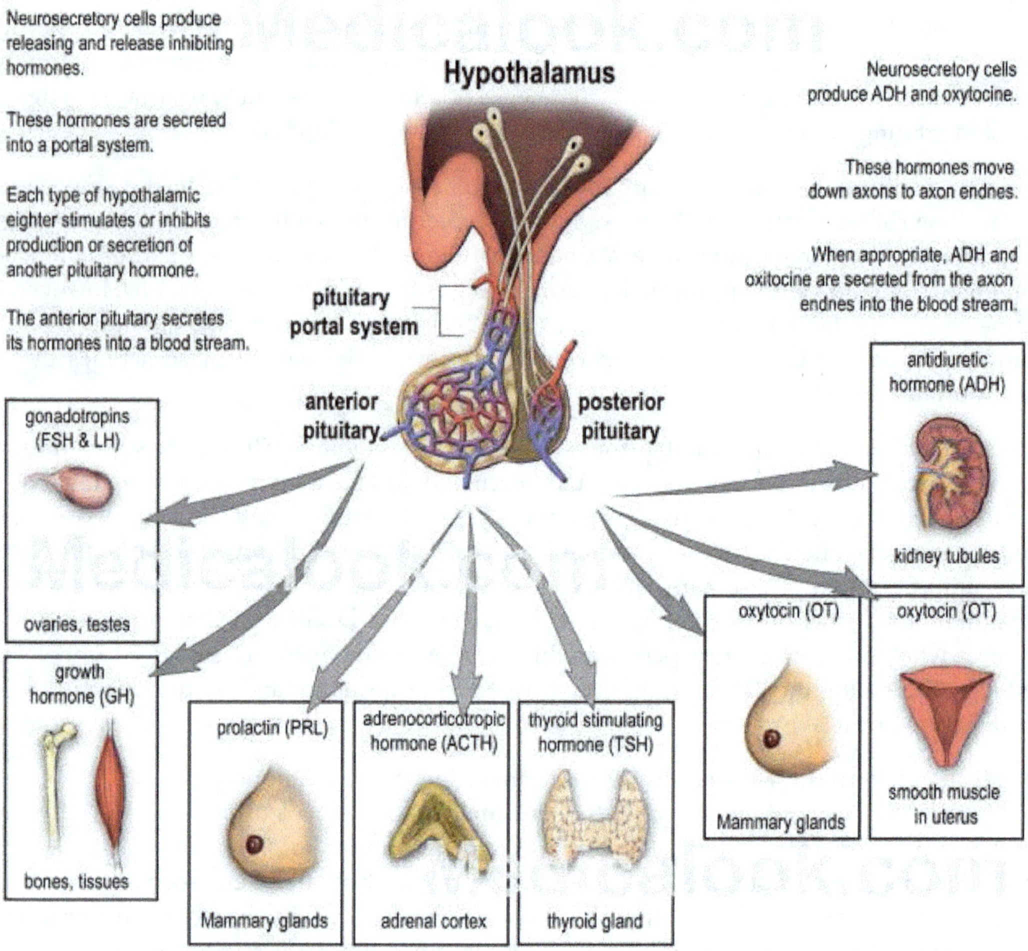

Figure 5. Pituitary hormone15

nerve injury varied and involved the olfactory nerve (66 cases), optic nerve (78 cases), oculomotor nerve (56 cases), trochlear nerve (eight cases), trigeminal nerve (four cases), abducent nerve (12 cases), facial nerve (48 cases), acoustic nerve [10 cases), glossopharyngeal nerve (eight cases), vagus nerve (six cases), accessory nerve (10 cases) and hypoglossal nerve (six cases) [21].

Environmental control equipment provides a means of controlling simple electrical equipment around the house such as the ability to turn the television, lights and other equipment on and off, and the ability to answer the telephone, open the door and adjust the bed. Such independence can be very important to an individual who is otherwise entirely dependent on a third party. The application of relatively simple technology can sometimes make a dramatic difference to level of independence. For example, a number of devices are available that enable a severely disabled person to drive a motor vehicle. These can vary from simple hand controls (switches) to more complex joystick steering with voice controlled accessory equipment (Figure 6]. Overall, those with severe physical disabilities need the support of a rehabilitation expert, which in turn will have access to the necessary wide range of multidisciplinary expertise, facilities and equipment.

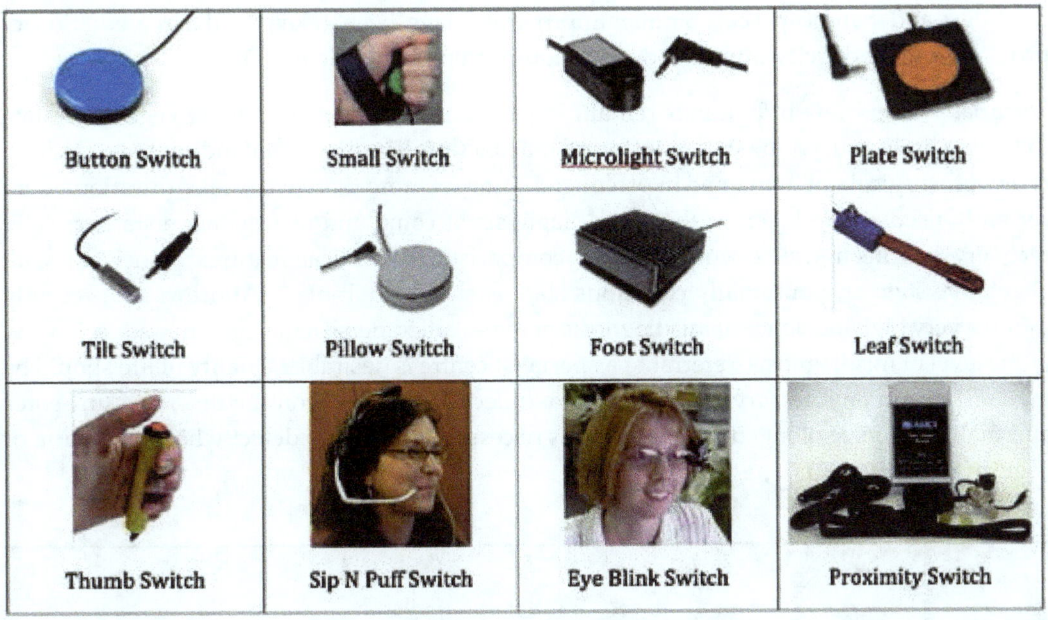

Figure 6. Adaptive devises

Following head injury, a variety of important cognitive impairments can be observed. The commonest are those associated with attention deficits, problems with concentration, memory and perception, information processing speed and problem solving. Normal recovery of neuropsychological difficulties can take place over a prolonged period of time and certainly up to two years post-injury. Obviously, this can be a complex set of impairments and consequent disabilities need to be assessed by a clinical neuropsychologist. It is somewhat controversial whether neuropsychological intervention can actually promote recovery, but there is little doubt that coping strategies can be designed that will effectively reduce disability. There have been very few randomized trials in this field and such trials are likely inappropriate when one is dealing with so many variables. The use of well-designed single case studies is a methodology that is probably best pursued in this area. Most work has been conducted in the field of memory disorders [21].

Rehabilitation can be divided into those techniques involving internal strategies and those dependent on external resources. Internal strategies, for example, can involve the use of various mnemonic techniques such as the use of imagery, methods to organize information in particular sequences (e.g., the PQRST technique), as well as other techniques that involve the use of acronyms, rhymes and systematic queuing. An alternative or even coexistent strategy is to devise interventions for reducing the handicapping effects of amnesic problems. Some may appear simple and obvious, such as planned use of a personal organizer with electronic alarm systems, colour codes around the house or a rigid use of lists, memos and diaries.

However, there is no doubt that such techniques, whilst not influencing memory impairment, can certainly reduce the effects of such impairment and have positive benefits in terms of disability and handicap [22]. Similar approaches have been taken to the remediation of problem solving deficits, attention deficits and perceptual problems [23]

Fortunately, very few individuals remain in prolonged coma or prolonged vegetative state following brain injury. One study [24] found that 0.6% of all brain-injured individuals admitted to a neurosurgical unit remained in prolonged coma (of more than two weeks' duration). Care certainly needs to be taken in the early diagnosis of coma and/or vegetative state, as later recovery has been well documented. A comparison of clinical features associated with vegetative state and minimally conscious state is shown in Table 2. Andrews [25] recently found a very high incidence of misdiagnosis in the so called persistent vegetative state. In view of the level of misdiagnosis, referral to a specialist centre is desirable. Quality of life should be maximized and unnecessary complications avoided, particularly contractures, pressure sores and malnutrition. Prolonged reassessment is necessary in order to detect when some form of cognitive recovery is taking place.

Condition	Consciousness	Sleep /wake	Motor Function	Auditory Function	Visual Fixation	Communication	Emotion
Coma	None	Absent	Reflex and postural responses only	None	None	None	None
Vegetative State	None	Present	Postures or withdraws from noxious stimuli Occasional non purposeful movement	Startle Brief orienting to sound	Startle Brief visual Fixation	None	None Reflexive crying or smiling
Minimally Conscious State	Partial	Present	Localizes noxious stimuli Reaches for objects Holds or touches objects in a manner that accommodate size and shape Automatic movements (e.g., scratching)	Localizes sound location Inconsistent command following	Sustained visual fixation Sustained inconsistent but intelligible verbalization or gesture	Contingent vocalization Inconsistent but intelligible verbalization or gesture	Contingent smiling or crying

Table 2. Comparison of clinical features associated with vegetative state and minimally conscious state

Regrettably, there are a number of case studies that illustrate instances of cognitive recovery when attendants, staff and relatives believed the individual to have still been in a vegetative state. This stage is critical and requires patience and more recovery time. The rehabilitation team should dedicate their specialized skills and techniques to get away from their conditions. The rehabilitation team can apply the appropriate evidence-based pharmacological and non-pharmacological methods. For example, to recover from awareness medication like amantadine, sensory modality assessment and rehabilitation technique (SMART) and coma recovery programme–revised (CRS-R) can be utilized. The rehabilitation team might consider that the involvement of a psychologist or specialized neuropsychology is preferable to the involvement of a psychiatrist.

Many TBI patients are required to undergo appropriate counselling and psychotherapy. Many people with TBI develop behavioural problems in the short-term, particularly whilst emerging from a coma or during the phase of posttraumatic amnesia. A few individuals develop persistent and severe behavioural problems and can be a source of extreme disruption on the acute or rehabilitation ward, and certainly a source of major difficulty for the family. Eames and colleagues [26] stated that the application of behavioural management techniques could be effective in ameliorating difficult behaviour and in improving functional independence levels, as well as improving compliance with physical therapy even years after injury. Staff at a rehabilitation unit should have a degree of expertise in the management of behavioural problems; nevertheless, those with severe and persistent difficulties should be referred to appropriate psychiatric or specialized behavioural units.

The use of drug therapy in the management of such behaviours is best avoided, but in practise, this is unavoidable. Certainly, the use of sedative anxiolytics or psychotropic medication is generally unhelpful and may even worsen behaviour. Occasionally such intervention is essential, because of the proximity of vulnerable people of TBI or because of extreme pressure on staff time and resources. There is very little good quality literature on this subject; however, some studies have indicated an improvement in aggression and episodic dyscontrol by use of serotoninergic anti-depressant Trazodone [27] or the anti-convulsant Carbamazepine [28]. Other authors advocate the use of lithium or beta-blockade with Metoprolol [29]. If TBI patients became severely agitated, some advocate the use of Buspirone, which is chemically distinct from other anxiolytics.

For negative behaviours, some improvement is occasionally noticed following the use of dopamine agonists. A few authors continue to use stimulants such as Dexamethetamine or methyl phenidate, but such medication should be used with caution and only by those with some experience in the field. Other behavioural problems can be less troublesome but nonetheless give rise to marital stress, social isolation and often unemployment. Such problems can include egocentricity, poor judgment, lack of initiation, reduced achievement drive, lethargy, disinterest, lack of depth of feeling, irritability, aggressiveness, reduced tact and increase or decrease in sexual interest. Alongside these problems, both in the patient and the carer, can be the presence of associated mood disorders, particularly depressive illness and anxiety [30]. It is essential for the multidisciplinary team to recognize such problems and treat them appropriately.

There is no evidence that depressive illness responds less well in the context of acquired brain injury than in the context of endogenous depression. Thus, standard approaches, either psychological or pharmacological, should be used as aggressively as needed. Even if some of these problems are not remediable, they should be recognized and explained to the injured individual's family and colleagues. The immediate family will often benefit from counselling and supportive psychotherapy. Nowadays, before initiating pharmacotherapy or psychotherapy, patients should be screened to rule out any history of constipation, retention urine, infection, fracture and musculoskeletal illness. Levy et al. [31] stated that numerous studies have examined the use of medications in the treatment of agitation of post-TBI patients, but that there is limited evidence to help guide the clinician. Thus, the prescription of pharmacotherapy must be closely monitored and a multidisciplinary approach combining both pharmacological and non-pharmacological interventions may be necessary.

In the US, a number of studies have shown the efficacy of an employment support scheme. In such schemes, a trained rehabilitator accompanies the individual back to work and further rehabilitation will take place in the workplace, allowing an opportunity for specific goal orientated re-entry as well as an opportunity for education of the employer and work colleagues. It is regrettable that many rehabilitation facilities feel their job to be completed after the patient has been discharged back home, perhaps having received a follow up after the passing of a few months.

The best long-term outcome in those of working age is to return to their pre-accident employment situation. In many countries, little attention is paid to employment rehabilitation. Such rehabilitation rarely take place at all, or if it does, is the responsibility of a completely separate government department that likely lacks the necessary expertise for the management of those with brain injury problems. Following TBI recovery, rushing back to work too quickly is not advisable. If this happens, symptoms that were on the mend might flare up once more. A period of retraining may be required and adaptations to the workplace may be needed.

If an individual can return to work it will serve as a boost to their self-esteem and independence, particularly from a financial point of view. Such re-employment will clearly be of overall benefit to the state in terms of reduced benefits and may even enable the carer to return to employment as well. Wehman and colleagues [32] have clearly demonstrated the effectiveness of the supported employment programme. In his study forty-one [41] head injured people were included in the initial study;Only 36% of referred clients had achieved any competitive postinjury employment, compared with 91% of the same group who were competitively employed before injury. A job retention rate of 71% was reported, with most jobs in warehouse, clerical, and service-related occupations. This group presented a mean period of seven years from injury and thus the chances of spontaneous recovery were minimal.

The improved integration of employment professionals with health and social service professionals must be a priority in the future. At present, simulator-based education programmes have a strong scientific basis. Virtual reality driving simulation rehabilitation training (Figures 7 and 8) has shown promising results with respect to retraining driving performance and behaviour among military personnel recovering from TBI [33]. This is a new development in advanced driving solutions for disabled individuals after TBI or stroke and spinal cord injury, employing a fully immersive car driving simulator ideally suited for driver assessment and rehabilitation application.

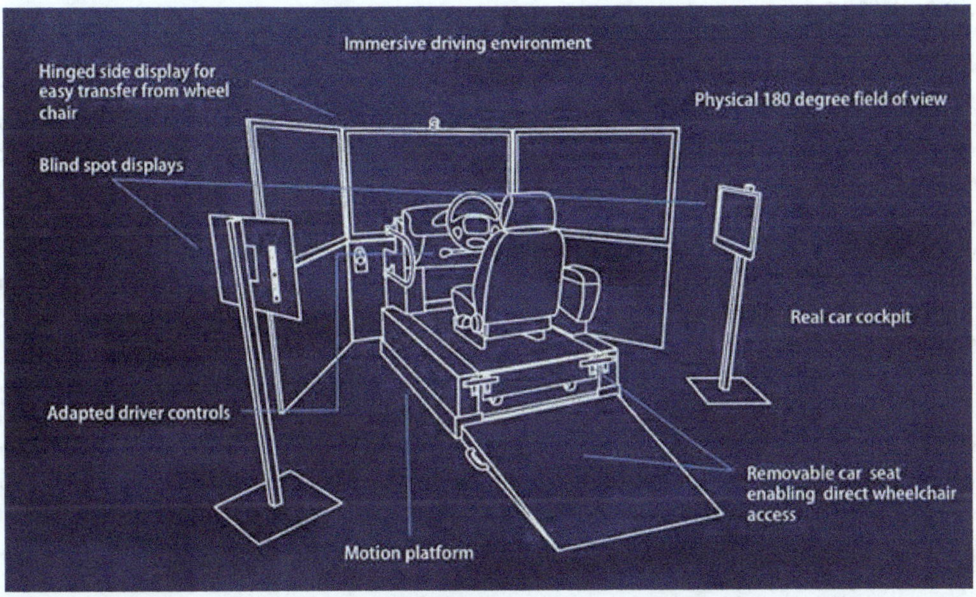

Figure 7. Virtual reality driving simulation rehabilitation training

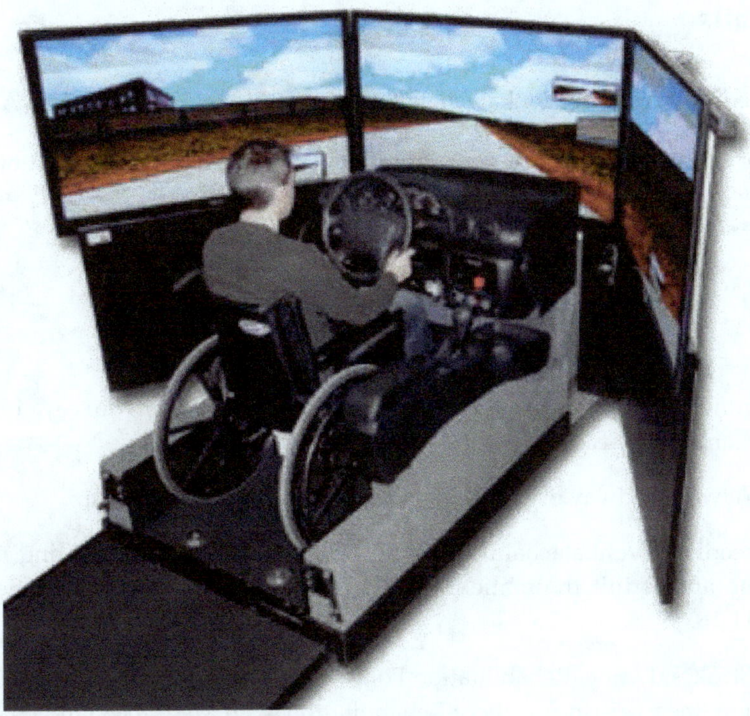

Figure 8. Virtual reality driving simulation rehabilitation training

3. Conclusion

TBI is a diverse disorder of major public health significance. Rehabilitation services, matched to the needs of people with TBI, as well as community-based nonmedical services are required to optimize outcomes over the course of recovery. Both the person with TBI and their social support networks should have access to rehabilitation services through the entire course of recovery, which will continue for many years after the injury. The services required will change as the person's needs change over time. Survivors of severe TBI face the challenge of resuming a meaningful life for themselves and their families. However, severe TBI is not curable and medical and rehabilitation management may not ultimately be able to provide the improvement desired by the patient and his/her family.

In summary, TBI rehabilitation is a recognized subspecialty of neurorehabilitation and there is increasing awareness of its important role in early management for all severities of injury. While evidence for its effectiveness and specific interventions is limited, emerging therapies need to be subjected to rigorous research. The families of TBI survivors, particularly the severely injured, young TBI patients and those in a vegetative state accept most of the social and societal burdens of long-term care. It is crucial to bear in mind that prevention of TBI is vital, as there remains no cure for the sequelae of either moderate or severe TBI.

Author details

Wafa Al Yazeedi, Loganathan Venkatachalam, Somaya Al Molawi and Fatma Al Kuwari

Department of Physical Medicine & Rehabilitation, Hamad Medical Corporation, Doha, Qatar

References

[1] Data from the National Hospital Ambulatory Medical Care Survey, 1995-1996. National Center for Health Statistics.

[2] https://www.headway.org.uk/rehabilitation-after-brain-injury.aspx

[3] Al Yazeedi W, Venkatachalm L, Georgievski AB. Factors influencing rehabilitation outcome after adult traumatic brain Injury in Qatar. Qatar Medical Journal, 2010, 19(1): 11-16.

[4] urner-Strokes, Lynne. Rehabilitation Following Acquired Brain Injury: National Clinical Guidelines. British Society of Rehabilitation. Clin Med. 2004 Jan-Feb;4(1):61-5.

[5] Barnes MP. Rehabilitation after traumatic brain injury. Br. Med. Bull.1999; 55(4): 927-43.

[6] Blackerby WF. Intensity of rehabilitation and length of stay. Brain In., 1990, 4:167-73.

[7] Cope DN, Hall K. Head injury: benefit of early intervention. Arch Phys Med Rehabil., 1982, 63:433-7.

[8] Aronow HU. Rehabilitation effectiveness with severe brain injury: translating research into policy. Head Trauma Rehabil., 1987, 2:24-36.

[9] McKinlay WW, Brooks DN, Bond LR et al. The short term outcome of severe blunt head injury as reported by relatives of the injured persons. NeurolNeurosurg Psychiatry, 1981, 44:527-33.

[10] Oddy M, Humphrey M, Uttley D. Stresses upon the relatives of head injured patients. Br Psychiatry, 1978, 133: 507-13.

[11] Simpson DM, Alexander DN, O'Brien CF et al. Botuhnum toxin type A in the treatment of upper extremity spasticity: a randomised, double-blind, placebo controlled trial. Neurology, 1996, 46:1306-10.

[12] Yablon SA, Agana BT, Ivanhoe CB et al. Botuhnum toxin in severe upper extremity spasticity among patients with traumatic brain injury: an open labelled trial. Neurology, 1996, 47:939-44.

[13] Dejerne A, Ceillier A. Para-osteo-arthropathies des paraplegiques par lesion medullaire; etude clinique et radiographique. Ann Med., 1918, 5:497.

[14] Orzel JA, Rudd TG. Heterotopic bone formation: clinical, laboratory and imaging correlation. J Nucl Med., 1985, 26: 125-132.

[15] Rogers RC. Heterotopic ossification in severe head injury: a preventive programme. Brain Inj., 1988, 2:169-73.

[16] Bader DL (Ed) Pressure Sores – Clinical Practice and Scientific Approach. London: MacMillan, 1990.

[17] Lipides J, Diokno AC, Lowe BS et al. Follow-up on sterile, intermittent self-catheterization.J.urol /1974, 111:184-7.

[18] Urban RJ, Harris P, Masel B. Anterior hypopituitarism following traumatic brain injury. Brain Inj., 2005, 19(5):349-58.

[19] http://www.worldhealth.net/pdf/Gordon_Thera10.pdf

[20] Jin H, Wang S, Hou L, Pan C Li, B Wang, H Yu. Clinical treatment of traumatic brain injury complicated by cranial nerve injury. Injury, 2010, 41(9):918-23.

[21] Wilson B, Moffat N. The Clinical Management of Memory Problems London: Croom Helm, 1984.

[22] Wilson BA, Baddeley A, Evans J, Shiel A. Errorless learning in the rehabilitation of memory impaired people. Neuropsychol Rehabil., 1994, 4:307-26.

[23] Gianutsos R. Cognitive rehabilitation a neuropsychological speciality comes of age. Bram Inj., 1991, 5:353-68.

[24] Briccolo A, Turazzi S, Fenot HG. Prolonged post-traumatic unconsciousness. Neurosurg., 1980, 52:625-34.

[25] Andrews K, Murphy L, Munday R, Littlewood C. Misdiagnosis of the vegetative state, a retrospective study in a rehabilitation unit. BMJ, 1996, 313:13-6.

[26] Eames P, Cotterill G, Kneale TA et al. Outcome of intensive rehabilitation after severe brain injury: a long term follow-up study. Bram Inj., 1996, 10:631-50.

[27] Simpson DM, Foster D. Improvement in organically disturbed behavior with Trazodone treatment. Clin Psychol. 1986, 47:191-3.

[28] Foster HG, Hillbrand M, Chi CC. Efficacy of Carbamazepine in assaultive patients with frontal lobe dysfunction. Prog Neuropsychopharmacol Biol Psychiatry, 1989, 13:865-74.

[29] Mattes JA. Metoprolol for intermittent explosive disorders. Am J Psychol., 1985, 142:1108-9.

[30] Gualtien CT. Pharmaco therapy and the neurobehavioral sequelae of traumatic brain injury. Bram In., 1988, 2:101-29.

[31] Levy M, Berson A, Cook T, Bollegala N, Seto E, Tursanski S, Kim. Treatment of agitation following traumatic brain injury: a review of the literature. NeuroRehabilitation, 2005, 20(4):279-306.

[32] Wehman P, Kreutzer JS, West MD et al. Return to work for persons with traumatic brain injury: a supported employment approach. Arch Phys Med Rehabil., 1990, 71:1047-52.

[33] Cox DJ, Davis M, Singh H, Barbour B, Nidiffer FD. Driving rehabilitation for military personnel recovering from traumatic brain injury using virtual reality driving simulation: a feasibility study. Mil Med., 2010, 175(6):411-6.

7

Management of Traumatic Brain Injury in the Intensive Care Unit

Farid Sadaka, Tanya M Quinn,
Rekha Lakshmanan and Ashok Palagiri

1. Introduction

Traumatic brain injury (TBI) is a major source of death and severe disability worldwide. In the USA alone, this type of injury causes 290, 000 hospital admissions, 51, 000 deaths, and 80, 000 permanently disabled survivors [1, 2]. TBI occurs in two phases, primary and secondary brain injury. The primary injury results from the direct physical impact to the brain parenchyma resulting in structural and shearing injury of neurons, injury to vessels, and interruption of neurochemical processes. This leads to hemorrhage, edema, compression of intracranial structures. Primary injury is unalterable after the time of the trauma.The secondary injury, on the other hand, is characterized by a cascade of events that starts within minutes of the primary injury. As in ischemia –reperfusion injuries, the acute post-injury period in TBI is characterized by several pathophysiologic processes that start in the minutes to hours following injury and may last for hours to days. These result in further neuronal injury and are termed the secondary injury. The causes of the secondary injury can be evaluated by those that occur of the systemic or extracerebral level and those that occur on the cellular level. On the systemic level contributing factors include hypoxia, hypotension, hypercapnia, acidosis and hyperglycemia [3, 4].While the cellular mechanisms of secondary injury include all of the following: apoptosis, mitochondrial dysfunction, excitotoxicity, disruption in ATP metabolism, disruption in calcium homeostasis, increase in inflammatory mediators and cells, free radical formation, DNA damage, blood-brain barrier disruption, brain glucose utilization disruption, microcirculatory dysfunction and microvascular thrombosis [5-8]. All this leads to development of cerebral edema, blood-brain barrier disruption, vasospasm, increase in volume of bleeding and contusions, and intracranial hypertension.TBI patients, like other patients with brain injury, need multidisciplinary approach (neurointensivists, neurologists, neurosurgeons, and specialized nurses, respiratory therapists, physical therapists, nutritionists, etc.) for improved outcomes. Mortality and functional outcomes in all brain injured patients, including TBI patients improve when monitored and managed in neuroICUs and by neurointensivists [9-12]. This chapter will focus on the management of TBI patients in the intensive care unit.

2. Neurological assessment

The most widely used and most studied coma scale to date is the Glasgow coma scale (GCS) (Figure 1), first described by Teasdale and Jennett in 1974 and revised in 1976 with the addition of a sixth point in the motor response subscale for "withdrawal from painful stimulus" [13, 14]. The GCS was initially intended to assess level of consciousness after TBI in a Neurosurgical Intensive Care Unit (Neuro-ICU) [13].The GCS was broadly accepted as an instrument to classify the severity of TBI because it was easy to use and reproducible. It was used to classify the severity of TBI as mild (GCS 13-15), moderate (GCS 9-12), and severe (GCS 8 and below) [15, 16]. Since then it has become the gold standard against which newer scales are compared. As a result, the GCS was incorporated into several scoring systems, including the APACHE II [17], the Simplified Acute Physiology Score (SAPS) and SAPSII [18], the Revised Trauma Score (RTS) [19], the Circulation, Respiration, Abdomen, Motor, Speech scale (CRAMS) [20], the Traumatic Injury Scoring System (TRISS) [21], and A Severity Characterization of Trauma (ASCOT) scale [22], all of which are used to score the severity and predict outcome of TBI. However, the reliability of GCS in predicting patient outcomes is unsatisfactory, especially with regard to the verbal component. As a result, Widjicks et al. published a new scoring system in 2005, the Full Outline of UnResponsiveness (FOUR) score (Figure 2), a newer scale, developed to provide a more comprehensive assessment [23]. The FOUR score includes additional information not assessed by the GCS like brainstem reflexes, visual tracking, breathing patterns, and respiratory drive [23] (Figure 2). It is also more practical for evaluating critically ill intubated patients, as it does not depend on an evaluation of the verbal response. It has already been validated in various populations of comatose patients, including TBI patients [24-30]. While GCS lacks the ability to identify subtle changes in alteration of consciousness, the FOUR score assesses four variables: eye response, motor response, brainstem reflexes, and respiration pattern (Figure 2). The acronym also reflects the number of categories and the maximum number of potential points in each category, making it fairly simple to use and remember. In addition, the FOUR score can account for the intubated patient and can also differentiate between a locked-in state and a vegetative state, via the addition of testing eye tracking, thus incorporating midbrain and pontine functions, effectively allowing the examiner to localize lesions. Another advantage for the FOUR score is that is gives all components equal weight, making it linear which is ideal for a coma scale compared to the GCS score is weighted toward motor responses. The GCS scale does offer the benefit of rapid evaluation in the emergency department, it is readily reproducible by multiple personal, from nursing staff to trauma surgeons, and gives a rapid assessment of the severity of injury. This is likely attributable to its long standing application in the field, which makes it second nature for many to communicate the information. More studies are needed to favor one over the other. For now, using either GCS or FOUR score for initial neurological assessment as well as follow up neurologic checks is acceptable.

Best eye response (E)	Spontaneous--open with blinking at baseline	4
	Opens to verbal command, speech, or shout	3
	Opens to pain, not applied to face	2
	None	1
Best verbal response (V)	Oriented	5
	Confused conversation, but able to answer questions	4
	Inappropriate responses, words discernible	3
	Incomprehensible speech	2
	None	1
Best motor response (M)	Obeys commands for movement	6
	Purposeful movement to painful stimulus	5
	Withdraws from pain	4
	Abnormal (spastic) flexion, decorticate posture	3
	Extensor (rigid) response, decerebrate posture	2
	None	1

Figure 1. Glasgow Coma Scale

3. Intracranial pressure monitoring

Intracranial hypertension develops commonly in acute brain injury related to trauma [31, 32]. Raised Intracranial pressure (ICP) is an important predictor of mortality in patients with severe TBI, and aggressive treatment of elevated ICP has been shown to reduce mortality and improve outcome (32-39). Guidelines for the Management of Severe TBI, published in the Journal of Neurotrauma in 2007 [4] make a Level II recommendation that ICP should be monitored in all salvageable patients with a severe TBI (Glasgow Coma Scale [GCS] score of 3–8 after resuscitation) and an abnormal computed tomography (CT) scan. ICP monitoring is also recommended in patients with severe TBI and a normal CT scan if two or more of the following features are noted at admission: age over 40 years, unilateral or bilateral motor posturing, or systolic blood pressure < 90 mm Hg (Level III recommendation). In comatose TBI patients with an abnormal CT scan, the incidence of ICH was 53–63% [40]. Patients with a normal CT scan at admission, on the other hand, had a relatively low incidence of intracranial hypertension (13%). However, within the normal CT group, if patients demonstrated at least two of three adverse features (age over 40 years, unilateral or bilateral motor posturing,

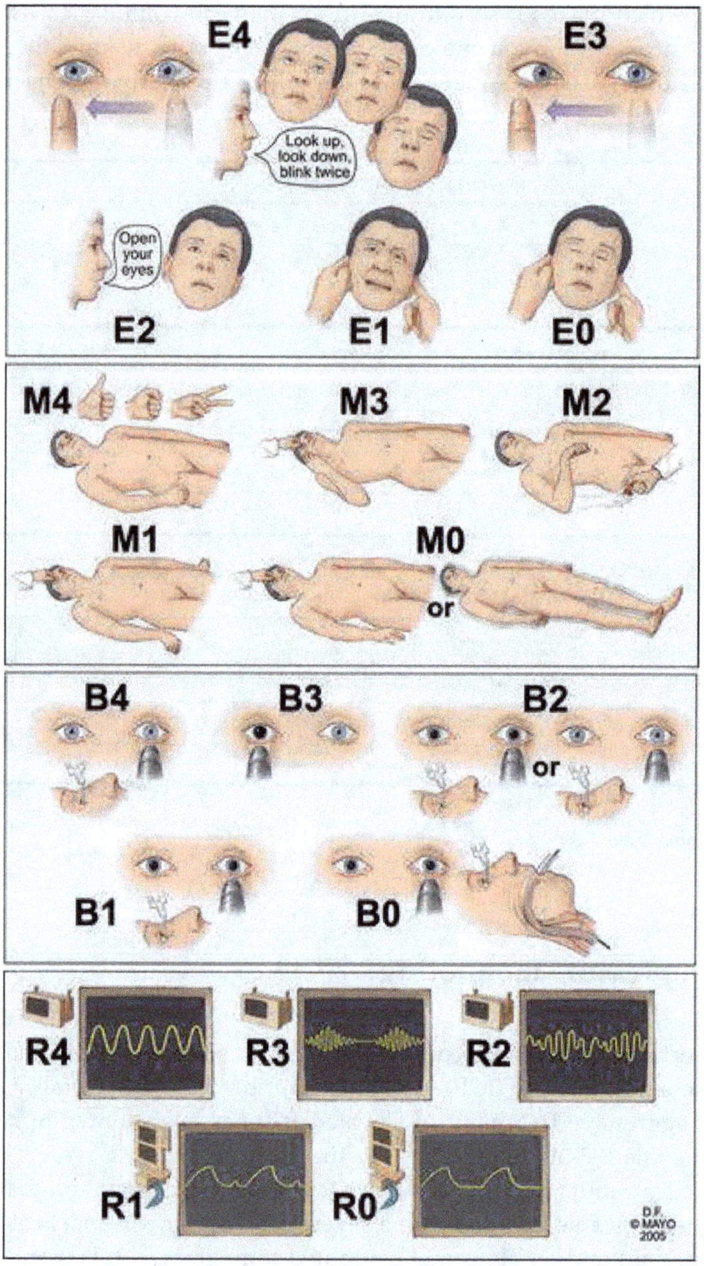

Figure 2. Full Outline of UnResponsiveness (FOUR) score. Eye response: E4 eyelids open or opened, tracking, or blinking to command; E3 eyelids open but not tracking; E2 eyelids closed but open to loud voice; E1 eyelids closed but open to pain; and E0 eyelids remain closed with pain. Motor response: M4 thumbs-up, fist, or peace sign; M3 localizing to pain; M2 flexion response to pain; M1 extension response to pain; and M0 no response to pain or generalized myoclonus status. Brainstem reflexes: B4 pupil and corneal reflexes present; B3 one pupil wide and fixed; B2 pupil or corneal reflexes absent; B1 pupil and corneal reflexes absent; and B0 absent pupil, corneal, and cough reflex. Respiration pattern: R4 not intubated, regular breathing pattern; R3 not intubated, Cheyne-Stokes breathing pattern; R2 not intubated, irregular breathing; R1 breathes above ventilatory rate; and R0 breathes at ventilator rate or apnea.

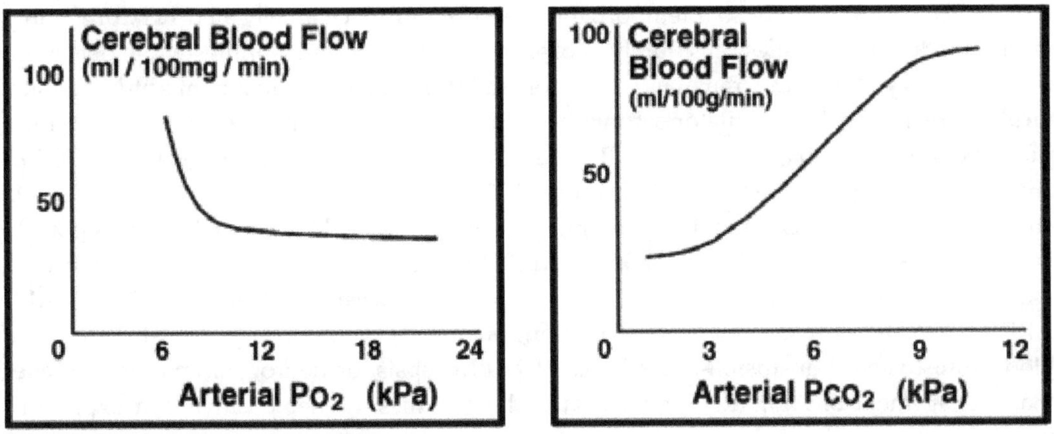

Figure 3. Oxygen tension and carbon dioxide effects on Cerebral Blood flow

or systolic BP < 90 mm Hg), their risk of intracranial hypertension was similar to that of patients with abnormal CT scans [4]. ICP is a strong predictor of outcome from severe TBI [33, 34, 36, 41-43]. Because of this, ethically a randomized trial of ICP monitoring with and without treatment is unlikely to be carried out. Similarly, a trial for treating or not treating systemic hypotension is not likely. Both hypotension and raised ICP are the leading causes of death in severe TBI. Furthermore, several studies have shown that patients who do not have intracranial hypertension or who respond to ICP-lowering therapies have a lower mortality than those who do not respond to therapy [5-12, 44-47]. As a result, Guidelines for the Management of Severe TBI recommend that treatment should be initiated with ICP thresholds above 20 mm Hg (level II) as well as target a cerebral perfusion pressure (CPP) within the range of 50-70 (level III) [4]. Prevention and/or treatment of intracranial hypertension is commonly accomplished by employing a progression of therapeutic approaches that are efficacious in controlling ICP and uniformly believed to be easily applied with minimal or rare negative side effects. These measures include(but are not limited to): elevation of the head of the bed, avoiding hypotension, hypoxia, and hypercapnea or prolonged hypocapnea, intravenous sedation and analgesia, administration of hyperosmolar agents (mannitol, hypertonic saline), and CSF drainage [4].

4. Oxygenation and ventilation

Hypoxia (PaO2 < 60 mmHg or O2 saturation < 90%) worsens secondary brain injury and thus significantly worsens outcome in patients with TBI [48, 49]. In addition, duration of hypoxemia (median duration ranging from 11.5 to 20 min) was found to be an independent predictor of mortality [50]. Elevated Carbon dioxide dilates the cerebral blood vessels, increasing the volume of blood in the intracranial vault and therefore increasing ICP [51]. On the other hand, hyperventilation leads to cerebral vasoconstriction, and thus can result in cerebral ischemia, despite possible improvements in CPP and ICP [52]. Thus, hyperventilation is recommended only as a temporizing measure to reduce an elevated ICP, preferably not below 30 mmHG unless absolutely necessary and only for few minutes while determining an etiology of the intracranial hypertension and initiating other treatment options or surgical intervention. The ventilator settings should be adjusted to maintain normoxia with a pulse oximetry (SpO2) around 95% or PaO2 around 80 mm Hg and eucapnia with PaCO2 of 35 to 40 mm Hg (in patients with chronic CO2 retention, such as COPD patients, CO2 should be maintained close to their baseline CO2 and normal pH). (Figure 3) At this point it is worth mentioning acute lung injury (ALI) and acute respiratory distress syndrome (ARDS). The incidence of ALI/ARDS in TBI is reported between 10 % and 30 % [53, 54]. ALI/ARDS could develop secondary to aspiration, pneumonia, pulmonary contusion, massive blood transfusion, transfusion-related ALI (TRALI), sepsis, or neurogenic pulmonary edema. Management of ALI/ARDS entails low tidal volumes, higher positive end expiratory pressure, and permissive hypercapnea [55]. However, as mentioned above, hypercapnea (> 40 mmHG) is contraindicated in TBI patients with intracranial hypertension. One needs to balance need for low tidal volume and CO2 levels, and thus frequent ABG measurements is warranted.

5. Blood pressure and cerebral perfusion

Hypotension (SBP < 90 mm Hg) can worsen secondary injury in TBI and is associated with worsening mortality and neurologic outcomes [56, 57]. In TBI patients from the Trauma Coma Data Bank, early hypotension occurred in 34.6% of patients with severe traumatic brain injury and was shown to double the mortality rate (55% versus 27%). Late hypotension (in the ICU) occurred in 32% of patients. For patients whose only hypotensive episode occurred in the ICU, 66% died or were vegetative survivors compared with 17% of patients who never had a hypotensive episode [56]. We recommend IVF resuscitation to maintain euvolemia, using either invasive (e.g. CVP or pulmonary capillary wedge pressure) or noninvasive methods (e.g. Echocardiogram or NICOM-noninvasive cardiac output monitoring) to measure either static (CVP) or dynamic (Stroke volume index variation) surrogates of intravascular volume and hemodynamics. Hypotonic, hyponatremic, and sugar containing fluids should be avoided. If patient is euvolemic and remains hypotensive, then vasopressors should be started to maintain adequate blood pressure. Cerebral perfusion pressure is defined as mean arterial pressure (MAP) minus ICP (CPP = MAP – ICP). CPP < 60 mm HG should be avoided since it is associated with poor outcomes in patients with TBI [58]. Both 60 mmHg and 70 mm Hg are cited in the literature as the threshold above which CPP should be maintained. However, as reported earlier, the Guidelines for the Management of Severe Traumatic Brain injury recommend maintaining CPP between 50-70 mmHg [4]. In our patients, when the neurologic status is stable with a normal ICP, aggressive measures do not need to be taken as long as CPP >50 mmHg. Conversely, in patient's where exam is poor or ICP has been elevated/required treatment, then would recommend CPP >60 mmHg since the risk of secondary injury developing is more imminent in these patients. In the absence of cerebral ischemia, aggressive attempts to maintain CPP above 70 mmHg with fluids and vasopressors should be avoided because of the risk of ARDS [59].

6. Hyperosmolar therapy

Brain parenchyma is 80% water, and thus brain volume is very responsive to changes in water content. A hyperosmolar agent creates a gradient for water to move from brain parenchyma to the intravascular space across the blood-brain barrier (BBB). As a result, the effectiveness of a hyperosmolar agent depends on the extent it is prevented from crossing the BBB. Both mannitol and hypertonic saline posses this property and will be discussed in this section. Mannitol is given in a 20% or 25 % solution in boluses of 0.25 to 1.0 g per kilogram of body weight at intervals of 2, 4, 6, or more hours. In addition to the osmotic properties of mannitol, , it also lowers blood viscosity which leads to increase cerebral blood flow resulting in cerebral vasoconstriction (autoregulation), which in turn reduces cerebral blood volume and thus intracranial pressure [60]. In patients with impaired cerebral autoregulation, aggressive use of mannitol could result in increased ICP. As this implies, for mannitol to be fully effective, the blood brain barrier must be intact. In patients where the BBB is not intact, mannitol crosses the BBB and can draw fluid into brain resulting in an increase in ICP [61, 62], hence concentrations of mannitol should be assessed before each dose. Instead of measuring actual mannitol, an easier and more practical way is to measure serum osmolarity or osmolar gap (measured – calculated serum osmolarity) before infusing mannitol. Because of the above as well as to minimize risk of acute kidney injury, Mannitol should thus not be given if serum osmolarity is more than 320 mOsm/Kg H2O or osmolar gap > 10. Side effects of mannitol include hypotension, hypovolemia, hypokalemia, hyperkalemia, and acute kidney injury [63, 64]. Mannitol is contraindicated in patients with renal failure. Hypertonic saline increases serum osmolarity directly rather than by inducing osmotic dieresis, as well as by viscosity-related cerebral vasoconstriction [65]. It is used in a 3% solution infusion or in boluses of approximately 150 ml, in a 7.5% solution in 75-ml boluses, or in a 23.4% solution in 30-ml boluses every 2, 4, 6, or more hours. Serum osmolarity and serum sodium should be checked before dosing hypertonic saline. Hypertonic saline should not be given if serum Na is more than 160 mmol/liter. Side effects of hypertonic saline include fluid overload secondary to intravascular volume expansion, acidosis, hypokalemia, and hyperchloremia. There is a potential for development of central pontine myelinolysis with rapid increase in serum Na concentration, however, this phenomenon has not been documented in this scenario of management of intracranial hypertension. The question remains as to which one, mannitol or hypertonic saline, is superior? Recent evidence including two metanalysis, suggest that hypertonic saline may be more effective than mannitol in reducing ICP [66-69], however, high quality studies comparing the agents, while accounting for side effects and contraindications are lacking. Furthermore, it is very important to take into consideration patient characteristics, such as volume status, renal function, hemodynamic status, sodium levels, etc.., when choosing the appropriate hyperosmolar agent. Hyperosmolar therapy should be weaned gradually rather than stopped abruptly in the days to follow.

7. Refractory intracranial hypertension: Therapeutic hypothermia and barbiturate coma

Refractory intracranial hypertension (RICH) is defined as intracranial pressures that exceed 25 mm Hg for 30 minutes, 30 mm Hg for 15 minutes, or 40 mm Hg for 1 minute despite tier 1 and tier 2 therapies [70]. Tier 1 therapies include head of patient's bed at or more than 30 degrees, adequate sedation and analgesia, and adequate CSF draining if ICP is monitored by ventriculostomy. Tier 2 therapies include adequate hyperosmolar therapy (mannitol or hypertonic saline or both), mild hyperventilation (pCO2 goal of 30 – 35 mmHg), and neuromascular blockade. RICH occurs in approximately 15% of patients with traumatic brain injury [70]. If it is not aggressively treated, RICH can result in cerebral herniation and death.High-dose barbiturate administration is recommended to control elevated ICP refractory to maximum standard medical and surgical treatment (level II) [3]. High-dose barbiturates have been scarcely studied for this indication. In 2004, the Cochrane Injuries Group performed a systematic review of the barbiturate RCTs. In the only two studies examining the effect on ICP, the relative risk for refractory ICP with barbiturate therapy was 0.81 (95% CI 0.62–1.06). Concerning this indication, the Cochrane group concluded: "There is no evidence that barbiturate therapy in patients with acute severe head injury improves outcome. Barbiturate therapy results in a fall in blood pressure in one of four treated patients. The hypotensive effect of barbiturate therapy will offset any ICP lowering effect on cerebral perfusion pressure" [71]. Significant side effects of barbiturates include hypotension, arrhythmias, immunosuppression, hepatotoxicity, fever and injection site reactions. The Guidelines for the Management of Severe TBI recommend that more studies are needed to identify alternative agents for this indication - "elevated ICP refractory to standard therapy" [3]. Albeit small, there are more RCT evaluating the effect of therapeutic hypothermia on ICH in severe TBI (13 studies) than for barbiturates; all consistently demonstrating that hypothermia is effective in controlling ICP (This is reviewed in more detail elsewhere : Farid Sadaka, Christopher Veremakis, Rekha Lakshmanan and Ashok Palagiri (2013). Therapeutic Hypothermia in Traumatic Brain Injury, Therapeutic Hypothermia in Brain Injury, Dr. Farid Sadaka (Ed.), ISBN: 978-953-51-0960-0, InTech, DOI: 10.5772/48818. Available from: http://www.intechopen.com/books/therapeutic-hypothermia-in-brain-injury/therapeutic-hypothermia-in-traumatic-brain-injury). Complications from hypothermia include electrolyte imbalances, increase in incidence of infections, thrombocytopenia, coagulopathy, arrhythmias (especially bradycardia), pancreatitis, and rebound ICH (during re-warming). In one extensive review [72], Povlishock et al showed that posttraumatic hypothermia followed by slow rewarming appeared to provide maximal protection in terms of traumatically induced axonal damage, microvascular damage and dysfunction, contusional expansion, intracranial hypertension, and neurocognitive recovery. In contrast, hypothermia followed by rapid rewarming not only reversed the protective effects associated with hypothermic intervention, but exacerbated the traumatically induced pathology and its neurologic consequences. Povlishock's review concluded that the rate of posthypothermic rewarming is an important variable in assuring maximal efficacy following the use of hypothermic intervention. The most challenging issue appears to be rebound ICP during re-warming. We suggest that re-warming only be considered if the patient's ICP is stable and <20mmHg for at least 48 hours, and, thereafter implemented at a rate not faster than 0.1 -0.25°C per hour. Surgical management of TBI patients such as Decompressive hemi-craniectomy or bilateral craniectomy are discussed in more detail in chapter http://www.intechopen.com/books/traumatic-brain-injury/surgical-treatment-of-severe-traumatic-brain-injury. Please refer to figure 4 for protocolized step-wise approach to ICP management.

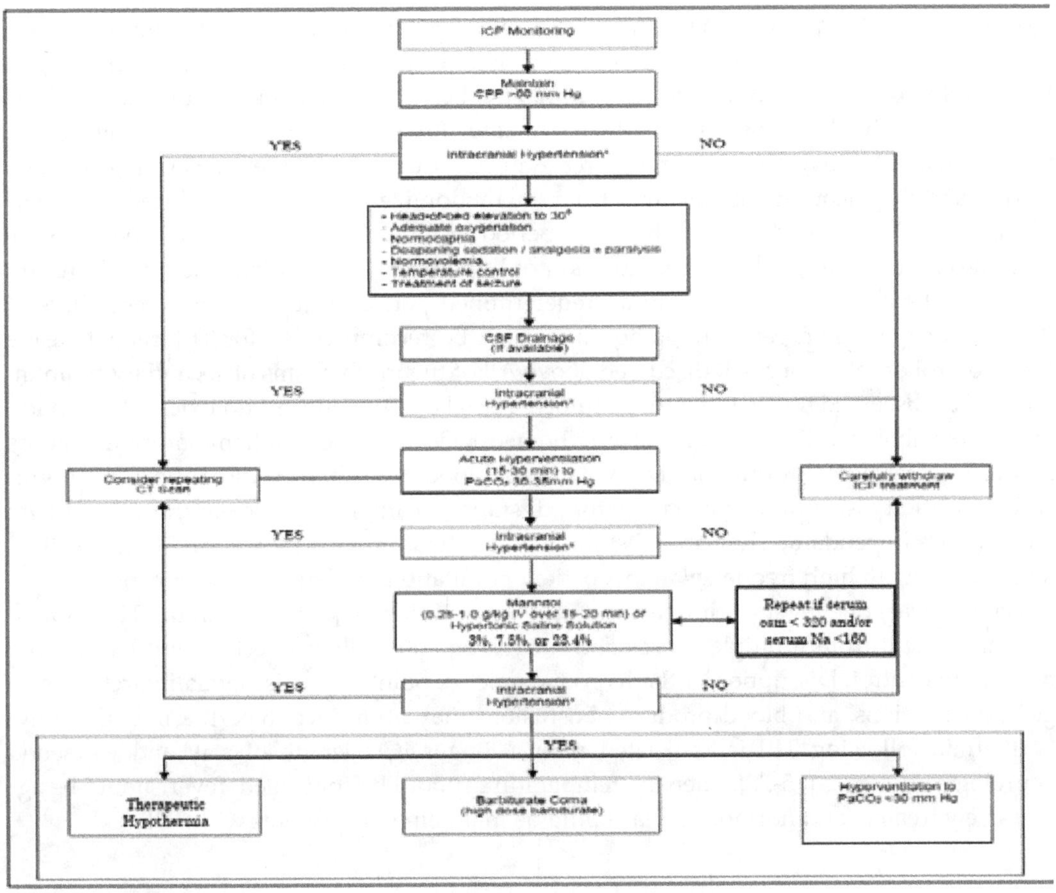

Figure 4. Stepwise approach to management of intracranial hypertension.

8. Temperature modulation and normothermia

Aside from role of hypothermia in ICP control in patients with refractory intracranial hypertension, therapeutic hypothermia has also been studied as a primary neuroprotectant in patients with severe TBI, based on the fact that early administration of TH could halt the secondary injury processes discussed above, and thus possibly improve outcome. This topic is reviewed in more detail elsewhere : Farid Sadaka, Christopher Veremakis, Rekha Lakshmanan and Ashok Palagiri (2013). Therapeutic Hypothermia in Traumatic Brain Injury, Therapeutic Hypothermia in Brain Injury, Dr. Farid Sadaka (Ed.), ISBN: 978-953-51-0960-0, InTech, DOI: 10.5772/48818. Available from: http://www.intechopen.com/books/therapeutic-hypothermia-in-brain-injury/therapeutic-hypothermia-in-traumatic-brain-injury. In short, although single-center studies were encouraging, multicenter trials with early administration of hypothermia for a defined period of time irrespective of ICP have almost uniformly been negative except maybe for patients undergoing craniotomy for hematoma evacuations. However, hypothermia was maintained for a fixed duration of only 48 hrs, and ICP elevations mainly occurred during and after rewarming. These results suggest that a period of 48 hours of hypothermia may be too short to have a beneficial effect on outcome. A standardized one size fit all may be inappropriate. The rate of rewarming plays an important role as well as pointed above.The rebound increase in ICP during and after rewarming in these studies and the encouraging outcomes from the randomized studies that induced hypothermia early and continued it throughout the period of intracranial hypertension point to the realization that individualizing the duration of hypothermia to fit a patient's ICP in future trials may be a better strategy than a predetermined period of hypothermia regardless of ICP. As for now, therapeutic hypothermia cannot be recommended for TBI patients aside from control of refractory ICP discussed above.All of the mechanisms of secondary brain injury in TBI discussed above (apoptosis, mitochondrial dysfunction, excitotoxicity, disruption in ATP metabolism, disruption in calcium homeostasis, increase in inflammatory mediators and cells, free radical formation, DNA damage, blood-brain barrier disruption, brain glucose utilization disruption, microcirculatory dysfunction and microvascular thrombosis) are temperature dependant. They are all stimulated and exacerbated by fever [73]. In addition, fever occurs with high frequency in this patient population, with up to 68% of patients experiencing at least one fever during their intensive care unit stay [74]. Fever in the TBI population may result from multiple causes and for reasons other than infection and has proven difficult to control. Disruption of the hypothalamic set point, tissue ischemia/infarction, surgery, medications, and blood product transfusions may all induce hyperthermia. Early hyperthermia following TBI is associated with a longer ICU length of stay and worsened neurologic outcomes [75-77]. Thereby, temperature should be controlled, fever should be aggressively treated, and normothermia should be maintained in patients with TBI.

9. Nutrition and glucose control

TBI, especially severe TBI, can cause increase metabolism and can create a hypercatabolic state that results in rapid depletion of nutrition reserves, as well as worsening immune function and morbidity [78, 79]. In TBI patients, adequate nutrition that is started early after injury is associated with enhanced immunity, decreased infectious morbidity, shortened length of hospitalization, improved neurological recovery and reduced mortality [80, 81]. Brain trauma foundation recommends that patients should be fed to attain full caloric replacement by day 7 post-injury [3]. American Society for Parenteral and Enteral Nutrition

(ASPEN) for nutrition support in critically-ill adult patients suggest that enteral nutrition should be started within the first 24–48 h following admission, as long as patients are hemodynamically stable [82]. The European Society for Parenteral and Enteral Nutrition (ESPEN) recommends initiating enteral nutrition within 24 h if possible [83]. Despite popular belief, recent evidence reiterates that bowel sounds and passing flatus or stool are not required for the initiation of enteral nutrition[82]. In circumstances when early enteral nutrition cannot be initiated, parenteral nutrition should be strongly considered.There is no question that hyperglycemia is associated with worse outcome in brain injured patients [84, 85]. Hypoglycemia leads to deprivation of the brain of its fuel which can lead to compromised brain energy metabolism and worsen the already existent brain injury, especially during the increase in glucose utilization and brain energy demand observed after TBI [86, 87]. However, the optimal target for systemic glucose control is not known. In patients with severe brain injury, tight systemic glucose control (80–120 mg/dL) was associated with reduced cerebral extracellular glucose availability and increased prevalence of brain energy crisis, which in turn correlates with increased mortality [88]. Intensive insulin therapy may thus impair cerebral glucose metabolism after severe brain injury. Based on the existing low quality evidence, the most recent guidelines from the Society of Critical Care Medicine (SCCM) suggest that blood glucose (BG) ≥ 150 mg/dL should trigger initiation of insulin therapy for most patients admitted to an ICU with the diagnosis of TBI, titrated to achieve BG values absolutely < 180 mg/dL, to minimize the adverse effects of hyperglycemia [89]. The guidelines also suggest that BG < 100 mg/dL be avoided during insulin infusion for patients with brain injury [89].

10. Anemia and transfusion

Hypoxia and hypotension worsen secondary brain injury and are important determinants of outcome in TBI patients. They both are associated with worse outcomes as discussed above. This could be the reason why many patients with TBI are still transfused to a hemoglobin threshold of 10 g/dl. Although red blood cells are an essential requirement for the transport of oxygen to the tissues, several problems are documented with red blood cells (RBC) transfusions such as infection, pulmonary complications such as transfusion-related acute lung injury (TRALI) and transfusion-associated circulatory overload (TACO), transfusion-related immunomodulation (TRIM) and multiorgan failure, and increased mortality [90]. Besides, there is no clear correlation between anemia and hypoxia or hypotension in TBI patients. In one retrospective study, linear regression showed that more days with hematocrit < 30% was associated with improved neurologic outcomes. In addition, transfusion of RBCs was significantly associated with worse outcomes [91]. In a subgroup analysis of a multicenter randomized controlled clinical trial involving 67 critically ill patients from the Transfusion Requirements in the Critical Care trial who sustained a closed head injury, patients were randomized to a restrictive RBC transfusion strategy (Hb 7.0 g/dL and maintained between 7.0 and 9.0 g/dL) or a liberal strategy (Hb 10.0 g/dL and maintained between 10.0 and 12.0 g/dL). This study was unable to detect significant improvements in mortality with a liberal as compared with a restrictive transfusion strategy in critically ill trauma patients with moderate-to severe TBI [92]. Guidelines for transfusion developed by EAST (Eastern Association for Surgery of Trauma) and the American College of Critical Care Medicine (ACCM) of the Society of Critical Care Medicine (SCCM) state that there is no benefit of a "liberal" transfusion strategy (transfusion when Hb is <10 g/dL) in patients with moderate-to-severe TBI [93]. Large multicenter prospective studies are needed to evaluate the effects of anemia and RBC transfusion in patients with TBI.

11. Deep venous thrombosis

The application of chemical venous thrombo-embolism (VTE) prophylaxis traumatic brain injury patients has been long been guided by the dogma of physicians practicing under assumptions rather than evidenced based guidelines. This has resulted in the blanket denial of the use of any chemical DVT prophylaxis up until more recent years, despite the common knowledge that trauma patient are at high risk for development of venous thromboembolic events. The overwhelming fear associated with propagating the intracranial injury has also limited the number of studies until recently. Most of the data that is currently applied to support the safety of chemical prophylaxis has been extrapolated from studies that were performed looking that the risks of post-operative hemorrhage in elective craniotomy patients. In 1998 Agnelli et. al. compared the use of enoxaparin combined with compression stockings to patients treated with compression stockings alone and found a significant reduction in the number of VTE without any increase in hemorrhage after elective neurosurgery [94]. This study and others like it opened the door for further application and research in the area of traumatic brain injury. The current formal recommendation by the Guidelines for the Management of Severe Traumatic Brain Injury 2007 state that the use of low-molecular weight heparin or low dose unfractionated heparin should be used in combination with mechanical prophylaxis, but there is an increased risk for expansion of intracranial hemorrhage. There is insufficient evidence to support recommendations regarding the preferred agent, dose, or timing [4].The lack of guidelines to follow has prompted many institutions to develop their own guidelines based on extrapolated data and to record and report their experiences. In 2010, clinicians at McGill University published their findings, which showed an acceptable VTE control rate without increased risk of expanding intracranial hemorrhage [95]. The general principles that predominate in the use of chemical VTE prophylaxis are the following: 1) patients not expected to go to the operating room in the next 24 hours for intracranial procedure 2) no evidence of systemic coagulopathy 3) 2 stable CT scans. All guidelines should be applied with the consideration of the injuries of the specific patient in question and altered as seen appropriate for the situation. The first phase of a randomized, double-blind study involving the early use of enoxaparin in trauma patients was just published in 2012 [96]. The study found at 2.3% higher rate of progression in the patients treated with enoxaparin over placebo, however, none were clinically significant. DEEP-II is intended to evaluate the efficacy of this VTE prevention and DEEP-III will apply to moderate-risk patients. A recently published systematic review and meta-analysis of the use of early chemical VTE prophylaxis in TBI patients found that it reduced the risk of VTE without progression of intracranial hemorrhage [97]. While there is certainly the need for more studies to quantify the risk associated with the early use of chemical VTE prophylaxis, there is evidence that supports the appropriate application in traumatic brain injury patients at high risk for developing DVT. Although we cannot not provide official recommendations, dosage, or timing of administration, it is used in our institution.

12. Conclusion

TBI is a devastating injury and often these patients would require monitoring and treatment in intensive care unit. Management of TBI patients requires multidisciplinary approach, frequent close monitoring and judicious use of multiple treatments to lessen secondary brain injury and improve outcomes. There is a lot of opportunity for further research in TBI, including but not limited to multimodal monitoring, and therapeutics to further improve outcomes in this very common mechanism of brain injury.

Author details

Farid Sadaka*, Tanya M Quinn, Rekha Lakshmanan and Ashok Palagiri

*Address all correspondence to: farid.sadaka@mercy.net

Mercy Hospital St. Louis/St. Louis University, Critical Care Medicine/Neurocritical Care, St. Louis, USA

The authors report no conflicts of interest. All authors declare that No competing financial interests exist. All authors report that no potential conflicts of interest exist with any companies/organizations whose products or services may be discussed in this article.

References

[1] Dombovy ML, Olek AC (1997) Recovery and rehabilitation following traumatic brain injury. Brain Inj 11(5):305-18.

[2] Rutland-Brown W, Langlois JA, Thomas KE, Xi YL (2006) Incidence of traumatic brain injury in the United States, 2003. J Head Trauma Rehabil 21: 544 - 48.

[3] Bader, MK. (2006) Recognizing and Treating Ischemic Insults to the Brain: The Role of Brain Tissue Oxygen Monitoring. Crit Care Nurs Clin N Am 18: 243-256.

[4] Brain Trauma Foundation; American Association of Neurological Surgeons; Congress of Neurological Surgeons; Joint Section on Neurotrauma and Critical Care,

AANS/CNS. Guidelines for the management of severe traumatic brain injury. J Neurotrauma 2007; 24 (Suppl 1):1-117.

[5] Small DL, Morley P, Buchan AM (1999) Biology of ischemic cerebral cell death. Prog Cardiovasc Dis 42:185–207.

[6] Dietrich WD, Atkins CM, Bramlett HM (2009) Protection in animal models of brain and spinal cord injury with mild to moderate hypothermia. J Neurotrauma 26(3): 301-12.

[7] Chesnut RM (1995) Secondary brain insults after head injury: clinical perspectives. New Horiz 3:366-75.

[8] Unterberg AW, Stover JF, Kress B, Kiening KL (2004) Edema and brain trauma. Neuroscience 129:1021-9.

[9] Mirski MA, Chang CW, Cowan R (2001) Impact of a neuroscience intensive care unit on neurosurgical patient outcomes and cost of care: evidence-based support for an intensivist-directed specialty ICU model of care. J Neurosurg Anesthesiol 13(2):83-92.

[10] Diringer MN, Edwards DF (2001) Admission to a neurologic/neurosurgical intensive care unit is associated with reduced mortality rate after intracerebral hemorrhage. Crit Care Med 29(3):635-40.

[11] Varelas PN, Conti MM, Spanaki MV, Potts E, Bradford D, Sunstrom C, Fedder W, Hacein Bey L, Jaradeh S, Gennarelli TA (2004) The impact of a neurointensivist-led team on a semiclosed neurosciences intensive care unit. Crit Care Med 32(11):2191-8.

[12] Varelas PN, Eastwood D, Yun HJ, Spanaki MV, Hacein Bey L, Kessaris C, Gennarelli TA (2006) Impact of a neurointensivist on outcomes in patients with head trauma treated in a neurosciences intensive care unit. J Neurosurg 104(5):713-9.

[13] Teasdale G, Jennett B (1974) Assessment of coma and impaired consciousness. A practical scale. Lancet 2:81–4.

[14] Teasdale GM, Jennett B (1976) Assessment and prognosis of coma after head injury. Acta Neurochir 34:45–55.

[15] Rimel RW, Giordani NP, Barth JT, Jane JJ (1982) Moderate head injury: completing the spectrum of brain trauma. Neurosurgery 11: 344–351.

[16] Rimel RW, Jane JA, Edlich RF (1979) An injury severity scale for comprehensive management of central nervous system trauma. JACEP 8: 64–67.

[17] Knaus WA, Draper EA, Wagner DP, Zimmerman JE (1985) APACHE II: a severity of disease classification system. Crit Care Med 13:818–29.

[18] Le Gall JR, Lemeshow S, Saulnier F (1993) A new Simplified Acute Physiology Score (SAPS II) based on a European/North American multicenter study. JAMA 270:2957–63.

[19] Gormican SP (1989) CRAMS scale: field triage of trauma Champion HR, Sacco WJ, Copes WS, Gann DS, Gennarelli TA, Flannagan ME. A revision of the trauma score. J Trauma 29:623–9.

[20] Gormican SP (1982) CRAMS scale: field triage of trauma victims. Ann Emerg Med 11:132–5.

[21] Boyd CR, Tolson MA, Copes WS (1987) Evaluating trauma care: the TRISS method. Trauma Score and the Injury Severity Score. J Trauma 27:370–8.

[22] Champion HR, Copes WS, Sacco WJ, Frey CF, Holcroft JW, Hoyt DB, Weigelt JA (1996) Improved predictions from a severity characterization of trauma (ASCOT) over Trauma and Injury Severity Score (TRISS): results of an independent evaluation. J Trauma 40:42–8. discussion 48–9.

[23] Wijdicks EF, Bamlet WR, Maramattom BV, Manno EM, McClelland RL (2005) Validation of a new coma scale: the FOUR score. Ann Neurol 58(4):585–93.

[24] Iyer VN, Mandrekar JN, Danielson RD, Zubkov AY, Elmer JL, Wijdicks EF (2009) Validity of the FOUR score coma scale in the medical intensive care unit. Mayo Clin Proc 84(8): 694–701.

[25] Stead LG, Wijdicks EF, Bhagra A, Kashyap R, Bellolio MF, Nash DL, Enduri S, Schears R, William B. (2009) Validation of a new coma scale, the FOUR score, in the emergency department. Neurocrit Care 10(1):50–4.

[26] Wolf CA, Wijdicks EF, Bamlet WR, McClelland RL (2007) Further validation of the FOUR score coma scale by intensive care nurses. Mayo Clin Proc 82(4):435–8.

[27] Fugate JE, Rabinstein AA, Claassen DO, White RD, Wijdicks EF (2010) The FOUR score predicts outcome in patients after cardiac arrest. Neurocrit Care 13(2):205-10.

[28] Weiss N, Mutlu G, Essardy F, Nacabal C, Sauves C, Bally C, Houbert M, Lecorre C, Germack V, Demeret S, Pierrot-Deseilligny C, Bolgert F (2009) The French version of the FOUR score: a new coma score. Rev Neurol 165:796–802.

[29] Akavipat P (2009) Endorsement of the FOUR score for consciousness assessment in neurosurgical patients. Neurol Med Chir 49:565–71.

[30] Sadaka F, Patel D, Lakshmanan R (2012) The FOUR score predicts outcome in patients after traumatic brain injury. Neurocrit Care 2012 16(1):95-101.

[31] Miller JD, Becker DP, Ward JD, Sullivan HG, Adams WE, Rosner MJ. Significance of intracranial hypertension in severe head injury. J Neurosurg 1977; 47:503–516.

[32] Miller JD, Dearden NM, Piper IR, Chan KH. Control of intracranial pressure in patients with severe head injury. J Neurotrauma 1992; 9(suppl 1):S317–S326.

[33] Marmarou A, Anderson PL, Ward JD, Choi SC, Young HF. Impact of ICP instability and hypotension on outcome in patients with severe head trauma. J Neurosurg 1991; 75(suppl):59–66.

[34] Ghajar J, Hariri RJ, Patterson RH. Improved outcome from traumatic coma using only ventricular cerebrospinal fluid drainage for intracranial pressure control. Adv Neurosurg 1993; 21:173–177.

[35] Juul N, Morris GF, Marshall SB, Marshall LF. Intracranial hypertension and cerebral perfusion pressure: influence on neurological deterioration and outcome in severe head injury. The Executive Committee of the International Selfotel Trial. J Neurosurg 2000; 92:1– 6.

[36] Becker DP, Miller JD, Ward JD, Greenberg RP, Young HF, Sakalas R. The outcome from severe head injury with early diagnosis and intensive management. J Neurosurg 1977; 47:491– 502.

[37] Patel HC, Menon DK, Tebbs S, Hawker R, Hutchinson PJ, Kirkpatrick PJ. Specialist neurocritical care and outcome from head injury. Intensive Care Med 2002; 28:547–553.

[38] Steiner T, Ringleb P, Hacke W. Treatment options for large hemispheric stroke. Neurology 2001; 57:S61–S68.

[39] Qureshi AI, Geocadin RG, Suarez JI, Ulatowski JA. Long-term outcome after medical reversal of transtentorial herniation in patients with supratentorial mass lesions. Crit Care Med 2000; 28:1556 –1564.

[40] Narayan RK, Kishore PR, Becker DP, Ward JD, Enas GG, Greenberg RP, Domingues Da Silva A, Lipper MH, Choi SC, Mayhall CG, Lutz HA 3rd, Young HF (1982) Intracranial pressure: to monitor or not to monitor? A review of our experience with severe head injury. J Neurosurg 56: 650–659.

[41] Lundberg N, Troupp H, Lorin H (1965) Continuous recording of the ventricular-fluid pressure in patients with severe acute traumatic brain injury. A preliminary report. J Neurosurg 22:581–590.

[42] Marshall LF, Smith RW, Shapiro HM (1979) The outcome with aggressive treatment in severe head injuries. Part I: the significance of intracranial pressure monitoring. J Neurosurg 50:20–25.

[43] Narayan RK, Greenberg RP, Miller JD, Enas GG, Choi SC, Kishore PR, Selhorst JB, Lutz HA 3rd, Becker DP (1981) Improved confidence of outcome prediction in severe head injury. A comparative analysis of the clinical examination, multimodality evoked potentials, CT scanning, and intracranial pressure. J Neurosurg 54:751–762.

[44] Eisenberg HM, Frankowski RF, Contant CF, Marshall LF, Walker MD (1988) High-dose barbiturate control of elevated intracranial pressure in patients with severe head injury. J Neurosurg 69: 15–23.

[45] Howells T, Elf K, Jones P, Ronne-Engström E, Piper I, Nilsson P, Andrews P, Enblad P (2005) Pressure reactivity as a guide in the treatment of cerebral perfusion pressure in patients with brain trauma. J Neurosurg 102:311–317.

[46] Saul TG, Ducker TB (1982) Effect of intracranial pressure monitoring and aggressive treatment on mortality in severe head injury. J Neurosurg 56:498–503.

[47] Timofeev I, Kirkpatrick P, Corteen E, Hiler M, Czosnyka M, Menon DK, Pickard JD, Hutchinson PJ (2006) Decompressive craniectomy in traumatic brain injury: outcome following protocol-driven therapy. Acta Neurochir Suppl 96:11–16.

[48] Stochetti N, Furlan A, Volta F (1996) Hypoxemia and arterial hypotension at the accident scene in head injury. J Trauma 40:764–767.

[49] Auer RN (2001) Non-pharmacologic (physiologic) neuroprotection in the treatment of brain ischemia. Ann N Y Acad Sci 939:271-82.

[50] Jones PA, Andrews PJ, Midgley S, Anderson SI, Piper IR, Tocher JL, Housley AM, Corrie JA, Slattery J, Dearden NM (1994) Measuring the burden of secondary insults in head injured patients during intensive care. J Neurosurg Anesthesiol 6:4–14.

[51] Paul RL, Polanco O, Turney SZ McAslan TC, Cowley RA. (1972) Intracranial pressure responses to alterations in arterial carbon dioxide pressure in patients with head injuries. J Neurosurg 36:714-720.

[52] Coles JP, Minhas PS, Fryer TD, Smielewski P, Aigbirihio F, Donovan T, Downey SP, Williams G, Chatfield D, Matthews JC, Gupta AK, Carpenter TA, Clark JC, Pickard JD, Menon DK (2002) Effect of hyperventilation on cerebral blood flow in traumatic head injury: clinical relevance and monitoring correlates. Crit Care Med 30(9): 1950-1959.

[53] Holland MC, Mackersie RC, Morabito D, Campbell AR, Kivett VA, Patel R, Erickson VR, Pittet JF (2003) The development of acute lung injury is associated with worse neurologic outcome in patients with severe traumatic brain injury. J Trauma 55:106-111.

[54] Bratton SL, Davis RL (1997) Acute lung injury in isolated traumatic brain injury.Neurosurgery 40:707-712.

[55] The Acute Respiratory Distress Syndrome Network (2000) Ventilation with lower tidal volumes as compared with traditional tidal volumes for acute lung injury and the acute respiratory distress syndrome. N Engl J Med 342:1301-1308.

[56] Chesnut RM, Marshall SB, Piek J, Blunt BA, Klauber MR, Marshall LF. (1993) Early and late systemic hypotension as a frequent and fundamental source of cerebral ischemia following severe brain injury in the Traumatic Coma Data Bank. Acta Neurochir Suppl (Wien) 59:121–5.

[57] Manley G, Knudson MM, Morabito D, Damron S, Erickson V, Pitts L (2001) Hypotension, hypoxia, and head injury: frequency, duration, and consequences. Arch Surg 136:1118-1123.

[58] Clifton GL, Miller ER, Choi SC, Levin HS (2002) Fluid thresholds and outcome from severe brain injury. Crit Care Med 30:739–745.

[59] Robertson CS, Valadka AB, Hannay HJ, Contant CF, Gopinath SP, Cormio M, Uzura M, Grossman RG (1999) Prevention of secondary ischemic insults after severe head injury. Crit Care Med 27:2086–2095.

[60] Muizelaar JP, Wei EP, Kontos HA, Becker DP (1983) Mannitol causes compensatory cerebral vasoconstriction in response to blood viscosity changes. J Neurosurg 59:822-8.

[61] Marshall LF, Smith RW, Rauscher LA, Shapiro HM (1978) Mannitol dose requirements in brain-injured patients. J Neurosurg 48:169-172.

[62] Wise BL, Perkins RK, Stevenson E, Scott KG (1964) Penetration of C14-labelled mannitol from serum into cerebrospinal fluid and brain. Exp Neurol 10:264-270.

[63] Better OS, Rubinstein I, Winaver JM, Knochel JP (1997) Mannitol therapy revisited (1940-1997). Kidney Int 52:886-94.

[64] Manninen PH, Lam AM, Gelb AW, Brown SC (1987) The effect of high dose mannitol on serum and urine electrolytes and osmolality inneurosurgical patients. Can J Anaesth 34:442-446.

[65] Hijiya N, Horiuchi K, Asakura T (1991) Morphology of sickle cells produced in solutions of varying osmolarities. J Lab Clin Med 117:60–66.

[66] Vialet R, Albanèse J, Thomachot L, Antonini F, Bourgouin A, Alliez B, Martin C (2003) Isovolume hypertonic solutes (sodium chloride or mannitol) in the treatment of refractory posttraumatic intracranial hypertension: 2 mL/kg 7.5% saline is more effective than 2 mL/kg 20% mannitol. Crit Care Med 31:1683–1687.

[67] Battison C, Andrews PJ, Graham C, Petty T (2005) Randomized, controlled trial on the effect of a 20% mannitol solution and a 7.5% saline/6% dextran solution on increased intracranial pressure after brain injury. Crit Care Med 33:196–202.

[68] Kamel H, Navi BB, Nakagawa K, Hemphill JC 3rd, Ko NU (2011) Hypertonic saline versus mannitol for the treatment of elevated intracranial pressure: A meta-analysis of randomized clinical trials. Crit Care Med 39:554–559.

[69] Mortazavi MM, Romeo AK, Deep A, Griessenauer CJ, Shoja MM, Tubbs RS, Fisher W (2012) Hypertonic saline for treating raised intracranial pressure: Literature review with meta-analysis. J Neurosurg 116:210–221.

[70] Censullo JL, Sebastian S (2003) Pentobarbital sodium coma for refractory intracranial hypertension. J Neurosci Nurs 35(5):252-62.

[71] Roberts I (2005) Barbiturates for acute traumatic brain injury. The Cochrane Library Volume 4.

[72] Povlishock JT, Wei EP (2009) Posthypothermic rewarming considerations following traumatic brain injury. J Neurotrauma 26:333–340.

[73] Polderman,Kees H (2008) Induced hypothermia and fever control for prevention and treatment of neurological injuries. Lancet 371: 1955–69.

[74] Albrecht RFII, Wass CT, Lanier WL (1998) Occurrence of potentially detrimental temperature alterations in hospitalized patients at risk for brain injury. Mayo Clin Proc 73(7):629–35.

[75] Geffroy A, Bronchard R, Merckx P, Seince PF, Faillot T, Albaladejo P, Marty J (2004) Severe traumatic head injury in adults: which patients are at risk of early hyperthermia? Intensive Care Med 30(5):785–90.

[76] Suz P, Vavilala MS, Souter M, Muangman S, Lam AM (2006) Clinical features of fever associated with poor outcome in severe pediatric traumatic brain injury. J Neurosurg Anesthesiol 18(1):5– 10.

[77] Diringer MN, Reaven NL, Funk SE, Uman GC (2004) Elevated body temperature independently contributes to increased length of stay in neurologic intensive care unit patients. Crit Care Med 32(7):1489–95.

[78] Charrueau C, Belabed L, Besson V, Chaumeil JC, Cynober L, Moinard C (2009) Metabolic response and nutritional support in traumatic brain injury: evidence for resistance to renutrition. J Neurotrauma 26(11):1911–20.

[79] Krakau K, Omne-Ponten M, Karlsson T, Borg J (2006) Metabolism and nutrition in patients with moderate and severe traumatic brain injury: a systematic review. Brain Inj 20(4):345–67.

[80] Sacks GS, Brown RO, Teague D, Dickerson RN, Tolley EA, Kudsk KA (1995) Early nutrition support modifies immune function in patients sustaining severe head injury. JPEN J Parenter Enteral Nutr 19(5):387–92.

[81] Ha°rtl R, Gerber LM, Ni Q, Ghajar J (2008) Effect of early nutrition on deaths due to severe traumatic brain injury. J Neurosurg 109(1):50–6.

[82] McClave SA, Martindale RG, Vanek VW, McCarthy M, Roberts P, Taylor B, Ochoa JB, Napolitano L, Cresci G; A.S.P.E.N. Board of Directors; American College of Critical Care Medicine; Society of Critical Care Medicine (2009) Guidelines for the provision and assessment of nutrition support therapy in the adult critically ill patient: Society of Critical Care Medicine (SCCM) and American Society for Parenteral and Enteral Nutrition (A.S.P.E.N.). JPEN J Parenter Enteral Nutr 33(3):277–316.

[83] Kreymann KG, Berger MM, Deutz NEP, Deutz NE, Hiesmayr M, Jolliet P, Kazandjiev G, Nitenberg G, van den Berghe G, Wernerman J; DGEM (German Society for Nutritional Medicine), Ebner C, Hartl W, Heymann C, Spies C; ESPEN (European So-

ciety for Parenteral and Enteral Nutrition) (2006) ESPEN guidelines on enteral nutrition: intensive care. Clin Nutr 25 (2):210–23.

[84] Rovlias A, Kotsou S (2000) The influence of hyperglycemia on neurological outcome in patients with severe head injury. Neurosurgery 46:335–342; discussion 42–43.

[85] Jeremitsky E, Omert LA, Dunham CM, Wilberger J, Rodriguez A (2005) The impact of hyperglycemia on patients with severe brain injury. J Trauma 58:47–50.

[86] Hayes RL, Katayama Y, Jenkins LW, Lyeth BG, Clifton GL, Gunter J, Povlishock JT, Young HF (1988) Regional rates of glucose utilization in the cat following concussive head injury. J Neurotrauma; 5:121–137.

[87] Bergsneider M, Hovda DA, Shalmon E, Kelly DF, Vespa PM, Martin NA, Phelps ME, McArthur DL, Caron MJ, Kraus JF, Becker DP (1997) Cerebral hyperglycolysis following severe traumatic brain injury in humans: A positron emission tomography study. J Neurosurg; 86:241–251.

[88] Oddo M, Schmidt JM, Carrera E, Badjatia N, Connolly ES, Presciutti M, Ostapkovich ND, Levine JM, Le Roux P, Mayer SA (2008) Impact of tight glycemic control on cerebral glucose metabolism after severe brain injury: a microdialysis study. Crit Care Med 36(12):3233-8.

[89] Jacobi J, Bircher N, Krinsley J, Agus M, Braithwaite SS, Deutschman C, Freire AX, Geehan D, Kohl B, Nasraway SA, Rigby M, Sands K, Schallom L, Taylor B, Umpierrez G, Mazuski J, Schunemann H (2012) Guidelines for the use of an insulin infusion for the management of hyperglycemia in critically ill patients. Crit Care Med 40(12): 3251-76.

[90] Sadaka F (2012) Red Blood Cell Transfusion in Sepsis: A Review. J Blood Disord Transfus S4:001.

[91] Carlson AP, Schermer CR, Lu SW (2006) Retrospective evaluation of anemia and transfusion in traumatic brain injury. J Trauma 61:567–571.

[92] McIntyre LA, Fergusson DA, Hutchison JS, Pagliarello G, Marshall JC, Yetisir E, Hare GM, Hébert PC (2006) Effect of a liberal versus restrictive transfusion strategy on mortality in patients with moderate to severe head injury. Neurocrit Care 5:4–9.

[93] Napolitano LM, Kurek S, Luchette FA, Anderson GL, Bard MR, Bromberg W, Chiu WC, Cipolle MD, Clancy KD, Diebel L, Hoff WS, Hughes KM, Munshi I, Nayduch D, Sandhu R, Yelon JA, Corwin HL, Barie PS, Tisherman SA, Hebert PC; EAST Practice Management Workgroup; American College of Critical Care Medicine (ACCM) Taskforce of the Society of Critical Care Medicine (SCCM) (2009) Clinical practice guideline: red blood cell transfusion in adult trauma and critical care. J Trauma 67(6): 1439-42.

[94] Agnelli G, Piovella F, Buoncristiani P, Severi P, Pini M, D'Angelo A, Beltrametti C, Damiani M, Andrioli GC, Pugliese R, Iorio A, Brambilla G (1998) Enoxaparin plus

compression stokings compared with compression stockings alone in the prevention of venous thromboembolism after elective neurosurgery. New Engl. J. Med 339: 80-85.

[95] Dudley RR, Aziz I, Bonnici A, Saluja RS, Lamoureux J, Kalmovitch B, Gursahaney A, Razek T, Maleki M, Marcoux J (2010) Early Venous Thromboembolic Event Prophylaxis in Traumatic Brain Injury with Low-Molecular-Weight Heparin: Risks and Benefits. J of Neurotrauma 27: 2165-2172.

[96] Phelan HA, Wolf SE, Norwood SH, Aldy K, Brakenridge SC, Eastman AL, Madden CJ, Nakonezny PA, Yang L, Chason DP, Arbique GM, Berne J, Minei JP (2012) A randomized, double-blinded, placebo-controlled pilot trial of anticoagulation in low-risk traumatic brain injury: The Delayed Versus Early Enoxaparin Prophylaxis I (DEEP I) study. J Trauma Acute Care Surg 73(6):1434-1441.

[97] Jamjoom, A. A B., Jamjoom, A. B. (2013) Safety and Efficacy of Early Pharmacological Thromboprophylaxis in Traumatic Brain Injury: Systematic Review and Meta-Analysis. J of Neurotrauma 30:1-9.

8

Physiotherapeutic Procedures for the Treatment of Contractures in Subjects with Traumatic Brain Injury (TBI)

Fernando Salierno, María Elisa Rivas,
Pablo Etchandy, Verónica Jarmoluk, Diego Cozzo,
Martín Mattei, Eliana Buffetti,
Leonardo Corrotea and Mercedes Tamashiro

---

1. Introduction

Contractures limit free joint movement and are common a consequence of traumatic brain injury. They interfere with activities of daily living and can cause pain, pressure areas, and result in unsightly deformities [1 - 4], affecting patient quality of life and increasing institutionalization rates. Contractures also cause significant secondary impairment which ultimately interferes with the rehabilitation process. Their treatment is therefore an integral part of physical recovery. Before effective intervention can take place, therapists must first determine both the primary cause as well as the specific structures involved. Several different therapeutic modalities exist to treat them, and choice of which to apply will depend on each individual case [5].

The aim of this chapter therefore is to review currently available physical therapy techniques for the treatment of contractures and for prevention of deformity development, in subjects suffering traumatic brain injury (TBI).

2. Generalities

Contractures are a common complication of traumatic brain injury and may occur in up to 84% of cases [4, 6]. The most commonly affected joints are: the hip, shoulder, ankle, elbow and knee, with a significant percentage of patients developing contractures in five or more joints [4].

For purposes of this chapter, we define contracture as any degree of loss in joint range of motion restricting activities of daily living[4]. Movement restriction is not limited only to joints, but will also affect many other body structures including skin, subcutaneous tissue, muscles, tendons, ligaments, joint capsules, vessels and nerves [7].

Contractures are characterized by reduced range of motion (ROM) and increased stiffness. The increased resistance to stretch caused by changes in the mechanical properties of tissues is due to both neurally and non-neurally mediated factors [8, 9]. Non-neural factors include changes in mechanical properties of tissue resulting from stress deprivation, and may be secondary to orthopedic injury, heterotopic ossification, use of a splint or plaster, pain, paralysis, severe spasticity or any disorder that restricts movement. [10]. Contractures also produce structural changes within muscles; myofibril shortening and loss of sarcomeres are often observed, as well as relative increase in connective tissue causing loss of elasticity.

Neural factors are of central origin and cause muscle overactivity. They generate spasticity, increasing interdigitation between actin and myosin, thus reducing muscular concentric contraction range and producing rigidity, as a result of the absence of monosynaptic reflex inhibition [9, 11].

3. Evaluation and diagnosis

Evaluation of patients with head trauma includes examination of joint range of motion, looking for possible contractures. Prior to physical exam, it is important to record general patient posture (decortication, decerebration, etc.) and clinical condition, and especially to register any hyperexcitability such as spasms or clonus triggered by intense stimulation in patients with sensory impairment.

Joints should be observed at rest in order to establish whether muscle overactivity or flaccidity is present; next, voluntary movement should be examined, and presence of dystonia when changing positions recorded, if elicited [12]. These findings are important because contracture development in patients with TBI is related to presence of spasticity and/or dystonia[13]. Joint examination is performed systematically, mobilizing each joint manually and passively. In patients able to follow verbal commands and perform active movements, it is important to encourage them to move each segment to the widest possible range.

Once manual examination has been completed, findings in individual joints should be recorded including quality of resistance and end feel, which refers to examiner perception of a barrier to further motion when exerting passive ROM. For better diagnosis or evaluation, passive range of motion may be measured using an instrument such as a goniometer or applying other objective methods. The universal goniometer (UG) is simple and easy-to-use. Result reliability is acceptable, but only after appropriate user training and always applying standardized measuring methods [14, 15].

When loss of range of motion is detected, differential diagnosis needs to be established between lack of range due to motor deficit (muscle overactivity) or resulting from structural alterations. Clinical assessment of hypertonia can be conducted using a well-established rating scale, the Modified Ashworth Scale. However therapists should be aware that this scale does not distinguish between soft tissue and neural contributions to hypertonia [16]. To make this differential diagnosis, the contracture segments need to be re-mobilized at different speeds in order to unmask muscle overactivity, which if present, can be rated using the Modified Tardieu Scale. This scale is widely used because it renders both quantitative and qualitative measurement of spasticity. Its validity has been studied and has demonstrated high intra and inter-rater reliability when using a standardized protocol. It is highly reliable for assessing spasticity in hamstrings, rectus femoris, gastrocnemius, soleus and tibialis anterior muscles in adults with neurological injury. It has also shown very good intra rater reliability for elbow flexors [17 - 18].

Other important factors that need to be considered in the individual patient and factored into the therapeutic decision-making process include: periods of prolonged bedrest, presence of subcortical lesions, and decreased levels of awareness or lack of voluntary activity in the presence of muscle overactivity, as they are all indicators of greater lesional complexity. Yarkony et al. postulate contracture as clinically evident when coma extends beyond three weeks [4]. Severity of contracture is also generally more pronounced in patients with brainstem lesions and treatment usually begins later and will require more time to achieve gains in ROM [19].

Therefore, one can expect coma patients to suffer greater structural changes in muscle tissues both because of worse neurological status as well as absence of voluntary movement countering effects of immobility.

Motor control and presence of spasticity are important. For example, if no underlying motor control is present and spasticity is not reduced after contracture treatment, probability of sustaining improvement is poor [19]. In contrast, presence of voluntary motor control in muscles antagonist to the contracture, increase the likelihood of maintaining any ROM gain [20].

Cognitive impairment will also influence rehabilitation therapy choice. Sometimes, cognitive impairment may interfere with patient ability to cooperate and interpret pain[19].

Similarly, patients presenting preserved cognitive status, voluntary motor control and minimal or no muscle overactivity, will attain better treatment outcomes.

Once a thorough evaluation has been completed, a treatment plan can be individually designed and the most appropriate technique chosen to treat or prevent contracture. Treatment should be specifically adapted to each patient and will require constant reassessment in light of changes occurring in the course of recovering from head injuries. See table 1.

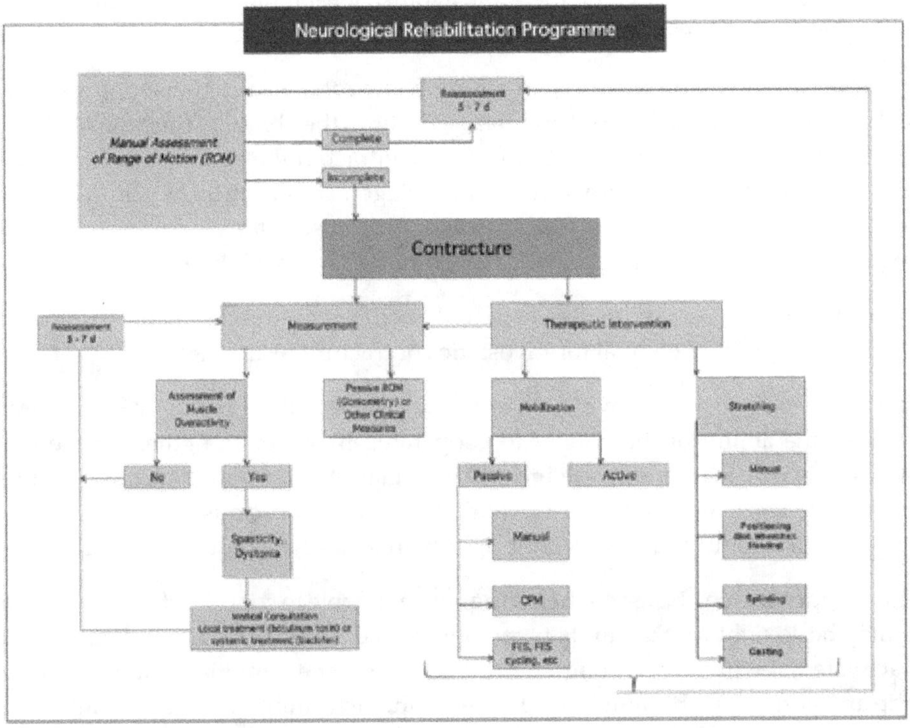

Table 1. Clinical reasoning and therapeutic choice for the contracture. CPM, continuous passive motion. FES, functional electrical stimulation. 5 – 7d, 5 - 7days.

4. Therapeutic modalities

Stretch is one of the most widely used techniques for treatment and prevention of contractures. Its aim is to increase joint mobility and it can be self-administered or applied manually by therapists. Splints, positioning programs or casts changed at regular intervals (serial casting) can also be used. All methods involve mechanical elongation of soft tissues during varying lengths of time. Some can only be applied for short periods, such as manually applied elongations, performed for only a few minutes at a time. Others, such as splints and plasters are used to stretch muscles for longer periods, and sometimes to provide uninterrupted elongation for days or even weeks.

5. Stretching

Research in physiotherapy and neurophysiology has led to the development of some alternatives to passive stretching. Cherry[10] described four approaches to reduce contractures, namely: activating or strengthening the weak agonist, local inhibition, general inhibition and passive lengthening, some of which may be used simultaneously.

The first approach involves activating or strengthening the weak agonist opposing the tight muscle. If tissue innervation is intact and the agonist has the ability to function at all, a double benefit will be gained by improving its ability to contract. If the agonist becomes stronger, it will be able to counter the contracture of the antagonist and pull the joint through more complete range. Also, the contracted muscle (antagonist) will be reciprocally inhibited, allowing itself to be stretched because the stretch reflex is also inhibited.

If the weak agonist can be activated and strengthened, better muscle balance around the joint may result, reducing the potential for myostatic contracture recurrence.

Selection of a technique to strengthen the weak muscle will depend on the nature of the problem and the ability of the patient to cooperate. Effective strengthening methods that employ resistance or load on muscle include maximal resistance in diagonal spiral patterns and progressive resistance exercises. Methods that use unconscious automatic responses to activate the weak agonist require eliciting righting reactions and equilibrium responses.

The second approach may be used when an agonist is unable to contract at all, or the antagonist muscle may be so tight that attempts to strengthen the agonist fail. Also, even if the agonist can be activated, it will move through more complete range of motion if the stretch reflex of the tight antagonist can be inhibited. In this approach, inhibition of the tight muscle is considered. The propioceptive neuromuscular facilitation techniques, such as contraction-relaxation or hold-relax may be used to inhibit the tight muscle selectively, so it will tolerate being stretched without immediate activation of the stretch reflex.

Local inhibition is useful for localized tightness, especially within one muscle group at a single joint, such as after plaster immobilization following injury or surgery. Techniques generating inhibition to the contracted muscle include vibration of the opposite muscle group, prolonged icing and hold-relax, used in traditional rehabilitation.

A third approach to reduce hypertonus, in a single limb or throughout the whole body, consists in allowing tight spastic muscle groups to relax and be lengthened. Some concepts as neuro-developmental treatment (NDT) consider that movement control is achieved in an integrated way when the nervous system works cooperatively. For example the organization of postural systems require interaction between external forces (gravity), body mechanics and kinetics, multisensory inputs, and adaptative responses to voluntary movements. Therefore, inhibition of hypertonus is best when the patient participates actively.

The fourth approach is passive lengthening. If passive lengthening is selected as the appropriate alternative, there are two techniques that may be applied. One involves manual passive stretching and the other prolonged holding of the desired position at the point of maximum tolerated length of the contracted muscle.

Passive stretching is likely to be most effective in individuals whose stretch reflex is inhibited by cortical effect or by peripheral nerve injury.

Adaptative equipment may enable an individual to function more readily in certain positions, for example use of a prone standing board for hip and knee extension, to align lower limb joints in weight bearing patients with lower limb flexor problems. Also, positions for sitting, sleeping, and other daily activities, useful in correcting contracture, can be adopted and held for prolonged periods.

Other techniques of passive lengthening include standing, orthosis, splints and casts with prolonged holding. All require close monitoring (see below). Generally, patients with head trauma present severe injuries. It is very common to find extremely weak agonist muscles to work with, or to attempt to generate antagonist tone inhibition on. When these techniques are employed it is important to consider that any increase in range obtained by forced motion will be lost unless it is maintained by active motion or by use of supportive devices.

6. Standing

TBI patients can be supported while standing using a tilt table, standing frame and\or knee extension splints. Regular standing in the correct position will maintain sufficient range of dorsal flexion of the ankle joint for walking when the patient reaches that stage but, if he has not been made to get out of bed from the beginning; his Achilles tendon may have already shortened [21]. In our experience, the first option for patients with more severe motor deficits or disorders of consciousness is the tilt table. Special attention must be paid to the knee and ankle. If the knee has full range, it should be positioned in slight flexion or in a neutral stance. The ankle must be able to bear sufficient weight on the rearfoot without causing tissue damage or increasing muscle overactivity.

The second option is the standing frame. Patient can be supported in upright position by a solid frame with padded struts in front of his knees to keep them extended and a broad strap behind his hips to prevent them from flexing. Using the standing frame may be useful when the patient has regained consciousness and is able to extend his trunk actively, because it is then possible for him to stand for longer periods.

The third option is standing assisted by the therapist, recommended for patients with better functional status and trunk control. If necessary, extension knee splints can be used to prevent lower limbs from giving way due to lack of motor activity. Knee extension splints should reach from about 8 cm below the ischial tuberosity to 4cm above the malleoli. Made of a firm posterior shell of plaster of Paris or some other hard material, knee-extension splints will need to be bandaged in place with two 10cm wide crepe bandages to give adequate support and maintain optimal leg positioning. Patient should be lying in supine position while therapist bandages on the splints, to be able to correct any inward or outward rotation of the limb [21].

When the patient has marked spasticity in the plantar flexors of the foot, standing upright is often the only way in which therapists can maintain range of ankle dorsiflexion and prevent shortening of the Achilles tendon [21].

In case of equinus deformity that does not allow the heel to contact the ground, a posting on the foot, AFO (anke-foot orthosis) or shoe is needed. Posting entails construction of an interface between the aligned foot and the ground to optimize heel loading and hip and knee alignment while standing or walking (filling in the space under the heel when the ankle is positioned in plantarflexion) [22].

When standing the patient up, one must consider alignment of the pelvis in the frontal plane, since use of a post will be shorten contra-lateral limb length. This must be compensated with an additional pad under the contra-lateral heel, high enough to correct pelvic alignment.

There is evidence to support placing patients in the standing position to prevent loss of calf muscle length. In severe brain trauma cases where little functional recovery is expected, maintaining patient physical condition is challenging. In this context, long term effects of supported standing to maintain muscle length appear more important. Although often prescribed, effectiveness of standing programmes carried out over months or even years remains unknown. Standing may prevent small losses of ankle dorsiflexion, but clinical importance of these effects is uncertain. Future studies should investigate standing in a wider range of settings. Evaluating potential multidimensional effects of standing using standardized measures would provide greater insight and be more effective than studies focused on a single outcome [23].

7. Splinting – Orthosis

Use of splinting for both prevention and reduction of contractures is recommended following traumatic brain injury [24]. Alternatively, orthosis also reduces contractures through prolonged low-load stretch, maintaining joints lengthened [25]. Therapists who apply a biomechanical treatment rationale recommend splinting both to prevent as well as manage length-associated changes in muscles and connective tissue.

7.1. Types of splints and outcome

Splints of various forms, often combined with other passive and/or active tissue 'stretching' procedures (e.g. passive movements, positioning, weight-bearing), are the treatment of choice for physiotherapists. General goals of therapy seek to inhibit/reduce increased muscle tone and/or elongate shortened soft tissues. In the case of some splints, an additional goal may be improving/maintaining appropriate biomechanical limb positioning during (later) functional activity retraining, such as walking [24].

Elongation effects obtained can be sustained by using splints overnight. Advantages to wearing a night splint are: overnight intervention which allows therapy time to be spent on active retraining of everyday tasks, ease of application, and perhaps most importantly, continued long term use after discharge from hospital. The main disadvantage is the risk of pressure sores, particularly when patients have poor vascular supply and/or sensation in the affected areas [26]. It is important for the therapist to monitor splint use with the interdisciplinary team. When indicating a night orthosis, patient tolerance and adherence to use should be closely controlled. In the presence of adverse effects the splint should be removed immediately and its indication reassessed.

A published case report illustrating lower limb orthosis implementation described use of a static adjustable ankle orthosis, placed after administration of a phenol nerve block in conjunction with stretching, strengthening and functional mobility training. The adjustable orthosis was applied to provide low-load prolonged stretch of the ankle and address apparent soft tissue shortening, and the phenol nerve block was administered to address ROM limitations secondary to muscle spasm [27]. Positive results reported in this case would support orthosis as an addition to standard physical therapy stretching regimens in patients with brain injury.

Other published evidence indicates that overnight splinting of an affected ankle in subjects with stroke appears to be as effective as standing on a tilt table in preventing contracture at the ankle [26].

In our experience an alternative intervention to prevent ankle contractures is use of an overnight splint. Although the ankle is not usually positioned in maximum dorsiflexion, the extra time spent in this position helps avoid contracture development.

Indication for upper limb splint placement is common, mostly at rest to keep the joint in extended position, thus halting further shortening.

According to Lannin [27], night splinting the hand in the functional resting position does not produce clinically useful effects in adults with acquired brain impairment who receive a daily stretching programme. In his discussion, the author postulates absence of effect after splint use may have been because routine motor training and upper limb stretch were maintaining muscle length. Therefore, additional stretching provided by the night splint may have been redundant.

Sometimes, therapists indicate additional electric stimulation and splinting for contracture management, but it is not clear if it is more effective than splinting alone after acquired brain injury [28].

7.2. Evidence and conclusion

There is insufficient evidence to either support or refute effectiveness of orthotic devices for contracture treatment or prevention. Further research is needed for better understanding of the influence of elongation on soft tissue, as well as with respect to timing, length of application and efficacy of splinting programmes. In conclusion, splinting options should be carefully analyzed in TBI patients as they may represent a clinically effective strategy when used appropriately.

8. Casting

Casts are a viable option for treating contractures after upper motor neuron injury in adults [19, 30]. These are non-removable external devices, made of plaster or casting tape, applied with intention to change structural or functional characteristics of the neuromuscular system [31]. Casting to control hypertonus (understood as increased resistance to passive movement as a result of spasticity and/or changes in muscular and connective tissue characteristics) was first described in the 1960's in the treatment of children with cerebral palsy [20, 32]. Later, casts were applied to adults with acquired brain injury with different therapeutic objectives. These goals include preventing loss of joint range, helping to cure pressure ulcers associated with severe spasticity, restoration of articular range (ROM) and muscle length, and inhibition of hyperexcitability [20].

Different theories have been proposed to explain underlying neurophysiological and mechanical mechanisms behind the positive effects of plasters, on hyperexcitability reflexes and mechanical changes [32].

The first hypothesis relates to neurophysiology. Plasters prevent changes in muscle length by eliminating excitatory input to muscle receptors, which in turn reduces spasticity. Prolonged elongation stimulates Golgi tendon organs and subsequently afferent Ib fibers, creating an inhibitory response in alpha motor neurons. Type II muscle afferents have also been postulated as inhibitors of alpha motor neurons following prolonged elongation [32]. Casts may also reduce spastic muscle tone through alleviation or reduction of tactile input, proprioceptive input, and temperature receptors. Uninterrupted contact provided by the cast, including the neutral pressure and heat generated, reduces excitability of alpha and gamma motor neurons at the spinal cord level [30 - 32].

A second hypothesis is based on biomechanics. It postulates that casts achieve low load elongation during prolonged periods, able to prevent and correct contractures. Casts are usually applied at the end of joint range of motion because prolonged stretch with low load, generating permanent changes in soft tissues. It has been well established that with prolonged immobilization, specific physiologic changes occur involving connective tissue and muscle remodeling. This remodeling is mediated by fibroblasts in response to physical forces. When a muscle is immobilized in a stretched position, the number and length of sarcomeres in series increases, thus changing the muscle tension / length ratio. Connective tissue is also extended through a process of disorganization of the fibrous matrix [30].

The third hypothesis refers to motor learning. It proposes that casts provide adequate support to proximal joints, until patient gains enough distal control [31]. The external stability provided by the cast to the limb is presumed to allow the patient to receive normal sensory input with appropriate weight bearing and normal reflex patterns, helping to develop normal movement and accommodation in the central nervous system [32].

8.1. Types of casts

Different casts used in TBI patient rehabilitation and described in the literature include: serial casts, inhibitive cast, drop out casts and bivalved casts [30]. Specific types of cast are important in treating contractures and indications will depend on patient characteristics and level of functional recovery.

Serial casting involves application and removal of a series of casts resulting in progressive range of motion increase with the introduction of each cast. Serial casting allows 24 hour a day elongation, with casts changed regularly to maintain gain as the joint becomes more mobile [33].

Inhibition cast. The purpose of an inhibitory cast application is to maintain a position, to reduce spasticity and facilitate improvements in motor function. Inhibitory casts seek to provide stability and inhibition to the treated joint. The inhibition may be achieved by normalizing proprioceptive input, joint alignment, and weight load. Effects of these casts do not seem to last long after they are removed; for this reason, inhibitory casts resulting in a positive impact on functional performance need to be followed by use of an inhibitory splint during a prolonged period [30].

Functional drop out casts are the combination of serial casting and inhibitory casts. When making a functional cast, a portion of a cylindrical cast is removed to allow the involved joint to move beyond the desired range, preventing the joint from pushing back toward the contracted position. This allows passive or active movement in the desired direction and allows the user to gain additional active range while using a cast. These casts also allow application of electrical stimulation or other facilitation techniques [30].

Bivalved casts are casts cut in two halves (front and back), which are then filled and padded at the edges to allow reapplication. Usually this is done when the patient has achieved the desired range and needs to maintain the new position. This is required when tone in the involved limb remains high and there is doubt whether a traditional splint will resist and keep the muscle in the desired position. Bivalved casts provide full contact and have the advantage that they can be removed for hygiene, inspection, active movement, and other dynamic activities [30].

The main indications for use of any type of plaster in general, and of serial casting in particular, is permanent limitation of range of motion [19], or immobility during muscle function only. If other disorders such as muscle weakness or overactivity of some kind are present, these will influence both plastering technique as well as length of treatment.

8.2. Application procedure

The cast-making process follows a basic preparation which adapts to any plastering technique, and consists first in the placement of soft materials such stockinette, foam and cast padding. to protect the skin and bony prominences and avoid friction and pressure points, followed by application of a plaster bandage (fiberglass and/or plaster cast) to achieve the necessary hardness to fix the limb in the desired position.

There two basic objectives sought after by the procedure: to place tension on the muscle and maintain the pressure during a pre established time period.

Tension levels will vary depending on which theory the therapy is based on. If we consider the biomechanics theory, plasters are applied on final range in order to gain maximum length. Neurophysiology-based theory considers tension levels should stretch the joint to within 5 degrees of final existing range. Variability in studies on angle used to make the cast range from 5° and 10° under full range, to neutral, to end of available range. This last option is the one with higher levels of evidence to support it [31]. In our experience, we prefer to use end of range for plaster application. The force applied to elongate the muscle is usually limited by patient pain threshold [31].

With respect to duration of application, it is highly variable, and will depend on the treatment objective and on how much time is needed to achieve the desired effect. There is significant discrepancy in the literature over total length of treatment between published studies [30]. Some publications suggest shorter implementation generates fewer complications and similar results [31].

Significant variation also exists in relation to length of time between cast changes. Duration of casting generally should reflect the pace at which the individual is making progress and the goals of the casting. Tardieu and Tardieu recommend lengthening via casting should be very gradual because careless application may result in muscle fiber break down, but they do not give specific time frames or guidelines. If the patient is experiencing slower progress or is at lower risk for breakdown or complications, casts can be left on longer between changes; this is particularly true if a cast is difficult to apply because of time constraints, cost, patient agitation, or patient need for medication during the switch. If the individual seems to be progressing rapidly or is at increased risk for skin breakdown, if the cast is damaged or wet, or if there is any other concern, it should be changed more frequently [30].

In a serial casting program, we start by placing an initial plaster at rest. This is applied with the extremity positioned at the end of the movement range, but easily reached without applying additional tension. Generally, we use 3 or 4 progressive casts [19]. Some authors such as Davies recommend 6 changes on average [21].

Authors suggest mobilizing passively through the entire range of motion available to maintain full mobility of all immobilized joints and then apply a new cast at a greater angle [23]. In contrast, Davies [21] does not mobilize in between casts, to avoid any chance on losing the range gained. Currently, there is no agreement on whether the extremity should or should not be mobilized between each change of plaster.

The last cast in the series is the supporting or positioning cast. It is cut in two halves making it bivalved, like an anterior-posterior splint [19]. This splint is used in the resting position for as long as deemed necessary until the patient improves and gradually stops using the equipment[19, 20]. If the patient´s muscles are still weak and present overactivity, it is important to continue using the device overnight [19].

Cast progression should be discontinued when there is no further gain of range. Although there is no consensus between authors on this point, some suggest that progression can be interrupted if no quantifiable gain is achieved after two consecutive applications. Others suggest stopping if there is no measurable gain (<5 ° measured with goniometer) in maximum range after three consecutive plaster changes. [20] If the team decides to end the application, it is important the patient be examined by a physician to consider the possibility of orthopedic surgery [20].

Therefore, application, duration and frequency of change will need to be individualized, defining for each protocol: timing, whether it will be a single plaster or several, how often casts will be changed, when joint range will be progressively increased and finally, total duration of single or serial casting [31].

8.3. Precautions, complications and contraindications

There are a number of precautions to consider before placing a cast. With respect to the patient it is important to take into account skin integrity, presence of fluctuating edema, decreased sensitivity, cognitive impairment and agitation [19, 30]. Therapist experience will contribute to establish level of existing complications and whether these can be managed and still continue with the cast. For some authors contracture treatment has priority over any skin condition, because they argue that it can help heal skin lesions [21]. Fluctuating edema and sensitivity disorders can be managed with frequent controls after application and if necessary the plaster may be removed at any time.

In cases of cognitive disorders and agitation, sedation or use of restraints have been described in the literature, so that the patient does not hurt himself or others during the placing of the plaster and is careful while wearing it [21].

Casting contraindications include: uncontrolled hypertension and/or elevated intracranial pressure, open wounds, external fixation or unresolved fractures, ligament injuries, need for access to check vital signs, recent episodes of autonomic dysreflexia, circulatory disorders such as deep vein thrombosis (DVT), acute inflammation, heterotopic ossification [19, 30, 33, 34], tone fluctuation or any unstable medical condition [31]. Some authors also exclude pregnant patients [34].

Adverse effects and/or complications should be considered. Close monitoring, assessing sensitivity, motion, blood flow, skin indemnity and the presence of inflammation is always recommended, checking for presence of vasoconstriction or discoloration of fingers or toes [33]. Temporary discoloration is quite common, but if it persists for more than 20 or 30 seconds, plaster should be removed and a new one applied [19]. It should be noted that patients often report less adverse effects than therapists [33].

In a study by Moseley, adverse effects reported included skin irritation, skin breakdown, pain, inflammation and dysautonomic events [31]. Inflammation and pain can be relieved by limb elevation, applying plaster with less tension and use of analgesia. Irritation and breakdown of skin are serious complications, and often require discontinuation. To avoid complications, patient selection is important together with careful monitor and regular plaster change (once to twice weekly)[33]. If patient develops pain cast may also need to be changed.

8.4. Complementary treatment

Casts are never applied as isolated intervention. Patients who are treated with casts usually also participate in multidisciplinary rehabilitation programs [33].

Techniques complementing treatment with casts include: mobilization, stretching, electrical stimulation, neurodinamics[21], mobility and strengthening exercises and any neuro-rehabilitation techniques such as NDT or PNF (propioceptive neuromuscular facilitation)

It is important to actively or passively mobilize joints adjacent to the cast as a routine practice, as many times a day as the therapist deems necessary.

Electrostimulation is mostly used with dropout techniques, and once the plaster is cut and bivalved can also be used to prevent atrophy or enhance voluntary motor activity.

Exercise plans are designed for each patient, to stimulate activity in paralyzed muscles and encourage voluntary motor control improvement [33].

For upper limb casts we recommend simultaneous exercises such as weight bearing activities, bilateral functional skill development, motor control training on muscles on the periphery of the cast, and voluntary isometric contraction of muscles included in the cast which can be contracted.

For lower limb casts, repetitive exercises are indicated to activate weak muscles in task-related training and improve strength and coordination. It is important that patients be helped to stand with supporting equipment, which will vary depending on motor reserve (tilt table, standing frame, or assisted by the therapist). In this manner patient is forced to use the affected limb. If the patient retains a good level of standing balance, exercises involving weight bearing on the affected limb can be considered, while other limbs perform swings or reaching for objects in the case of the upper extremity.

For subjects who respond minimally, treatment may focus on following simple commands to induce muscle activity in addition to the passive modalities mentioned before [33].

Physical therapists must consider a program of stretching, positioning and indication of night splints, or even use of splints during the day after removal of final cast [31].

Maintaining range gained with cast progression is difficult when muscle overactivity persists as a result of CNS injury and lack of motor control, or of voluntary activity in muscles antagonist to the contracture.

Another common combination is the application of progressive casts with botulinum toxin for muscle overactivity management. Toxin is often used as first line drug therapy for focal spasticity [34]. However, authors disagree on whether toxin use promotes or enhances cast effect [35]. One study attempted to determine whether serial casting combined with botulinum toxin reduced contracture development in calf muscles after severe head injury, and concluded cast alone was sufficient [34].

In the presence of severe or persistent dystonia pharmacological intervention may be required. Neurosurgery is another option to maintain gains obtained with serial casting [20].

The effectiveness of plasters has been compared to that of other therapeutic modalities in the TBI population. According to Moseley, casts are more effective in the short term than positioning for one hour a day to reduce elbow flexion contracture in patients with TBI, observing that treatment difference was not maintained over time [33]. Therefore, although serial casting is effective in reducing contracture deformity after acquired brain injury, and serial casting induces transient increase in range of motion, these effects are not maintained longterm [33].

8.5. Evidence and conclusion

There is insufficient evidence to support or refute the effectiveness of plasters in the upper limbs after an acquired brain injury. Although more evidence has been published for the lower limbs, systematic reviews on the use of casts also conclude there is lack of strong and consistent evidence to support their use in the lower limb [31].

Casts to improve passive joint range have a grade B level of recommendation, and for treatment of spasticity, a grade C. There is also lack of firm evidence therefore to recommend their use to improve function [32]. The development of clinical practice guidelines is limited because most studies are case series. One of the major limitations of research is the method selected for measuring results, very few studies use ROM measurement with controlled torque. For all the reasons mentioned above, authors disagree on when to prescribe casts, and on which approach to use and what underlying theory supports the indication. Currently, decisions on whether to use casts in patients with motor disorders due to CNS injury are based more on clinical judgment than on scientific evidence [31].

Finally, casts should be placed by experienced therapists in patients at early stages of their rehabilitation program. Associated complication rates will decrease as therapists get better at using the technique [19, 30, 34].

This treatment modality should always be part of a global and comprehensive rehabilitation program with a multifactorial vision of patient's deficits, in particular motor control, in order to maximize functional recovery [19, 30].

9. Case studies

Case 1: Patient with Traumatic Brain Injury and Bilateral Equinus

MC, a 47 year old male diagnosed with multiple trauma and severe TBI after a motor vehicle accident was admitted to the rehabilitation center 137 days post event.

Patient was conscious, oriented in time and space and able to communicate effectively. Physical examination showed mild quadriparesis and loss of trunk control. Superficial and deep sensitivity was preserved with generalized hyperreflexia and normal muscle tone.

Passive mobilization of the soleous and calf showed tension, shortening was observed in both lower limbs, and plantar flexion and contracture of both ankles detected. No signs of muscle overactivity (under the modified Tardieu scale) were found, ruling out presence of spasticity. Voluntary movement was also present in both ankles and feet.

Goniometric measurement with knees extended indicated a right ankle limitation of -24 ° to reach neutral right-angle position and - 34 ° on the left ankle. Ankles remained in plantar flexion even during weight-bearing while standing.

Given the absence of spasticity and the limited range of motion in both ankles, as a result of prolonged immobilization during the acute stage of treatment for multiple complications, the therapeutic team interpreted patient contracture responded to non-neural factors (muscle shortening, structural changes in connective tissue) and implemented the following therapeutic strategies

- Daily stretching in the standing position for 40-50 minutes, first on the tilt table and then using a standing frame.
- Electrical muscle stimulation (EMS) on gastronemius-soleus and pretibial muscles as adjunctive treatment, in order to generate elongation by reciprocal inhibition of both muscle groups, this was implemented while patient was standing and for 20 minutes in each leg.
- Manual passive stretching.

Patient quickly recovered skills such as sitting and standing independently, so the team decided to apply four serial casts (Fig. 1). These were changed every 7 to 14 days for a total program duration of two months.

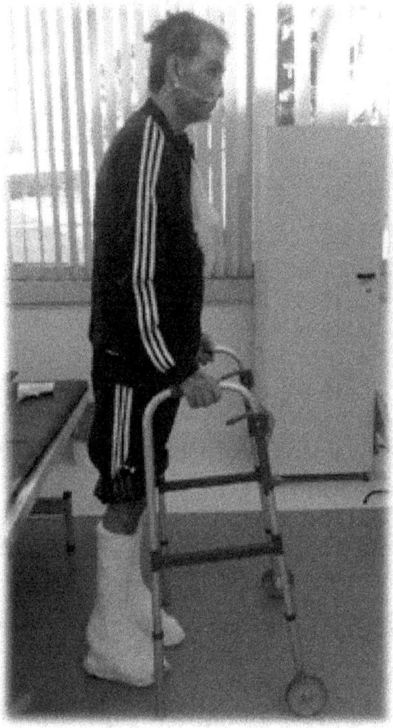

Figure 1. Independent standing with the first of the series of four casts.

Patient was allowed to rest for 2 days between casts, during which time he continued to stand using the standing frame with therapist assistance and received electro-therapy (Fig. 2).

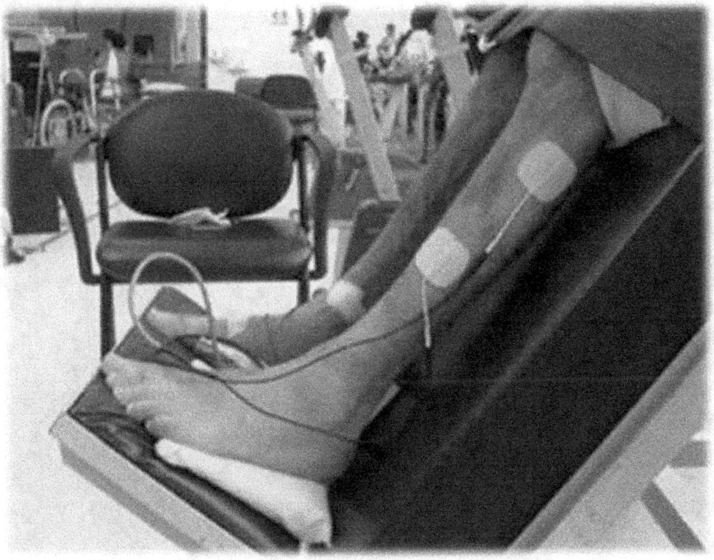

Figure 2. Stretching with electro-therapy on tilt table between casts.

While wearing the casts, patient performed lower limb weight-bearing exercises, balance and gait rehabilitation, with and without walking aids.

Serial cast result was positive with a ROM increase of -4 ° in the right ankle dorsi-flexion limitation, and of -10 ° in left ankle. Functional improvement was also achieved and patient was able to stand and walk unassisted, although use of a posting on both heels was required to compensate limited ankle range of motion (Fig. 3).

Case 2: Young adult with Traumatic Brain Injury and Multiple Contractures

CT, a 27 year-old man who suffered a traumatic brain injury as a result of a motor vehicle accident was referred to our rehabilitation center 53 days later. Imaging studies showed frontal and occipital hemorrhagic contusions had been treated with biparietal cranioplasty.

At time of admission patient was tracheostomized, evaluation of cognitive functioning showed level 3 function according to the Rancho Los Amigos Scale (localized response) and a score of 9/23 on the revised Coma Recovery Scale with visual pursuit, indicating a minimally conscious state. During physical examination, flexed global body posture and spastic flexor pattern was observed in all four limbs, with marked limitation in passive ROM and multiple contractures.

Goniometric measurement of right elbow movement indicated limitation in free range of motion from 10° to full flexion and in left elbow from 70° to full flexion. ROM could not been measured on wrists or hands because patient experienced pain during passive examination.

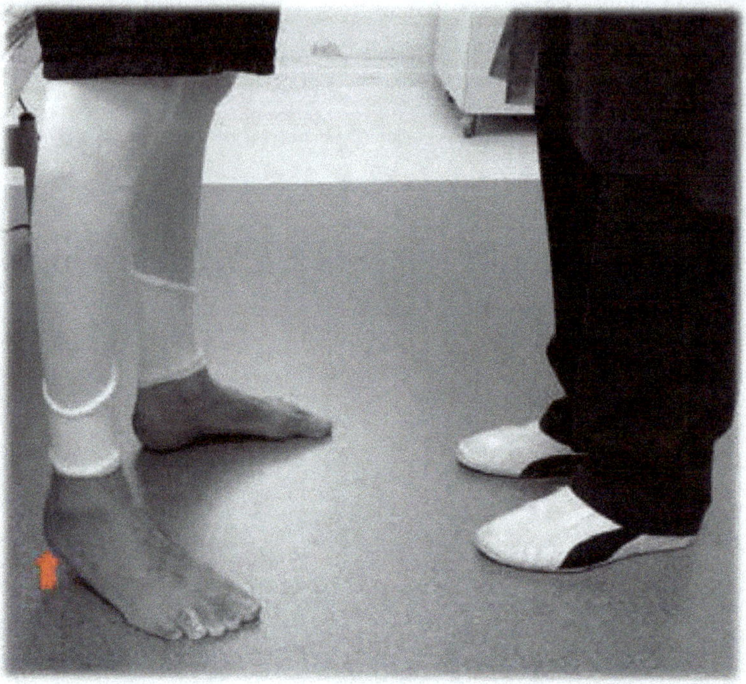

Figure 3. Standing unassisted post final cast without right heel contact on the floor.

Right wrist was extended and fingers flexed. Left wrist was in extreme flexion with metacarpophalangeal (MCP) joints in extension.

In the right lower limb severe hip limitation was present with free range of motion of 30° (from 60° to 90° of flexion), knee had short range of motion, only from 120 ° to full flexion and ankle presented plantar flexion with a 30° angle to reach right-angle neutral position.

In the left lower limb, hip presented severe contracture with range of motion limited to 45° (from 45° to 90° of flexion), knee had reduced range from 130° to full flexion and ankle did not reach the neutral position of (plantar flexion of 40°).

Muscle tone evaluated with the modified Ashworth scale showed a score of 3/4 for elbow flexors and hamstrings, although examination was difficult because of great lost of ROM and presence of heterotopic ossification in the right hip. Voluntary movement was present only in the right shoulder. Patient was admitted to the coma program to increase his level of awareness and receive multi-sensorial treatment (auditory, visual, etc.) to stimulate voluntary motor responses.

To manage contractures we developed the following treatment plan:

- Patient positioning, both in wheelchair and in bed. In the supine position a triangular foam cushion was used to hold legs in maximum possible knee extension and to prevent hip rotation (Fig. 4).

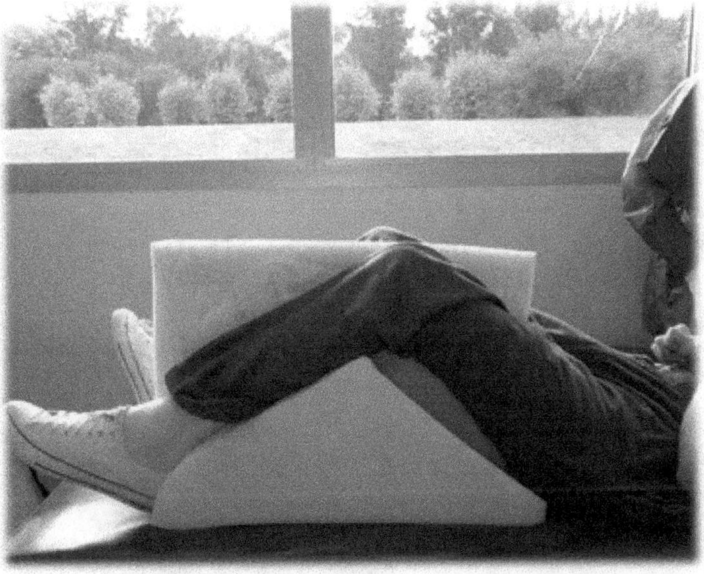

Figure 4. Positioning on bed.

- Manual passive stretching.
- Daily stretching postures achieved through use of the tilt-table, and prone positioning with adaptative equipment because of lack of range in both cases (Fig. 5).
- Knee extension splints were applied for night positioning and standing during therapy.

After two months, patient emerged from minimal consciousness and started a rehabilitation programme. Functional status showed trunk control with independent sitting and voluntary movement in lower limbs performed by imitation and procedural activities.

At this stage, patient muscle contractures were reassessed and a Baclofen pump test performed because of generalized muscle overactivity, with negative results. No changes were observed before or after the test. Given the favorable motor recovery a serial casting program was started for both knees, particularly because absence of spasticity and presence of voluntary movement favored a good outcome.

- Three progressive plasters were applied (changed every 4 to 6 days) on his left knee. The last cast was then bivalved. Initial goniometric measurement for the joint was 65º of flexion, and after final cast reached 40º of flexion. For right knee, initial measurement was 95º of flexion and reached 40º of flexion after six serial casts (lasting on average 6-8 days each). The fourth cast was a dynamic drop out cast. Three months after applying the last plaster, new ROM measurements showed further improvement, attaining 35º of flexion.
- During cast application, patient continued standing and carrying out prone activities. During the drop-out, he also worked on passive and active knee extension (Fig. 6 y 7).

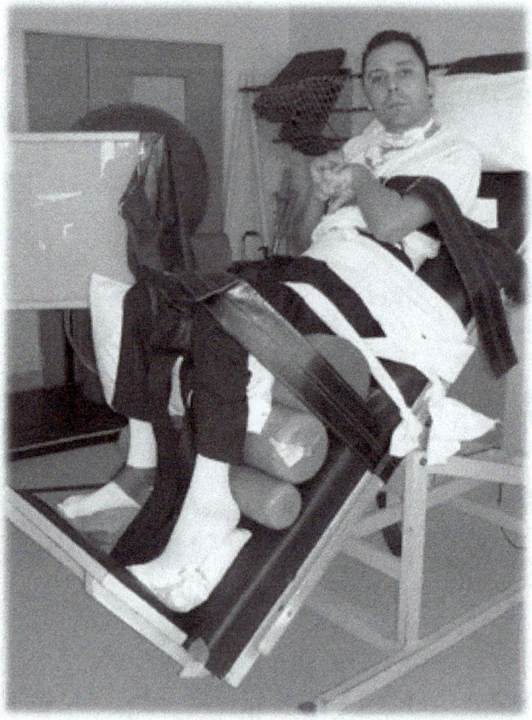

Figure 5. Standing on tilt table with adaptative equipment.

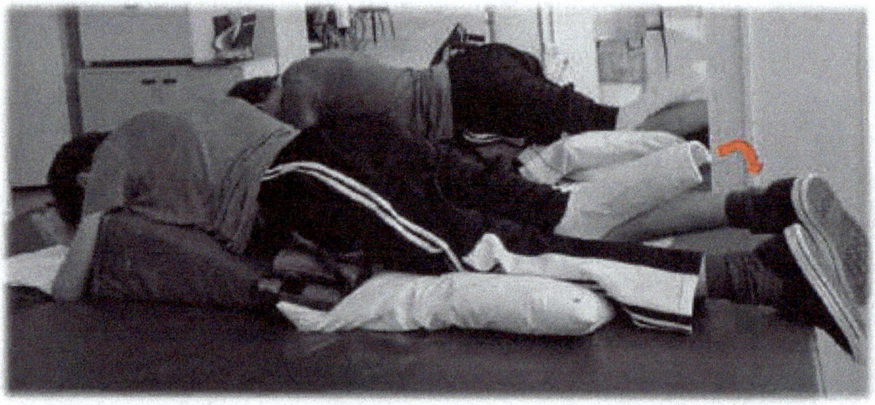

Figure 6. Prone position and exercise with Drop out cast in left knee.

- Electric stimulation was applied to the right quadriceps.

The cast allowed sufficient range to the knees to permit activity performance while standing, training of balance and for assisted walking with armrest support walker. Patient continued rehabilitation with favorable outcome (Fig. 8).

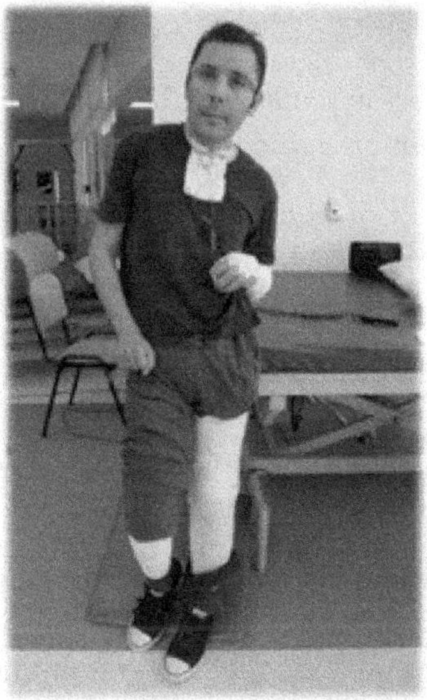

Figure 7. Supported standing with a knee extensor splint in the left leg and knee plaster in the right leg.

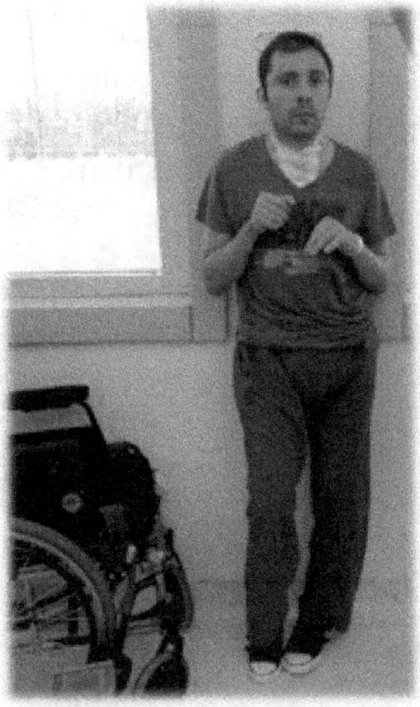

Figure 8. Standing as the final result of the progression of serial casting.

The right hip range limitation was solved surgically several months later. Currently, patient walks independently, requiring supervision for cognitive deficit. As for the upper limbs, right elbow regained normal mobility with conventional therapy and left elbow and wrist flexors required a tendon lengthening surgery.

10. Conclusion

The high prevalence of contractures in patients with head trauma limits functional therapy and presence of multiple complications often increases difficulty of rehabilitation implementation.

Contractures originate as a result of both neurologic disorders specific to central nervous system injuries and of non-neural disorders. These factors alter many anatomical structures that contribute to joint range loss.

While neurologic patients are always included in a comprehensive rehabilitation program, treatment of contractures requires special attention. The goals of the latter are to improve patient quality of life, reduce hospital stay and secondary complications, and promote better mobility and alignment, in order to recover maximum functional potential.

Several physiotherapy procedures exist for specific treatment of contractures, including stretching, positioning, splints and casts. All of them, to greater or lesser degree, involve placing anatomical structures in a position that respects or maintains normal joint range with varying duration of application. The techniques are usually combined with other therapeutic interventions to improve neurological dysfunction in its different presentations (weakness, paresis or paralysis and muscle overactivity). The variety of techniques available for treatment of contractures challenges physical therapists to gain better understanding of the principles on which the techniques are based and to develop skills in their application.

No single method renders final or full solution to contractures and all need further research to establish which procedures are most effective. All existing possibilities are commonly used in any rehabilitation program and represent the current tools until new procedures are developed. Research may also lead to the development of entirely new treatment modalities.

It is very important to address contracture management through a multidisciplinary team approach, and to train therapists for early detection as well as to assess degree of contracture. Treatment of contractures remains an active process conducted under constant monitoring, where team members can make use of different therapeutic procedures at appropriate times and adapt them to changes in clinical responses of each particular patient.

Author details

Fernando Salierno*, María Elisa Rivas, Pablo Etchandy, Verónica Jarmoluk, Diego Cozzo, Martín Mattei, Eliana Buffetti, Leonardo Corrotea and Mercedes Tamashiro

*Address all correspondence to: fsalierno@fleni.org.ar

Physical Therapy Department, FLENI Rehabilitation Institute, Escobar, Prov. de Buenos Aires, Argentina

References

[1] Harvey LA, Herbert RD. Muscle stretching for treatment and prevention of contracture in people with spinal cord injury. Spinal Cord. 2002 Jan; 40(1):1-9.

[2] Mollinger LA, Steffen TM. Knee flexion contractures in institutionalized elderly: prevalence, severity, stability, and related variables. Phys Ther. 1993 Jul; 73(7):437-44; discussion 444-6.

[3] Scott OM, Hyde SA, Goddard C, Dubowitz V. Prevention of deformity in Duchenne muscular dystrophy. A prospective study of passive stretching and splintage. Physiotherapy. 1981 Jun; 67(6):177-80.

[4] Yarkony GM, Sahgal V. Contractures. A major complication of craniocerebral trauma. Clin Orthop Relat Res. 1987 Jun; (219):93-6.

[5] Hellweg S, Johannes S. Physiotherapy after traumatic brain injury: a systematic review of the literature. Brain Inj. 2008 May; 22(5):365-73.

[6] Fergusson D, Hutton B, Drodge A. The epidemiology of major joint contractures: a systematic review of the literature. Clin Orthop Relat Res. 2007 Mar; 456:22-9.

[7] Botte MJ, Nickel VL, Akeson WH. Spasticity and contracture. Physiologic aspects of formation. Clin Orthop Relat Res. 1988 Aug; (233):7-18.

[8] Horsley AS, Herbert DR, Ada L. Four weeks of daily stretch has little or no effect on wrist contracture after stroke: a randomized controlled trial. Australian Journal of Physiotherapy. 2007; 53(4):239-245.

[9] Lieber RL, Steinman S, Barash IA, Chambers H. Structural and functional changes in spastic skeletal muscle. Muscle Nerve. 2004 May; 29(5):615-27.

[10] Cherry DB. Review of physical therapy alternatives for reducing muscle contracture. Phys Ther. 1980 Jul; 60(7):877-81.

[11] Farmer SE, James M. Contractures in orthopaedic and neurological conditions: a review of causes and treatment. Disabil Rehabil. 2001 Sep 10; 23(13):549-58.

[12] Yelnik AP, Simon O, Parratte B, Gracies JM. How to clinically assess and treat muscle overactivity in spastic paresis. J Rehabil Med. 2010 Oct; 42(9):801-7.

[13] Singer BJ, Dunne JW, Singer KP, Jegasothy GM, Allison GT. Non-surgical management of ankle contracture following acquired brain injury. Disabil Rehabil. 2004 Mar 18; 26(6):335-45.

[14] Van Trijffel E, van de Pol RJ, Oostendorp RA, Lucas C. Inter-rater reliability for measurement of passive physiological movements in lower extremity joints is generally low: a systematic review. J Physiother. 2010; 56(4):223-35. Review.

[15] Van de Pol RJ, van Trijffel E, Lucas C. Inter-rater reliability for measurement of passive physiological range of motion of upper extremity joints is better if instruments are used: a systematic review. J Physiother. 2010;56(1):7-17. Review.

[16] Pandyan AD, Johnson GR, Price CI, Curless RH, Barnes MP, Rodgers H. A review of the properties and limitations of the Ashworth and modified Ashworth Scales as measures of spasticity. Clin Rehabil. 1999 Oct; 13(5):373-83.

[17] Shabat E, Palit M, Fini NA, Brooks C, Winter A, Holland AE. Intra and inter-rater reliability of the Modified Tardieu Scale for the assessment of lower limb spasticity in adults with neurological injuries. Arch Phys Med Rehabil. 2013 Jul 11. pii: S0003-9993(13)00522-4. doi: 10.1016/j.apmr.2013.06.026. [Epub ahead of print]

[18] Singh P, Joshua AM, Ganeshan S, Suresh S. Intra-rater reliability of the modified Tardieu scale to quantify spasticity in elbow flexors and ankle plantar flexors in adult stroke subjects. Ann Indian Acad Neurol 2011;14(1):23-6

[19] Booth BJ, Doyle M, Montgomery J. Serial casting for the management of spasticity in the head-injured adult. Phys Ther. 1983 Dec;63(12):1960-6.

[20] Singer BJ, Gnanaketchumy M. Jegasothy, Kevin P. Singer, Garry T. Allison. Evaluation of Serial Casting to Correct Equinovarus Deformity of the Ankle After Acquired Brain Injury in Adults. Arch Phys Med Rehabil 2003;84:483-91

[21] Davies Patricia M. Starting Again: early rehabilitation after traumatic brain injury or other severe brain lesion. Springer-Verlag Berlin Heidelberg 1994.

[22] Cusick Beverly D. Serial Casting and Other Equinus Deformity Management Strategies for Children and Adults with Central Nervous System Dysfunction. Progressive GaitWays, LLC, 2010.

[23] Newman M, Barker K. The effect of supported standing in adults with upper motor neurone disorders: a systematic review. Clin Rehabil. 2012 Dec; 26(12):1059-77.

[24] Watson MJ. Do patients with severe traumatic brain injury benefit from physiotherapy? A review of the evidence. Physical Therapy Reviews 2001; 6: 233–249.

[25] Nuismer BA, Ekes AM, Holm MB. The use of low-load prolonged stretch devices in rehabilitation programs in the Pacific Northwest. Am J Occup Ther. 1997 Jul-Aug; 51(7):538-43.

[26] Robinson W, Smith R, Aung O, Ada L. Aust J Physiother. 2008; 54(1):33-8. No difference between wearing a night splint and standing on a tilt table in preventing ankle contracture early after stroke: a randomised trial.

[27] Blanton S, Grissom SP, Riolo L. Use of a static adjustable ankle-foot orthosis following tibial nerve block to reduce plantar-flexion contracture in an individual with brain injury. Phys Ther. 2002 Nov; 82(11):1087-97.

[28] Lannin NA, Horsley SA, Herbert R, McCluskey A, Cusick A. Splinting the hand in the functional position after brain impairment: a randomized, controlled trial. Arch Phys Med Rehabil. 2003 Feb;84(2):297-302.

[29] Leung J, Harvey LA, Moseley AM, Tse C, Bryant J, Wyndham S, Barry S. Electrical stimulation and splinting were not clearly more effective than splinting alone for contracture management after acquired brain injury: a randomised trial. J Physiother. 2012; 58(4):231-40.

[30] Stoeckman Tina. Casting for the Person with Spasticity. Top Stroke Rehabil 2001; 8(1):27-35.

[31] Lannin NA, Novak I, Cusick A. A systematic review of upper extremity casting for children and adults with central nervous system motor disorders. Clinical Rehabilitation 2007; 21: 963-976.

[32] Mortenson PA, Eng JJ. The Use of Casts in the Management of Joint Mobility and Hypertonia Following Brain Injury in Adults: A Systematic Review. Phys. Ther. 2003; 83:648-658.

[33] Moseley Anne M, Leanne M Hassett, Joan Leung, Jennifer S Clare, Robert D Herbert, Lisa A Harvey. Serial casting versus positioning for the treatment of elbow contractures in adults with traumatic brain injury: a randomized controlled trial. Clinical Rehabilitation 2008; 22: 406-417.

[34] Verplancke, S Snape, CF Salisbury, PW Jones, AB Ward. A ramdomized controlled trial of botulinum toxin on lower limb spasticity following acute acquired severe brain injury. Clinical Rehabilitation 2005; 19: 117 – 125

[35] Yaşar E, Tok F, Safaz I, Balaban B, Yilmaz B, Alaca R. The efficacy of serial casting after botulinum toxin type A injection in improving equinovarus deformity in patients with chronic stroke. Brain Inj. 2010;24(5):736-9.

9

Long-Lasting Mental Fatigue after Traumatic Brain Injury – A Major Problem most often Neglected Diagnostic Criteria, Assessment, Relation to Emotional and Cognitive Problems, Cellular Background, and Aspects on Treatment

Birgitta Johansson and Lars Rönnbäck

1. Introduction

Fatigue after traumatic brain injury (TBI) is common, but often overlooked. But for people fighting their fatigue after brain injury day after day, fatigue is a major problem. This post-injury mental fatigue is characterized by limited energy reserves to accomplish ordinary daily activities. Persons who have not experienced this extreme exhaustion which may appear suddenly, and without previous warning during mental activity, do not understand the problem. This is especially difficult to understand as the fatigue may appear even after seemingly trivial mental activities which, for uninjured persons, are regarded as relaxing and pleasant, as reading a book or having a conversation with friends. A normal, well-functioning, brain performs mental activities simultaneously throughout the day, but after a brain injury, it takes greater energy levels to deal with cognitive and emotional situations.

In this chapter, we highlight mental fatigue after TBI. In the case of long-lasting mental fatigue, it could be the only factor that keeps people from returning to the full range of activities that they pursued prior to their injury with work, studies and social activities. We describe mental fatigue and suggest diagnostic criteria and we also give a theoretical explanation for this. At the end of the chapter, we discuss treatment strategies and give some examples of possible therapeutic alternatives which may alleviate the mental fatigue.

Normally, the brain works in an energy-efficient manner and prominent energy reserves are present. This is due to well-functioning ion channel and amino acid transport systems and other effective physiological processes. After brain injury, some of these systems are down-regulated, and when mental energy requirements are high the physiological processes do not function to their full capacity; these cease to function efficiently with a resultant energy loss. This may be an explanation as to why the mental fatigue appears.

1.1. When does mental fatigue occur?

Annually, about 100-300/100 000 individuals sustain a TBI, and most of the injuries are mild in severity [1]. A majority of patients recover within one to three months following mild TBI [2, 3].

Fatigue is one of the most important long-lasting symptoms following TBI, and is most severe immediately after head injury. However it is difficult to arrive at any clear figure as to how common fatigue or, in particular, mental fatigue is. The reason for this is that different results have been obtained, and these are attributable to differences in definitions and differences in the methodology in the various studies. In follow-up studies, the frequency of prolonged fatigue varies from 16 up to 73 % [4-6]. There is no correlation between persistent fatigue and severity of the primary injury, age of the person at injury or time since injury [7, 8]. For those suffering from fatigue 3 months after the accident the fatigue remained relatively stable during longer periods [9]. In particular, for those subjects who were suffering from the syndrome one year after the accident improvement in the fatigue was limited [10].

In the above reports, fatigue is discussed in terms of a single construct, i.e. not differentiated between the physical or mental aspects. In this chapter, we consider mental fatigue as a separate construct and we discuss its relationship to cognitive and emotional symptoms.

1.2. Mental fatigue is not a separate diagnostic entity

Mental fatigue is not an illness, rather it represents a mental sequel, probably due to a disturbance of higher brain functions, either physical or psychological in origin. It is included in, and defined within the diagnoses Mild cognitive impairment (F06.7), Neurasthenia (F48.0) and Posttraumatic brain syndrome (F07.2) [11].

1.3. Typical characteristics of mental fatigue

A typical characteristic of pathological mental fatigue after TBI is that the mental exhaustion becomes pronounced during sensory stimulation or when cognitive tasks are performed for extended periods without breaks. There is a drain of mental energy upon mental activity in situations in which there is an invasion of the senses with an overload of impressions, and in noisy and hectic environments. The person feels that their brain is overloaded after a tiny load. Another typical feature is a disproportionally long recovery time needed to restore the mental energy levels after being mentally exhausted. The mental fatigue is also dependent on the total activity level as well as the nature of the demands of daily activities. Fatigue often fluctuates during the day depending on the activities carried out. Thus, this fatigue is a dynamic process with variations in the mental energy level. The fatigue can appear very rapidly and, when it does, it is not possible for the affected person to continue the ongoing activity. Common associated symptoms include: impaired memory and concentration capacity, slowness of thinking, irritability, tearfulness, sound and light sensitivity, sensitivity to stress, sleep problems, lack of initiative and headache [12].

For many persons, this mental fatigue is the dominating factor which limits the person's ability to lead a normal life with work and social activities. For most people, fatigue subsides after a period of time while, for others, this pathological fatigue persists for several months or years even after the brain injury has healed. Interestingly, however is that as many as 30% of family or friends interpreted fatigue as laziness [9].

Theories as to the mechanisms accounting for mental fatigue including our own theory, suggest that cognitive activities require more resources and are more energy-demanding after brain injury than usual [13, 14]. Thus, more extensive neural circuits are used in TBI victims compared to controls during a given mental activity [15]. This indicates an increased cerebral effort after brain injury.

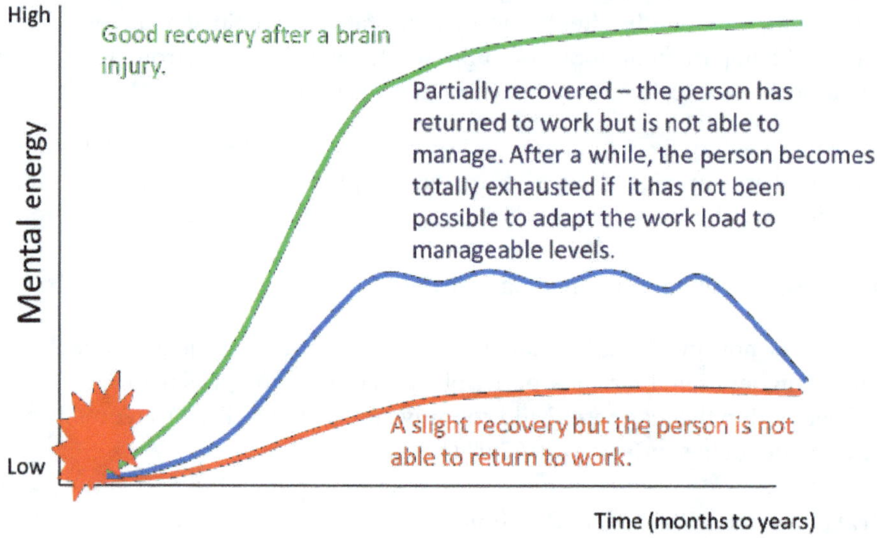

Figure 1. Schematic representation of recovery of mental energy after TBI. The green line represents a full recovery while the blue and red lines represent impaired recovery in terms of the mental energy levels. Persons whose recovery follows the blue line recover partially. On their return to work and daily activities, they are not able to manage and they become exhausted. Persons whose recovery follows the red line do not recover and are not able to return to work and daily activities.

Therapist Luann Jacobs describes mild TBI and the lack of energy and lack of endurance that many can experience. As they are able to do what is normal and what appears normal, they run the risk that their symptoms will be misunderstood [16].

"Mild brain injury is a real misnomer, as it conveys the idea that nothing much is a problem when quite the opposite is more often true. It is called "mild" because, in fact, the mildly brain injured can walk, talk, eat and dress independently, often times drive a car, shop, cook, go to school, or even work.

What the term fails to account for is the inherent limits of how often, for how long (endurance), and the all-important, how consistently (e.g., every day, once a week) these activities can be performed. Even more elusive is the concept of how many of these daily activities can be done sequentially in a given day as is normal in the lives of people who are not brain injured.

The fatigue they feel defies description, going far beyond and far deeper than anything a non-brain-injured person would consider profound exhaustion."

---

2. Theoretical explanation of mental fatigue

The cause of this extreme fatigue is not known. However, there are speculations that the symptom may be caused by dysfunction of the astrocytes, the most common supporting cells in the brain [17, 18]. As a consequence, nerve cell communications do not function properly.

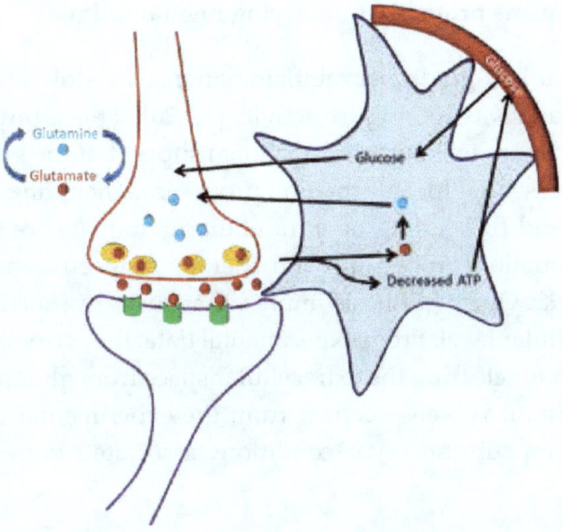

Figure 2. Schematic drawing of a synapse with glutamate as the transmitter and an astrocyte with processes surrounding the synaptic terminal. After being released from the presynaptic terminal (pre-syn; this is shown in red in the figure), glutamate interacts with glutamate recognizing receptors on the postsynaptic membrane (post-syn; shown in green in the figure). After stimulation of the postsynaptic neuron, glutamate is taken up by glutamate transporting systems on the astrocyte processes. Glutamate is converted to glutamine in the astrocyte and transported back to the presynaptic terminal where glutamine is converted back to glutamate. During this process, and with decreasing ATP levels as the signal, glucose is taken up from the blood to supply neurons and astrocytes with energy.

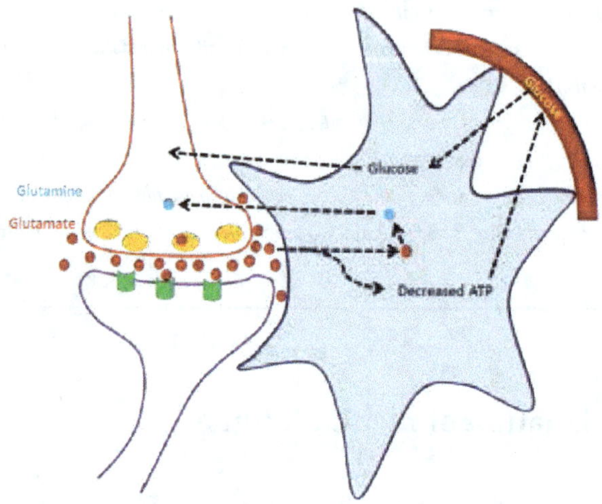

Figure 3. Following TBI there is a neuroinflammation with down-regulation of astroglial glutamate transport systems. If this state is not restored completely, there will be an impaired extracellular glutamate clearing with slightly increased extracellular glutamate levels, slight astrocyte swelling and impaired glucose uptake. Neuronal activity, if long-lasting, may result in energy crisis.

2.1. On cellular mechanisms probably underlying mental fatigue

Following TBI there is a low-grade neuroinflammation with down-regulation of astrocyte glutamate transporters and Na+/K+ ATPase activity [19, 20]. If these physiological systems are not restored completely there will be a dysfunctional support of the glutamate transmission. Glutamate signaling is essential for information processing, including learning and memory formation. Low levels and fine-tuning of extracellular glutamate are necessary to maintain high precision in information processing, and thereby high efficiency in the information handling within the CNS. Our hypothesis implies that such dysfunction could underlie the mental fatigue at the cellular level. From experimental data, the astroglial cells are considered the most important cells for clearing the extracellular space from glutamate during glutamate transmission. In addition, it is well-accepted from the experimental data that this clearing capacity is attenuated by substances or conditions associated with brain dysfunction or pathology (see [17]).

If the capacities of these processes are not fully restored, neuronal function is impaired in at least two ways: 1) extracellular glutamate levels increase upon neuronal activity leading to unspecific signaling and 2) lack of energy. In the event of a high mental load with high neuronal activity, these factors may lead to a metabolic collapse of neuronal circuits – we have previously called this a "dead-lock" situation, which may take a long time to restore.

We consider this metabolic failure as one probable explanation for the prominent and abrupt exhaustion that the TBI victims with mental fatigue can experience. The long restoring time at a cellular level corresponds to the long time it takes for the TBI victims to restore mental activity.

One way to restore this dysfunction is to stimulate Na^+/K^+-ATPase along the dopaminergic circuits which regulate attention and executive functions. Possible candidates are methylphenidate and the dopaminergic stabilizer OSU6162 (see below under the heading, 'Treatment').

3. Assessment of mental fatigue

There is an abundance of scales for assessing fatigue in general and several of these scales are designed for use in different diseases [21, 22]. The scales include questions relating to feelings of fatigue, perceived impact on activities, affective feelings and mental or cognitive effects. Many of the scales are self-reported on a Likert or an ordered scale, with the following response alternatives: Never, Sometimes, Regularly, Often or Always.

We have developed and used the Mental Fatigue Scale (MFS) during the last five years. We decided to construct this scale since we were not able to find an assessment scale adapted to mental fatigue. The MFS is a multidimensional questionnaire containing 15 questions. It incorporates affective, cognitive and sensory symptoms, duration of sleep and daytime variation in symptom severity. The questions concern the following: fatigue in general, lack of initiative, mental fatigue, mental recovery, concentration difficulties, memory problems, slowness of thinking, sensitivity to stress, increased tendency to become emotional, irritability, sensitivity to light and noise, decreased or increased sleep as well as 24-hour symptom variations. The questions in the scale are based on common activities and we have related the estimation to exemplified alternatives. It is also possible to provide estimations in-between two alternatives. The intention was to make the scale more consistent between individuals and also between ratings for the same individual. The exemplified alternatives can help the person to respond in a similar way despite the present state of fatigue or emotional state. The MFS is designed in a similar way as The Comprehensive Psychopathological Rating Scale (CPRS). The CPRS also includes exemplified alternatives and it is used to record changes in psychopathology over a comparatively short period [23]. The questions included in the MFS are based on symptoms described following longitudinal studies of patients with TBI, brain tumours, infections or inflammations in the nervous system, vascular brain diseases, and other brain disorders, which indicates that an acquired brain injury or disorder can result in similar symptoms [24-26]. The scale is free to use and can be downloaded at www.mf.gu.se (both in Swedish and English). We have transcribed one of the questions in the MFS, below:

Mental fatigue

Does your brain become fatigued quickly when you have to think hard? Do you become mentally fatigued from things such as reading, watching TV or taking part in a conversation with several people? Do you have to take breaks or change to another activity?

0	I can manage in the same way as usual. My ability for sustained mental effort is not reduced.
0.5	
1	I become fatigued quickly but am still able to make the same mental effort as before.
1.5	
2	I become fatigued quickly and have to take a break or do something else more often than before.
2.5	
3	I become fatigued so quickly that I can do nothing or have to abandon everything after a short period (approx. five minutes).

Figure 4 shows how healthy controls and subjects suffering from mild TBI, TBI and stroke have rated separate questions on the MFS. The brain injury victims were divided into different groups according to their total rating on MFS. When a person rates low on one question, the total rating on most of the separate questions will also be low, while persons rating high on one question on the MFS, will also rate most of the questions on a high level.

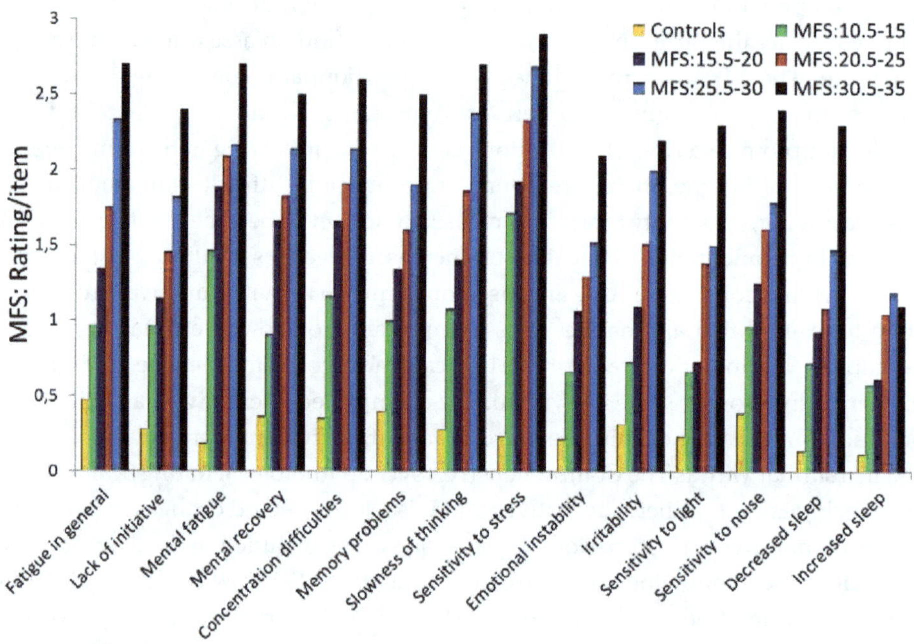

Figure 4. Rating on separate items on the Mental Fatigue Scale for controls and brain injured subjects. Brain injured subjects are divided into groups according to their total rating on MFS.

3.1. The use of MFS and results from the studies

The rating on MFS by healthy controls and people who suffered mild TBI or TBI did not reveal any significant differences between females and males, and there was no correlation between the results on MFS and age or education of the TBI victims (figure 5). Furthermore, we did not find any correlation for the TBI participants concerning time since injury and their rating on MFS. We have, in our studies worked with participants with mental fatigue lasting for six months or periods greater than six months. At this stage, we do not have any data relating to ratings early after TBI or mild TBI. This accounts for the fact that the rating may lack correlation to time since injury.

The control group rated MFS significantly lower than mild TBI and TBI victims. The participants included for the analysis were healthy controls and participants who had suffered mild TBI or TBI without major depression. The participants were between 20-67 years of age.

We recommend a cutoff score on the MFS at 10.5. A score of 10.5 on the MFS was found to deviate significantly from the control sample and is also above the 99th percentile for the control group. A score above 10.5 implies a problem for the person, although a serious problem is not always the case. However, such a score implies the need for the person to consider the current situation with their work and/or social life. The MFS had a high internal consistency and all separate items were rated significantly higher among brain injured subjects compared with healthy controls (see also figure 5).

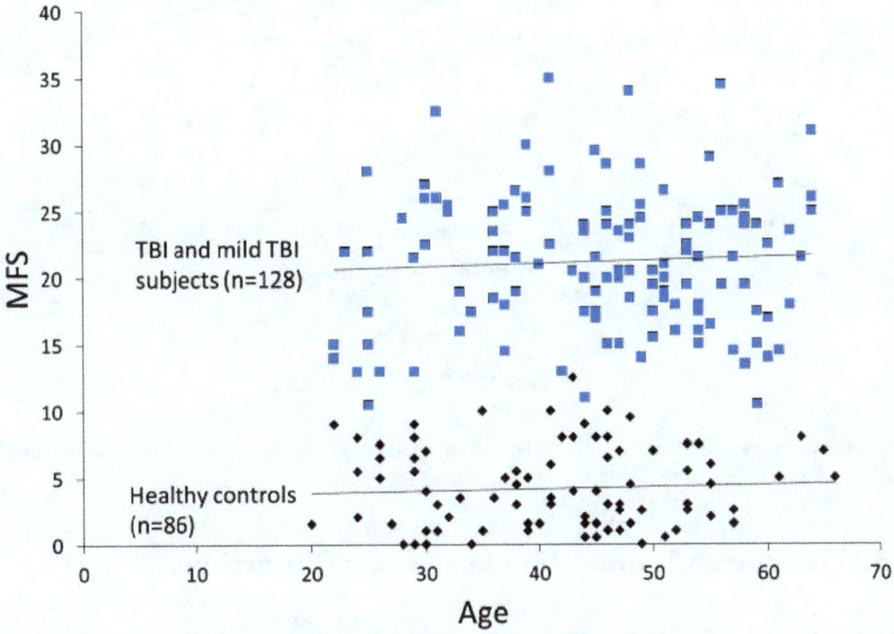

Figure 5. Correlation with age and rating on MFS for healthy controls and subjects with long-lasting mental fatigue after brain injury.

4. Mental fatigue and connection to cognitive functions

It has been proposed that subjective mental fatigue after TBI or mild TBI correlates to poor performance in attention tests and reduced processing speed [13, 27, 29-34]. We also found that information processing speed, attention and working memory were significantly reduced for the brain injury victims (both mild TBI and TBI) compared to controls. Furthermore, the tests correlated significantly to the results on the MFS (figure 6). Among the cognitive functions, processing speed was found to be a significant predictor for the rating on MFS [27].

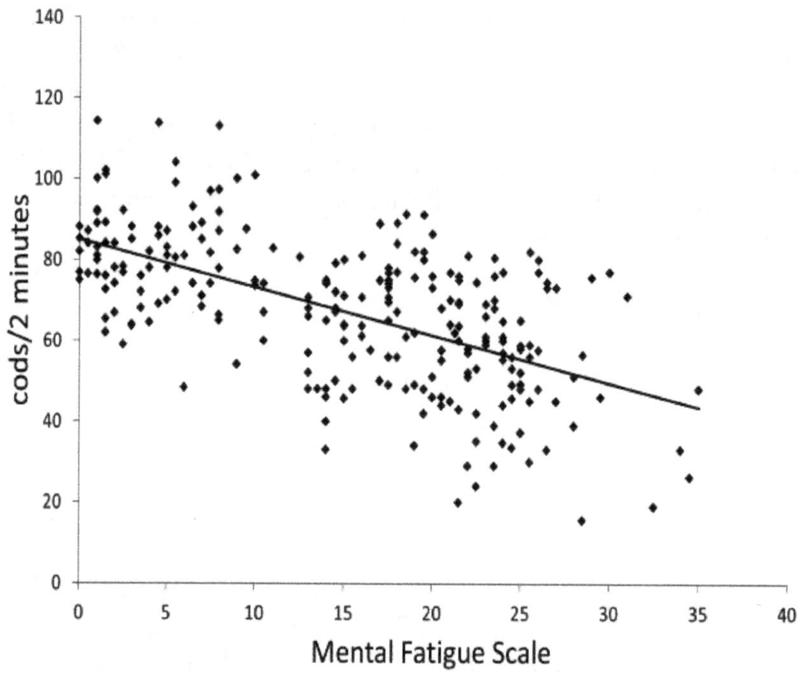

Figure 6. Correlation between Mental Fatigue Scale and information processing speed (Digit Symbol-Coding).

5. Mental fatigue and connection to emotional functions

In the population of TBI victims, depression is elevated although there is a wide variation in frequency, depending on methodological differences [35-37]. In our studies, we have included participants who complained of mental fatigue after TBI and we excluded subjects affected by major depression, as it was our intention to explore the mental fatigue component. Despite this, we found, with the use of the CPRS/MADRS, that there was an elevation in the rating of depression items for TBI subjects compared to controls. The CPRS scale includes both a depression and an anxiety scale [23, 38]. The CPRS depression scale is also called the Montgomery-Åsberg Depression Rating Scale (MADRS) [39].

However, there are overlapping items in the MFS and CPRS. The overlapping items include the following: lack of initiative, concentration difficulties, irritability and decreased sleep. With a factor analysis, the items were separated into a mental fatigue component and a depression and anxiety component. Irritability was placed in the depression-anxiety component and the other three items in the mental fatigue component. With an analysis using the new components, we found that by adjusting the mental fatigue component this removed the difference observed between the brain injured subjects and controls in the depression-anxiety component. However, by removing the depression-anxiety component this did not have an effect on the difference observed between the brain injured subjects and controls in the mental fatigue component.

In this subject sample, we were able to demonstrate that a significant effect on the difference observed between the brain injured subjects and controls in the scores for depression can result in an overestimation if the effect of the mental fatigue component is not taken into consideration. This indicates that mental fatigue and depression must be treated as separate constructs and it is also important to make this distinction for the purposes of therapeutic strategies.

6. Definition and diagnostic criteria for long-lasting mental fatigue

The diagnostic criteria for posttraumatic brain syndrome include most of the symptoms that are often present along with mental fatigue. However, we suggest mental fatigue to be a central symptom after a brain injury reflecting an inefficient support to the neuronal networks.

Mental fatigue is a lack of mental energy with impaired cognitive, emotional and sensory functioning. Mental fatigue is characterized by an unusual feeling of fatigue or malaise. There is a drain on the person's mental energy upon mental activity. The result is a diminished attention and concentration capacity. Situations which involve high levels of external cues and an overload of impressions are strenuous. Failing energy levels and excessively long recovery times are the result of over-exertion. The condition impairs the person's ability to function in their work, studies and gatherings with family and friends.

6.1. How to recognize long-lasting mental fatigue

- The mental fatigue has persisted for at least 1 month;
- The sum of scores from the MFS is 10.5 points or above.

Typical symptoms include:

- An unusually rapid drain of mental energy upon mental activity;

- Impaired attention and concentration capacity over time;
- Following over-exertion, a long recovery time disproportionate to the exertion level;
- Diurnal variation of the fatigue symptom with the fatigue often being better in the mornings and worse in the afternoons and evenings; variations from one day to the next;
- Usually one or several associated symptoms (see below):

The following additional or associated symptoms are common:

- Mood swings, irritability and stress intolerance;
- Trouble with memory;
- Sleep problems;
- Sensitivity to, or intolerance of light and loud noise;
- Headaches following over-exertion.

Sleep problems most often occur in the following way: either a shorter duration of sleep with interrupted wake-ups or sleeping more than usual. If the person becomes more mentally fatigued, the sleep will most often become worse, and if the person rests for some days the sleep can become improved again. The emotional load may increase the severity of the fatigue, but if mental fatigue exists, it will remain even once the emotional components, as depression or anxiety have been treated. However, it is important to treat the emotional problems. In this way, the mental fatigue may, to some extent be relieved.

6.2. If the fatigue is not acknowledged in time, this may result in the following

- A total and almost paralyzing fatigue;
- Longer periods of rest may be needed, often over several days;
- A worsening of symptoms over time;

6.3. Mental fatigue symptoms are often present in the following situations

- Situations in which there is an invasion of the senses with an overload of impressions, and noisy and hectic environments such as crowded events, also the hustle and bustle of shopping centers, and travelling by bus, etc.;
- Reading books and newspapers;
- Conversations with people – this becomes more of a struggle when more people are involved;
- Unexpected events.

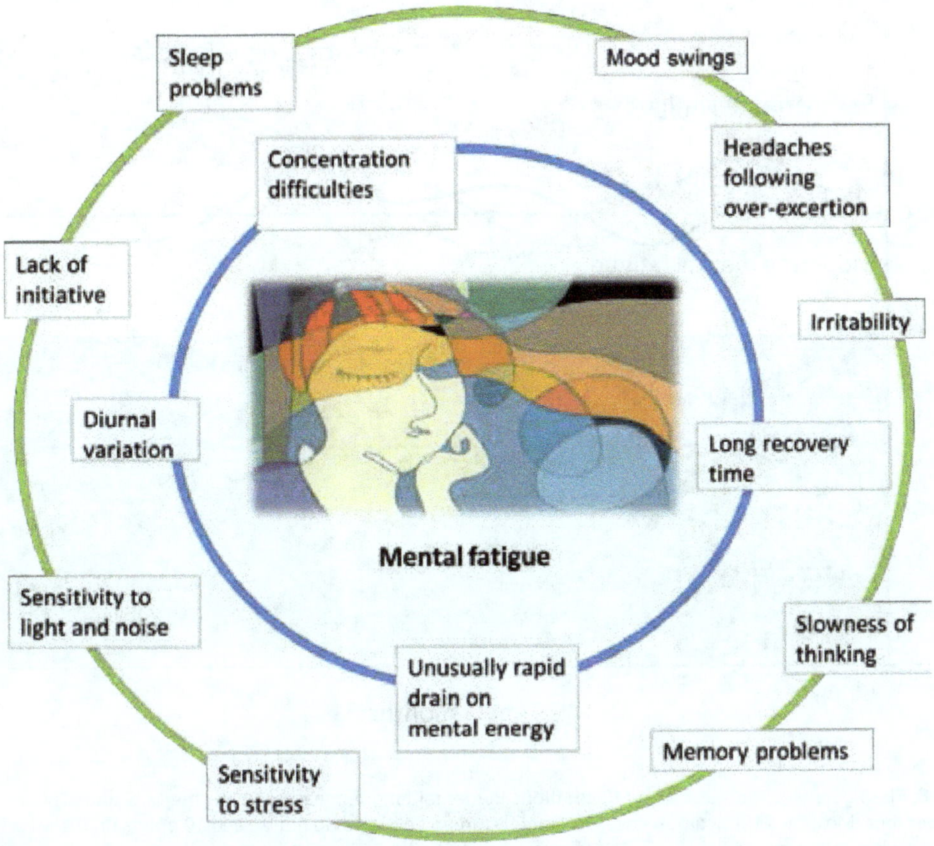

Figure 7. The figure illustrates mental fatigue. Characteristic symptoms are seen on the blue circle and associated symptoms on the green circle. (The figure in the middle is illustrated by Kristina Edgren Nyborg).

7. Treatment

There is currently no effective treatment for mental fatigue. For many people, there is an increased risk of doing too much and becoming even more fatigued. Today, the most important recommendations are to adapt to the energy available by doing one thing at a time, resting regularly and not overdoing things.

When mental fatigue is present, it is important to adapt work as well as daily activities to levels that the brain can manage. However, this is challenging for most people and it may take a long time, even years, to adapt to a sustainable level. It may also be difficult for the person to learn by himself/herself and it can take several years of considerable struggle, frustration, despair and depression, to find the right balance between rest and activity. Professional support is required but this can be hard or impossible to find especially when mental fatigue continues for many years.

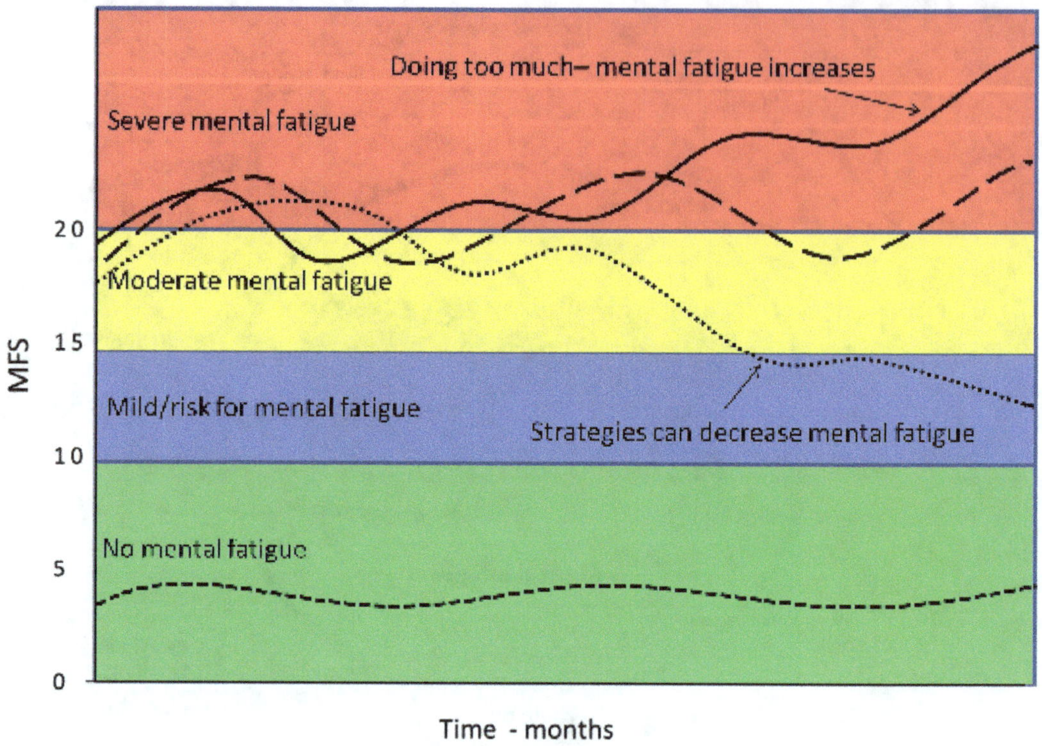

Figure 8. The figure illustrates levels and fluctuations in mental fatigue measured with the MFS after TBI and variations over time. Most mild TBI victims recover completely (green field) and do not exceed 10 points on the MFS. People within the blue, yellow or red fields suffer from metal fatigue to varying extents. It is also shown that treatment strategies decrease the mental fatigue, while over-exertion leads to increased rates on the MFS.

7.1. Treatment strategies

- Take regular breaks;
- Encourage rest before becoming over-tired;
- Try to work at a steady pace, taking one task at a time with short working periods, and prioritize the tasks;
- Plan the days' activities or the activities for the week in a diary or journal. Avoid over-exertion.

The use of strategies is important. By resting the brain as much as possible the mental energy will be alleviated. However, the brain and the individual also need positive experiences and stimulation to ensure wellbeing. It is difficult to achieve this balance between rest and stimulation.

7.2. Treatment studies for alleviating mental fatigue

When mental fatigue becomes a prolonged problem, it is essential to be able to alleviate the symptoms. We have reported on significantly reduced mental fatigue after treatment using the mindfulness-based stress reduction (MBSR) program [40, 41]. We have also reported on possible therapeutic strategies to reduce mental fatigue by means of pharmacological treatments, using neurostimulant substances as methylphenidate [42] which affects dopamine and norepinephrine signaling. We have also reported on a new substance not currently available on the market, (-)-OSU6162, which is a dopamine and serotonin stabilizer [43].

7.2.1. Mindfulness

The MBSR program was tested on TBI and stroke victims suffering from long-term mental fatigue [40]. MBSR is a clinically-effective

method for a wide range of conditions as stress, depression, pain, and fatigue after cancer, with the potential to help individuals to cope with their difficulties [44-47]. MBSR is also suggested to be linked to improvements in attention and cognitive flexibility [48] and also to changes in brain neuronal connectivity [49].

MBSR includes a range of both formal and informal practices. The intervention is based on Kabat Zinn's MBSR program [50]. The formal practices in MBSR are described by M. Cullen 2011 [51] and these include gentle Hatha yoga with an emphasis on mindful awareness of the body, a body scan designed to systematically, region by region, cultivate an awareness of the body without the tensing and relaxing of muscle groups associated with progressive relaxation, and sitting meditation with an awareness of the breath as well as a systematic widening of the field of awareness to include all four foundations of mindfulness: awareness of the body, feeling tone, mental states and mental contents. As such, the intention of MBSR is much greater than simple stress reduction. The program consists of eight weekly group sessions which are each approximately 2.5 hours long, one day-long silent-led retreat between sessions six and seven and home practice of about 45 minutes, six days a week. The participants receive guided instructions and CDs for home practice.

We found a significantly reduced mental fatigue after the MBSR program and participants improved their processing speed significantly compared to control on waitlist [40]. Improvement was independent of gender, time since injury and age. Another recent study with MBSR for mild TBI patients showed a similar result with significant improvement in quality of life, perceived self-efficacy, working memory and attention [52]. Furthermore, a small-scale study of 10 mild TBI subjects included in the MBSR program over a 12-week period also showed a significantly improved quality of life and decreased depression rating [53]. The effects were maintained one year later among the seven contactable participants. They also noted an improvement in reported energy levels at the follow-up [54]. However, after TBI, a short MBSR program over a 4-week period did not result in any cognitive or emotional changes [55].

The results demonstrate that mindfulness practice may be a therapeutic method well-suited to subjects suffering from mental fatigue after brain injury. One reason why MBSR was effective may be that this treatment offers strategies to better handle stressful situations appropriately and economize with mental energy. Despite the problem of ensuring that participants stay awake, which is one of the fundamental aspects of meditation, it was possible to adjust mindfulness to suit the needs of mental fatigue subjects and to improve their wakefulness as well as reducing their mental fatigue levels.

7.2.2. Methylphenidate

Methylphenidate inhibits dopamine and noradrenalin reuptake resulting in increased extracellular concentration of dopamine and noradrenalin [56]. Methylphenidate has been used for many years in the treatment of ADHD in children, in the first instance to increase wakefulness, attention and concentration capacity. Methylphenidate has also been tested on TBI victims with positive effects on information processing speed and, to some extent on working memory and attention [57-63]. Guidelines for use of methylphenidate for deficits of attention and processing speed after TBI have been suggested [64], while no such guidelines exist for fatigue following TBI.

In an open randomized study, methylphenidate significantly improved mental fatigue dose-dependently as assessed with the MFS [42]. The item, pain was also studied and we found that this item was rated high by most of the subjects in our study as the participants were recruited on the basis of the items, TBI and pain. However, no significant alleviation of pain was reported as a result of methylphenidate treatment. However, it is important to note that pain can hide posttraumatic brain injury symptoms or mental fatigue which is not always connected to the actual pain. We also found that there was no interaction between the pain and the mental fatigue in those participants treated with methylphenidate. These findings indicate that, not only is it necessary to treat patients for the pain for which they are primarily referred to the clinic, but also for the mental fatigue, if present.

Methylphenidate was well-tolerated by TBI subjects. However, tolerance of methylphenidate differed between subjects and we therefore recommend starting treatment with an initial low dose.

7.2.3. (-)-OSU6162

The monoaminergic stabilizer OSU6162 interacts with both dopaminergic and serotonergic systems. It appears to act as an antagonist on a binding site of the D2 receptor. More recent research has demonstrated that OSU6162 also exerts a stabilizing effect on serotonergic neuronal circuits, acting as a partial 5-HT2A agonist [65, 66].

In two randomized, double-blind and placebo-controlled studies we found statistically significant alleviation of mental fatigue after a stroke or TBI by OSU6162 during 4 weeks' treatment with active drug [43]. However, the numbers of patients in these studies were small (21 TBI and 19 stroke victims). Further studies are needed, with a larger number of patients and, in particular longer treatment periods as mental fatigue may be long-lasting. Adverse reactions were mild and could be avoided by dose adjustment. Several patients experiencing such adverse reactions expressed the wish to receive continued treatment with the drug.

Similar results were detected for methylphenidate and OSU6162. These drugs were shown to have the effect of both alleviating mental fatigue and increasing information processing speed.

8. Conclusions

Mental fatigue can become a prolonged and distressing problem after TBI having considerable effect on life and wellbeing. It is important to acknowledge and assess mental fatigue when discussing the options regarding therapeutic methods as the mental fatigue has been the result of a TBI.

After TBI, mental energy levels are failing, and the brain needs to rest. It is not possible to improve the mental energy with training in order to perform more mental activities. In fact, training with a view to resting the brain is what is important. Suitably-adapted and energy-saving strategies are important and most patients need support in order to achieve an enduring balance between activities and rest as this is difficult, it takes a long time and may be frustrating.

The treatment studies we reported on are aimed at helping the person to manage their life better. However, it is important to stress that there is a risk that the medication can compel the person to do more than is appropriate. The reason for this is that, most often they want to carry out activities in a similar way as before the injury and have been longing for the chance to be able to do this. The problem is that, for most persons suffering from long-term mental fatigue after TBI, the activity levels are close to the threshold of what they are able to sustain. This makes them susceptible if they increase their activity levels too much. With mindfulness most participants reported on more energy, but they also became more pleased and happy with life. Mindfulness also gave them a tool to use and they could take command over their own lives; how it is here and now, not longing for a better life or ruminating over what has been. This also saves energy! A combination with neurostimulants and mindfulness may be a good therapeutic strategy.

In the future, research is warranted for early treatment with the intention to reduce the development of long-term mental fatigue. We also need to better elucidate and carry out an in-depth analysis of mental fatigue.

Author details

Birgitta Johansson and Lars Rönnbäck

*Address all correspondence to: birgitta.johansson2@vgregion.se

Department of Clinical Neuroscience and Rehabilitation, Institute of Neuroscience and Physiology, Gothenburg University, Sweden

References

[1] Holm, L., et al., Summary of the WHO Collaborating Centre for Neurotrauma Task Force on Mild Traumatic Brain Injury. J Rehabil Med, 2005. 37(3): p. 137-141.

[2] Carroll, L.J., J.D. Cassidy, and P.M. Peloso, Prognosis of mild traumatic brain injury: results of the WHO collaborating Centre Task Force on Mild Traumatic Brain Injury. J Rehabil Med, 2004. 43(suppl): p. 84-105.

[3] Lundin, A., et al., Symptoms and disability until 3 months after mild TBI. Brain Injury 2006. 20(8): p. 799-806.

[4] Stulemeijer, M., et al., Recovery from mild traumatic brain injury: a focus on fatigue. J Neurol Neurosur Ps, 2006. 253(8): p. 1041-1047.

[5] Naalt, J.v.d., et al., One year outcome in mild to moderate head injury: the predictive value of acute injury characteristics related to complaints and return to work. J Neurol Neurosur Ps, 1999. 66: p. 207-213.

[6] O'Connor, C., A. Colantonio, and H. Polatajko, Long term symptoms and limitations of activity of people with traumatic brain injury: a ten-year follow-up. Psychological reports, 2005. 97: p. 169-179.

[7] Belmont, A., et al., Fatigue and traumatic brain injury. Ann Readapt Med Phys, 2006. 49: p. 283-288.

[8] Reitan, R.M. and D. Wolfson, The two faces of mild head injury. Arch Clin Neuropsych, 1999. 14(2): p. 191-202.

[9] Norrie, J., et al., Mild traumatic brain injury and fatigue: a prospective longitudinal study. Brain Injury, 2010. 24(13-14): p. 1528-15-38.

[10] Bushnik, T., J. Englander, and J. Wright, Patterns of fatigue and its correlates over the first 2 years after traumatic brain injury. Head Trauma Rehabil, 2008. 23(1): p. 25-32.

[11] ICD 10: International Statistical Classification of Diseases and Related Health (ICD-10-SE). 2nd edition ed. 2010, Stockholm.

[12] Rönnbäck, L. and B. Johansson, Long-Lasting Mental Fatigue After Recovery from Meningitis or Encephalitis - A Disabling Disorder Hypothetically Related to Dysfunction in the Supporting Systems of the Brain in Essential Notes in Psychiatry, V. Olisah, Editor. 2012, InTech: Rijeka, Croatia. p. 561-564.

[13] Azouvi, P., et al., Divided attention and mental effort after severe traumatic brain injury. Neuropsychologia, 2004. 42: p. 1260-1268.

[14] Zomeren, A.H.v. and W. van den Burg, Residual complaints of patients two years after severe head injury. J Neurosurg Psychiatry, 1985. 48(1): p. 21-28.

[15] Kohl, A.D., et al., The neural correlates of cognitive fatigue in traumatic brain injury using functional MRI. Brain Injury, 2009. 23(5): p. 420-432.

[16] Jacobs, L. Mild Brain Injury: Implications for Independence [cited 2013.

[17] Rönnbäck, L. and E. Hansson, On the potential role of glutamate transport in mental fatigue. J Neuroinflam, 2004. 1: p. 22.

[18] Rönnbäck, L. and B. Johansson, Long-lasting mental fatigue after traumatic brain injury or stroke – e new perspective 2012, Saarbrucken: LAP Lambert Academic Publishing

[19] Frencham, K.A.R., A.M. Fox, and M.T. Maybery, Neuropsychological studies of mild traumatic brain injury: a meta-analytical review of research since 1995. J Clin Exp Neuropsychol, 2005. 27(3): p. 334-351.

[20] Block, L., et al., A new concept affecting restoration of inflammation-reactive astrocytes. Neuroscience and Biobehavioral Reviews, 2013. in press.

[21] Christodoulou, C., The assessment of fatigue, in Fatigue as a window to the brain, J. DeLuca, Editor. 2005, The MIT Press: Cambridge, Massachusetts. p. 19-35.

[22] Dittner, A.J., S.C. Wessely, and R.G. Brown, The assessment of fatigue. A practical guide for clinicians and researchers. J Psychosomatic Res, 2004. 56: p. 157-170

[23] Åsberg, M., et al., A comprehensive psychopathological rating scale. Acta Psychiatr Scand 1978. 271(suppl): p. 5-27.

[24] King, N.S., et al., The Rivermead post concussion symptoms questionnaire: a measure of symptoms commonly experienced after head injury and its reliability. J Neurol Neurosur Ps, 1995. 24: p. 587-592.

[25] Lindqvist, G. and H. Malmgren, Organic mental disorders as hypothetical pathogenetic processes. Acta Psychiatr Scand, 1993. 88(suppl 373): p. 5-17.

[26] Rödholm, M., et al., Asteno-emotional disorder after aneurysmal SAH: reliability, symptomatology and relation to outcome. Acta Neurol Scand, 2001. 103: p. 379-385.

[27] Johansson, B., P. Berglund, and L. Rönnbäck, Mental fatigue and impaired information processing after mild and moderate traumatic brain injury. Brain Injury, 2009. 23(13-14): p. 1027-1040.

[28] Johansson, B., et al., A self-assessment questionnaire for mental fatigue and related symptoms after neurological disorders and injuries. Brain Injury, 2010. 24(1): p. 2-12.

[29] Belmont, A., N. Agar, and P. Azouvi, Subjective fatigue, mental effort, and attention dificits after severe traumatic brain injury. Neurorehabil Neural Repair, 2009. 23(9): p. 939-944.

[30] Ziino, C. and J. Ponsford, Selective attention deficits and subjective fatigue following traumatic brain injury. Neuropsychology 2006. 20: p. 383-390.

[31] Ziino, C. and J. Ponsford, Vigilance and fatigue following traumatic brain injury. J Int Neuropshychol Soc, 2006. 12(1): p. 100-110.

[32] Ashman, T.A., et al., Objective measurement of fatigue following traumatic brain injury. J Head Trauma Rehabil 2008. 23(1): p. 33-40.

[33] Park, N.W., M. Moscovich, and I.H. Robertson, Divided attention impairments after traumatic brain injury. Neuropsychologia 1999. 37(10): p. 1119-1133.

[34] Ponsford, J., et al., Long-term outcomes after uncomplicated mild traumatic brain injury: a comparison with trauma controls. J. Neurotrauma, 2011. 28: p. 937-946.

[35] Silver, J.M., J.W. Mc Allister, and D.B. Arciniegas, Depression and cognitive complaints following mild traumatic brain injury. Am J Psychiatry, 2009. 166(6): p. 653-661.

[36] Bombardier, C.H., et al., Rates of Major Depressive Disorder and Clinical Outcomes Following Traumatic Brain Injury. JAMA, 2010. 303(19): p. 1938-1945.

[37] Ashman, T.A., et al., Psychiatric challenges in the first 6 years after traumatic brain injury: Cross-sequential analyses of axis I disorder. Arch Phys Med Rehabil, 2004. 85(Suppl 2): p. S36-S42.

[38] Svanborg, P. and M. Åsberg, A new self-rating scale for depression and anxiety states based on the Comprehensive Psychopathological Rating Scale. Acta Psychiatr Scand, 1994. 89(1): p. 21-28.

[39] Montgomery, S.A. and M. Asberg, A new depression scale designed to be sensitive to change. Br J Psychiatry, 1979. Apr (134): p. 382-389.

[40] Johansson, B., H. Bjuhr, and L. Rönnbäck, Mindfulness-based stress reduction (MBSR) improves long-term mental fatigue after stroke or traumatic brain injury. Brain injury, 2012. 26(13-14): p. 1621-8.

[41] Johansson, B., H. Bjuhr, and L. Rönnbäck, Evaluation of an advanced mindfulness program following a mindfulness-based stress reduction program for participants suffering from mental fatigue after acquired brain injury. Mindfulness, DOI: 10.1007/S12671-013-0249-z.

[42] Johansson, B., et al., Evaluation of dosage, safety and effects of methylphenidate on posttraumatic brain injury symptoms with focus on mental fatigue and pain, Brain Injury, accepted.

[43] Johansson, B., et al., Placebo-controlled cross-over study of the monoaminergic stabiliser (−)-OSU6162 in mental fatigue following stroke or traumatic brain injury. Acta Neuropsychiatrica, 2012. 24(5): p. 266-274.

[44] Smith, B.W., et al., A pilot study comparing the effects of mindfulness-based and cognitive-behavioral stress reduction. J Altern Complement Med, 2008. 14(3): p. 251-258.

[45] Grossmana, P., et al., Mindfulness-based stress reduction and health benefits: A meta-analysis. Journal of Psychosomatic Research 57 (2004) 35–43, 2004. 57: p. 35-43.

[46] Kabat-Zinn, J., L. Lipworth, and R. Burney, The clinical use of mindfulness meditation for the self-regulation of chronic pain Journal of Behavioral Medicine, 1985. 8(2): p. 163-190.

[47] Carlson, L.E. and S.N. Garland, Impact of mindfulness-based stress reduction (MBSR) on sleep, mood, stress and fatigue symptoms in cancer outpatients International Journal of Behavioral Medicine 2005. 12(4): p. 278-285.

[48] Moore, A. and P. Malinowski, Meditation, mindfulness and cognitive flexibility. Consciousness and Cognition, 2009. 18: p. 176-186.

[49] Kilpatrick, L.A., et al., Impact of mindfulness-based stress reduction training on intrinsic brain connectivity. Neuroimage, 2011. 1(56): p. 290-298.

[50] Kabat-Zinn, J., Full catastrophe living: How to cope with stress, pain and illness using mindfulness meditation. 2001, London, 15th ed.: Piatkus Books.

[51] Cullen, M., Mindfulness-Based Interventions: An Emerging Phenomenon. Mindfulness, 2011. 2: p. 186-193.

[52] Azulay, J., et al., A Pilot Study Examining the Effect of Mindfulness-Based Stress Reduction on Symptoms of Chronic Mild Traumatic Brain Injury/Postconcussive Syndrome. Journal of Head Trauma Rehabilitation, 2013.28(4):323-331.

[53] Bedard, M., et al., Pilot evaluation of a mindfulness-based intervention to improve quality of life among individuals who sustained traumatic brain injuries. Disabil Rehabil, 2003. 25(13): p. 722-731.

[54] Bedard, M., et al., A Mindfulness-Based Intervention to Improve Quality of Life Among Individuals Who Sustained Traumatic Brain Injuries: One-Year Follow-Up. The Journal of Cognitive Rehabilitation, 2005. spring: p. 8-13.

[55] McMillan, T., et al., Brief mindfulness training for attentional problems after traumatic brain injury: A randomised control treatment trial Neuropsychological Rehabilitation, 2002. 12(2): p. 117-125.

[56] Leonard, B.E., et al., Methylphenidate: a review of its neuropharmacological, neuropsychological and adverse clinical effects. Hum Psychopharmacol Clin Exp, 2004. 19: p. 151-180.

[57] Alban, J.P., M.M. Hopson, and W. J, Effect on methylphenidate on vital signs and adverse effects in adults with traumatic brain injury. Am J Phys Med Rehabil 2004. 83: p. 131-137.

[58] Plenger, P.M., et al., Subacute methylphenidate treatment for moderate to moderately severe traumatic brain injury: A preliminary double-blind placebo-controlled study. 1996,77:536-540. Arch Phys Med Rehabil 1996. 77: p. 536-540.

[59] Speech, T.J., et al., A double-blind controlled study of methylphenidate treatment in closed head injury. Brain Injury 1993. 7(3): p. 333-338.

[60] Whyte, J., et al., Effects of methylphenidate on attentional function after traumatic brain injury: a randomized, placebo-controlled trial. American journal of Physical Medicine & Rehabilitation, 1997. 76(6): p. 440-450.

[61] Whyte, J., et al., Effects of methylphenidate on attention deficits after traumatic brain injury: a multidimensional, randomized, controlled trial. Am J Phys Med Rehabil, 2004. 83(6): p. 401-420.

[62] Willmott, C. and J. Ponsford, Efficacy of methylphenidate in the rehabilitation of attention following traumatic brain injury: a randomized, corssover, double-blind, placebo controlled inpatient trial. J Neurol Neurosur Ps, 2009. 80: p. 552-557.

[63] Kaelin, D.L., D.X. Cifu, and s.B. Matthie, Methylphenidate effect on attention deficit in the acutely brain-injured adult. Arch Phys Med Rehabil, 1996. 77(1): p. 6-9.

[64] Warden, D.L., et al., Guidelines for the pharmacologic treatment of neurobehavioral sequelae of traumatic brain injury. J Neurotrauma, 2006. 23(10): p. 1468-1501.

[65] Burstein, E.S., et al., II. In vitro evidence that (-)-OSU6162 and (+)-OSU6162 produce their behavioral effects through 5-HT2A serotonin and D2 dopamine receptors. J Neural Transm, 2011. 118(11): p. 1523-1533.

[66] Carlsson, M.L., et al., I. In vivo evidence for partial agonist effects of (-)-OSU6162 and (+)-OSU6162 on 5-HT2A serotonin receptors. J Neural Transm, 2011. 118(11): p. 1511-1522.

10

Prevention of Seizures Following Traumatic Brain Injury

Matthew J. Korobey

1. Introduction

Traumatic brain injury (TBI) is a devastating and complex disease state. Of the observed complications associated with TBI, the development of seizures following injury can be among the most challenging to manage. In addition to the direct effects on the brain, seizures following TBI lead to significant patient morbidity, with potential limitations on overall independence. Quality-of-life may also be adversely affected as the diagnosis of seizure carries the burden of extended exposure to anti-epileptic drugs. The use of these therapies often entails unfavorable medication related side-effects, frequent laboratory monitoring and dosage adjustments, as well as frequent physician visits. With these factors in mind, identification and prophylaxis of those at risk for post-traumatic seizures may provide significant improvement on patient outcomes.

2. Historical perspective

The association between head injury and seizures has long been observed. In the Hippocratic text, "On *Injuries of the Head*", wounds to the left temporal region were described as being associated with convulsion on the right side of the body. Later, Hippocratic surgeons noted that convulsions following head trauma were often a sign of impending fatality. [1] Interestingly, the reference to seizures was only in the immediate time frame surrounding the injury; chronic seizures were not noted to have been documented in those writings. [2] As medicine and neuroscience progressed, the recognition of the association between head trauma and the development of seizure disorder gradually began to grow. As an example, in the 14th century, the Italian physician Valescus de Tharanta described a patient who suffered a penetrating head wound which infiltrated into the pia mater and subsequently experienced seizures 7 to 8 times a day until death. [3] Approximately 150 years later, Berengarius da Carpi, an Italian physician and surgeon, documented that epileptic seizures developed approximately 60 days following a severe head wound which likely is the first documentation of post-traumatic epilepsy, or seizures occurring outside of the immediate post-injury period. This association was further strengthened by the writing of Duretus who reports his observations of a patient suffering a depressed skull fracture who developed seizures 6 years following injury. [1]

Despite the above observations, head injury failed to gain recognition as a *common* cause of epilepsy. Perhaps the first major medical publication noting this connection was book *"Epilepsy and Its Treatment"* in 1904 in which its author William Spratling specifically mentions trauma as an etiology for epilepsy. Spratling writes, "Traumatic lesions of the cranium and the cerebrum cause epilepsy without any predisposition to the disease", and he goes on to describe observed epileptic patterns in significant detail. [4]

The majority of our modern knowledge pertaining to seizures following TBI is derived from military literature. The Second World War, the Korean conflict, and the Vietnam War offered an extensive cohort from which to observe the effects of head trauma. While this data has provided tremendous insight, it does not translate well to head injuries in the civilian sector in regard to mechanism and potential complications. Recently, epidemiologic investigations have examined the impact of TBI and the frequency of post-traumatic seizures in civilians, yielding valuable information for this very different patient population.

3. Definitions

Post-traumatic seizure disorder is a broad term for new-onset seizures following TBI. This terminology fails to capture the distinct differences in etiology, incidence, outcome, and management of these seizures. It is these differences that necessitated the development of a classification system, separating the observed seizures into distinct diagnostic entities based on time of development. The first formal classification of post-traumatic seizures was suggested in 1939 when Elvidge proposed the observed seizures be separated into 3 distinct groups: immediate (within the first few hours following injury), delayed (occurring with 2 weeks of injury), and late (those occurring after a period of time). He further proposed that the immediate and delayed seizures be combined into a group of events termed early epilepsy which was felt to be distinctly different from late epilepsy. [5] This classification has been modified slightly, yet generally remains accepted to this day. The current accepted definitions adopted into practice today are:

- Immediate seizure: Seizures occurring less than 24 hours post injury.
- Early seizures: Seizures occurring less than 1 week post injury.
- Late seizure: Seizures occurring greater than 1 week post injury. [2] These seizures are considered "unprovoked" and are therefore considered epileptic in nature.
- Post-traumatic epilepsy: Recurrent late seizures, with no identifiable cause other then TBI

4. Epidemiology

The burden of post traumatic seizures (PTS) is often underestimated in relation to the overall incidence of epilepsy. A prevalence study by Hauser et al examined several characteristics of epileptic patients in Rochester, MN. Their results showed that approximately 20% of symptomatic disease and 5% of all epilepsies can be attributed to traumatic injury and that in patients less than the age of 65, brain trauma was the most frequently identified risk factor associated with the development of epilepsy. [6] In fact, trauma may be the primary cause of epilepsy in up to 30% of patients between the ages of 15 and 34. [2]

The incidence of seizures following TBI is commonly separated into two distinct categories; early seizures (occurring within 1 week of the index injury) and late (occurring greater than 1 week after the index injury). Each of these categories varies from the other in terms of incidence and risk factors.

The first major publication documenting the incidence of early PTS was presented in 1960. Jennett et al found that among 898 patients admitted with closed head injury, 4.2% experienced seizure within the first 7 days following the injury. [7] Approximately 20 years later, in a retrospective chart review of 2,747 head injury patients experiencing loss of consciousness, Annegers et all found the incidence of early seizure was 2.1%, and of those, 75% occurred in the first 24 hours following injury. [8] Desai et al reviewed the records of 702 patients with any degree of head trauma and found early seizure occurred in 4.1% of patients. [9] Annegers published a second retrospective chart review in 1998 after examining the records of 4,541 pediatric and adult head injury patients. This in-depth review reported the incidence of early PTS to be 2.6%. [10] Asikainen examined a group of 490 TBI patients (approximately 50% of patients studied were under the age of 16) admitted to a TBI rehabilitation facility. Early PTS were observed at an incidence of 16.4%, a number higher than what had been observed previously. The authors comment that there was a statistically significant relationship between the age at time of injury and occurrence of early PTS, as they reported that patients age 7 or younger experience early seizures at a rate of 30.8%, those ages 8 to 16 at a rate of 20%, and patients above the age of 16 at a rate of 8.4%. [11] These results mirrored findings in earlier studies in which pediatric head injury patients were more likely to experience early seizure, independent of the degree of head trauma as compared to adult patients with similar injuries. [7, 8]

Military data is the best source of information when assessing seizure risk following penetrating head injury. The Vietnam Head Injury Study (VHIS) provided valuable information regarding outcomes of patients with penetrating head wounds, including incidence of seizure. In this cohort, early PTS was observed at 4.3%. [12, 13]

While these studies offer useful insight into overall frequency of early PTS, there are limitations that must be addressed. The heterogeneity of the populations being assessed in the available literature makes generalization difficult. In the reports mentioned above, the characteristics of patients observed varies drastically based on severity of head injury, age distribution of the population observed, and mechanism of injury. In addition, the standard of care provided to the head injury patient has evolved and should be considered when assessing the occurrence of any disease sequelae. It must be noted that very little is mentioned in the epidemiologic literature about therapies provided to these patients. When evaluating the overall incidence of early PTS, these limitations must be taken into consideration.

Despite the above mentioned limitations, some of the most useful data gained from these epidemiologic studies is the identification of risk factors for early PTS. When looking at these risk factors as a whole and considering the various populations evaluated, several factors stand out. Age at the time of injury is associated with risk of early PTS, as younger patients are more likely to experience this complication than older patients. Jennett, as stated above, found that patients < 5 years of age were at increased risk of early PTS at any degree of head injury. Of the 75 patients in this age demographic, 9.4% developed early PTS while patients older than the age of 5 had in incidence rate of 3.8%. [7] Annegers et al. also identified children as being at higher risk of early PTS. The incidence of early PTS in patients <15 years of age was 30% while the rate was 10% in adult patients. [8] Similarly, Desai and Asikainen also found that younger patients had a greater risk of early PTS compared with older patients. [9, 11]

Severity of injury at the time of presentation has also been repeatedly associated with increased risk of early PTS. Early on, duration of post-traumatic amnesia (PTA), a guide to assessing the degree of brain injury as reported by Jennett, was found to be associated with an increased risk of early PTS. Approximately 11.7% of patients with PTA lasting greater than 24 hours were seen to have early PTS while those with shorter durations experienced early seizures at a rate of 2.7%. [7] Desai reported that focal deficit on admission and loss of consciousness (LOC)/PTA of more than 30 minutes following injury greatly increased the likelihood of early PTS. [9] It has also been shown that patients presenting with Glascow Coma Scale (GCS) scores of <10 have an increased risk of early PTS with an incidence as high as 20%. [14] Lee et al and Gilad et al examined the rates of PTS following mild head injury and found no increased incidence of seizure development than in the general population experiencing non-trauma related seizures further supporting the theory that severe head injuries pose a higher risk for PTS development. [15, 16] Skull fracture and penetrating head injury have been repeatedly shown to increase the risk of early PTS. Basilar skull fractures, specifically those that are depressed or in the temporal-parietal region, appear to infer the highest risk. [7, 9]

The presence of intracranial blood on radiographic imaging has also been positively associated with early PTS. It is observed that intracranial hemorrhage (ICH) may precede early PTS in up to 23% of patients while epidural/subdural hematoma and cortical contusion are seen in approximately 16% of such cases. [9, 14] Jennett utilized the presence of bloodstained cerebral spinal fluid (CSF) to infer the presence of ICH as cranial imaging at the time was very limited. In those with bloodstained CSF, early PTS were observed at a rate of 9.7% which is noted to be approximately double the incidence of patients observed in the entire series. [7] Additionally, a survey of approximately 3000 patients with severe closed head injury revealed that ICH was present in 66% of all patients experiencing early PTS. [17]

The incidence and risk factors for late PTS are significantly different than that of early PTS and must be described separately. The lowest incidence of late PTS reported was by Jennett at 10.2% whereas Caveness et al, in the VHIS, reported a rate of 27.9%. [7, 13] Annengers, having collected data on 2,747 patients, was able to compare the incidence of late PTS to the expected rate of new onset epilepsy. Using the age and sex-specific incidence rates for Rochester, Minnesota as a comparator, there was found to be a 3.6 fold increase in the risk of developing seizure disorder following head trauma. [8]

Several authors have assessed the duration of risk for the onset of late PTS and a strong trend has emerged from that data. The time-frame for the development of late PTS potentially extends several years post-injury. Salazar et al, utilizing data from the VHIS, found that 7% of all patients with late PTS reported their first seizure 10 or more years post injury while Annegers reports that in patients with moderate to severe TBI, the risk for late PTS extends as far as 20 years post injury. [10, 12] With the awareness of the extended risk for late PTS, it must be noted that more than half of all seizures occur within the 1 year following TBI and approximately 80% occurring within 2 years. [7, 12, 13, 18, 19]

Early PTS are found to be an important predictor of late PTS as Jennett reports a four-fold increase in late PTS if the patient seizes within 7 days of injury. [7] Annengers also found that in patients with moderate or severe TBI, early PTS were associated with an increased likelihood of late PTS. This was found not to be true in pediatric patients, mirroring the findings of Asikainen, who reported increasing age as predisposing factor for late onset seizures. [8, 11] Temkin and Englander report that the presence of intracranial blood, be that SDH or ICH, increases the risk of late seizure development some 400 times the expected rate seen in the general population. [14] Several investigators also report the severity of head injury, as stratified by GCS or an extended duration (most commonly > 24 hours) of PTA, exhibits a positive correlation with late PTS. [7, 10, 11, 13, 14, 19, 21]

Study Author	Population	N	Early Seizure %	Risk Factors Identified	Late Seizure %	Risk Factors Identified
Jennett and Lewin [7]	All admitted patients	896	4.2	Age<5, PTA >24 hours, skull fracture, ICH	10.2	Early PTS, PTA >24 hours, Depressed Skull fracture
Annengers et al. 1980 [8]	General population	2747	2.1	Age <15, severe injury	1.9	Moderate/ Severe TBI
Desai et al. [9]	All admitted patients	702	4.1	Age <16, focal defect, LOC/ PTA >30 minutes, skull fracture, ICH	Not assessed	Not assessed
Annegers et al. 1998 [10]	Gerneral population	4541	2.6	Not assessed	2.1	Early PTS, Cortical Contusion/ SDH, PTA >24hours
Asikainen et al. [11]	TBI Rehab	490	16.4	Age <8	24.8	Coma >24 hours
Englander et al. [20]	Severe TBI	647	3	Not Assessed	10.2	Early PTS, cortical contusion, dural penetration, multiple intracranial procedures, >5mm midline shift, evacuated SDH

Table 1. Incidence and Risk Factors for PTS

Early	Late
• Penetrating Head Injury	• Early PTS
• Age <16 years	• Advanced Age
• Severity of injury (GCS <10)	• Intracranial Blood
• Basilar Skull Fracture	• Severity of Injury
• Intracranial Blood	

Table 2. Risk Factors for PTS

5. Pathophysiology

The exact mechanisms surrounding the pathogenesis of PTS are still highly debated. Despite extensive animal modeling and basic science bench work, an accurate replication of human TBI has yet to be created. With the lack of an accurate model, the hypotheses found regarding PTS development must be taken in such context. [22]

The pathology surrounding the development of PTS is likely different based on the time of seizure onset, with different mechanisms playing a role in the development of early PTS and late PTS. Early PTS are often considered injury-induced or "provoked" and therefore cannot be considered epileptic. Following the initial insult of tissue deformation and compression, a cascade of events begins to take place almost immediately. Vascular damage and increased permeability of the blood brain barrier (BBB) are noted. [22, 23] Inflammatory cascades are drastically up-regulated leading to neuronal and glial swelling. Glial swelling may lead to impaired neuronal oxygen delivery and subsequent energy depletion leading to cellular death. Glutamate, an excitatory neurotransmitter, is released in high quantities. High concentrations of extracellular glutamate may stimulate ion channel activation and an intracellular flooding of calcium, followed by eventual cell death. [22, 23, 24] In any type of penetrating injury, direct neuronal damage due to cortical laceration, contusion, imbedded bone fragments, or retained foreign bodies becomes extraordinarily irritating to the injured brain and a potential focus for seizure activity. Also, the presence of intracranial blood has been found to predispose the TBI patient to early PTS. When extravasated blood undergoes hemolysis, hemoglobin is engulfed by macrophages which degrade the hemoglobin into hemosiderin and biliverdin. Hemosiderin is deposited into neuronal tissue. These pathogenic deposits initiate lipid peroxidation, damaging cell membranes, and inhibiting Na-K ATPase. [25, 26] The combination of these factors is profoundly pro-excitatory and likely predisposes the post TBI patient to seizures proximal to the time of injury.

The pathology of late PTS is considerably different and more controversial. There are three core theories of epileptogenesis in this setting, the kindling model, the fluid-percussion model, and the synaptic plasticity model. Each of these models attempts to describe the changes taking place in the brain during the latent period between the time of injury and onset of first late seizure.

The kindling theory of epileptogenesis is well validated in several animal models. Briefly, weak electrical stimulation is applied to specific, susceptible regions of the brain in rodents until a seizure occurrs. It has been found that over time, less stimulation was needed to initiate a seizure and this reduced threshold is a change that appears permanent over the remaining life of the animal. In the post-TBI human brain, it is thought that subclinical seizures due to structure changes or brain lesions will reduce the seizure threshold to a point in which epileptogenesis occurs. [27, 28] While this is well described in several animal models, the findings do not completely translate into human patients. Additionally, compounds traditionally assumed effective in controlling kindling type epilepsy (phenytoin, carbamazapime) have been shown to be ineffective preventing late PTS. [29]

The fluid-percussion model may more accurately help depict epileptogensis following TBI in humans. In animal-based experiments, a small hole is drilled into the skull of the animal, followed by the delivery of a fluid-wave percussion against the intact dura initiated by a pendulum impact on a fluid column. The seizures following this type of injury appear after a latent period, much like is seen in late PTS. Sustained hyperexcitablity was also observed in the region surrounding the injured neocortex and this excitability was associated with intense glial reactivity. [30] This reactivity may impair glutamate metabolism, exposing injured neurons to potentially toxic concentrations of this excitatory neurotransmitter. [31] This also mirrors late PTS in humans, as epileptiform activity seems to generate from the injured, hyperexcitable region of brain. [30]

The brain has the ability to adapt to injury through both changes in function and structural reorganization. [32, 33, 34] These changes are termed synaptic plasticity and are found to be an adaptive mechanism aiding in neurologic recovery. [35] During the recovery process, compensatory axons sprout, forming new adaptive neural pathways. While generally beneficial to recovery, these sprouts may, in some settings, become a focus for epileptic activity and may allow a seizure to impact relatively distant regions of the brain. [36] This "maladaptive plasticity" after TBI makes management of this potential pathology very challenging as not all plasticity is harmful. In using therapies that target the sprouting axons, there may be significant impairment in neurological recovery as "adaptive plasticity" would be targeted as well. [37, 38]

6. Impact

Post-traumatic seizures have a broad, sweeping impact on the lives of post-TBI patients. In addition to loss of independence from seizure restrictions (restricted driving privileges); psychological health, employment, quality of life, and mortality may also suffer.

Recurrent seizures are identified as an important cause of hospital readmission among patients with severe TBI. [39, 40] These readmissions are not always directly related to PTS as psychologically related admissions are seen to increase as well. It is understood that TBI patients often suffer from mood disturbances and behavioral abnormalities. Patients with PTS are increasingly sensitive to these disorders and there is a significant increase in the number of psychiatric related hospitalizations among patients with PTS as compared to those without. [41] Additionally, it has been found that irritability and aggressive, disinhibited behavior were observed to be more frequent and severe in rehabilitation patients with PTS as opposed to those not experiencing seizures. [41]

Post-traumatic seizures have been found to correlate with poorer outcomes and quality of life. In the *VHIS*, seizures following penetrating head injury were 1 of 7 impairments that were independently predictive of poor employment status. [42] Also, Asikainen reports that patients with PTS have inferior outcomes per Glasgow Outcome Scale (GOS) scores when compared to those without PTS. These results were mirrored by the findings of Mazzini, who also notes that PTS correlated with poorer GOS scores as well as several other neurobehavioral scales in TBI patients 1 year post injury. [11, 43]

Mortality is seen to be higher in patients with PTS in multiple reports, although it is unknown if there is a direct correlation. [44, 45, 46, 47] It is highly possible that the increase in the incidence of death is more likely related to the severity of the injury as opposed to the development of seizures. [48, 49]

7. Prevention of post-traumatic seizures

With the evolution of the association between head injury and seizure activity, as well as the recognition of the above discussed repercussions, came considerable efforts to develop preventative strategies against epileptic activity post TBI. Early studies, some dating back to the late 1940's, examined the use of anti-epileptic medication in patients with a variety of head injuries. Rapport and Penry noted that in three distinct series of head injured patients, the use of anti-epileptic medication seemed to reduce the incidence of seizure activity when compared to those not receiving such treatment. Their survey of American board certified neurosurgeons found that, at the time, only 14% of those polled typically used PTS prophylaxis. There were no specific professional recommendations for prophylactic treatment and most physicians at the time felt the evidence was considerably sparse. In fact, the most common reasoning for not treating prophylactically was uncertainty of appropriate indication for treatment. When a PTS prophylaxis regimen was initiated, the use of diphenylhydantoin was by far the most commonly used medication, followed the combination of phenobarbitol + diphenylhydantoin. [50]

Phenytoin, the most commonly utilized agent in the hydantoin class, is the most extensively studied PTS prophylaxis medication. Phenytoin is available intravenously (IV) and because of its high (80-90%) bioavailability, can be given orally (PO) as well. [51] The drug enters the brain rapidly and is redistributed throughout the body, being disbursed well throughout all tissues. [52] Phenytoin has a complex, and not yet fully understood, mechanism of action. It appears that the primary site of action for phenytoin is the motor cortex, where it inhibits the spread of seizure activity. Phenytoin has been observed to promote sodium efflux from neurons, stabilizing the neuron and increasing the cell's threshold against hyperexcitability caused by excessive stimulation or environmental changes capable of reducing membrane sodium gradient. [53] Phenytoin is complex kinetically, saturating its metabolism at clinically utilized dosing ranges. Consequently, small changes in dose can translate to large changes in plasma concentration, potentially leading to toxicity or loss of efficacy. Extensively bound to albumin, phenytoin plasma levels must be interpreted in the context of the patient's serum albumin concentration and if necessary, corrected for. Phenytoin levels are appropriately drawn as a "trough", approximately 30 minutes prior administering a dose and the optimal concentration maximizing efficacy and minimizing toxicity is between 10-20mcg/mL. [53]

The impact of phenytoin on the occurrence of PTS has been investigated repeatedly with variable results depending on trial design and outcome assessed. Wohns and Wyler investigated the effect of phenytoin for PTS prophylaxis as compared to no treatment in the seriesz in 62 patients with severe head injury. The dosing of phenytoin was not standardized, but most patients received a 1g load with a maintenance dose of 400mg/day. Therapy was continued for 1 year in the 50 patients managed with phenytoin and plasma concentrations were maintained between 10-20mcg/mL. There were no early PTS observed in this series but a marked difference in the incidence of late PTS was observed. Of the 50 patients treated with phenytoin for seizure prophylaxis, 10% had EEG confirmed late PTS, while those without prophylaxis experience late PTS at a rate of 50%. There was no statistical assessment of this data, but the authors hypothesized that phenytoin may offer some degree of protection from late PTS. [54]

Young et al was not able to confirm the findings of Wohns and Wyler. In a study assessing the effectiveness of phenytoin prophylaxis in preventing late PTS, patients at high risk (>15%) of developing late PTS were assigned to receive either PTS prophylaxis with phenytoin or matching placebo for a minimum of 18 months. There was no measurable difference in the rate of late PTS between groups, however; all patients in the phenytoin arm whom developed PTS had plasma concentrations <12mcg/mL, potentially explaining the lack of efficacy. [55]

The landmark trial demonstrating the efficacy of phenytoin in PTS prophylaxis was published by Temkin et al in 1999. Patients with severe TBI were randomized to receive phenytoin or placebo for 12 months unless adverse drug reactions necessitated early discontinuation. Those receiving phenytoin were loaded with 20mg/kg via IV infusion within 24 hours of injury. The follow-up dosing was not standardized, but an unblinded study-staff member followed frequent blood levels and adjusted phenytoin dosing as need to maintain high therapeutic serum concentrations. The effect of phenytoin on both early and late PTS was evaluated as patients were followed for a total of 24 months (12 months post discontinuation of study medication). Early PTS occurred at a rate of 3.6% ± 1.3 in those receiving phenytoin versus 14.6% ± 2.6 in the placebo group (p<0.001). This effect was seen in spite of early serum phenytoin concentrations being less than desired. Unfortunately, the rate of late PTS was unaffected by phenytoin therapy with no significant difference in the number of PTS events when compared with placebo after both 1 year (21.2% ± 3.6 vs. 15.7% ± 3.2; p>0.2) and 2 years (27.5% ± 4 vs. 21.%1 ± 3.7; p>0.2) of treatment. No difference in mortality was observed and treatment was generally well tolerated, although more patients in the phenytoin group needed to therapy discontinued secondary to medication related adverse events. [56]

A follow-up study, looking at the same data set, attempted to determine if PTS prophylaxis with phenytoin following TBI had any effect on neurocognitive and psychosocial recovery. All patients, independent of treatment arm, (phenytoin or placebo for 1y post TBI) received neuropsychological and psychosocial testing 1, 12, and 24 months post injury. Interestingly, at 1 month post injury, those treated with phenytoin performed significantly worse than those receiving placebo across most neuropsychological parameters. The difference seemed to vanish at the 1 year assessment, but it was noted that at the 2 year assessment, there was a small but widespread negative effect seen in patients treated with phenytoin. Additionally, the negative trend was also seen in patients receiving placebo that developed PTS and were subsequently started on phenytoin for the remainder of the study period. [57]

The above mentioned data set was utilized a third time in order to assess if treatment with phenytoin for 1 or 2 weeks as prophylaxis of early PTS was associated with changes in mortality or morbidity due to adverse drug events. Rash was the most commonly observed drug reaction. Hypersensitivity was rarely seen, occurring only in 0.6% of patients during the first week of therapy and increasing to 2.5% at the end of the second week. Of note, very few adverse reactions were reported in the first week of therapy, with no reports of fever and only one report of leukocytosis. No difference in mortality was observed between patients receiving phenytoin and those receiving placebo, but it was noted that if the patient experienced early PTS, the risk of death increased significantly independent of the treatment arm ($p=0.03$ RR 2; 95% CI 1.1-3.7). [58] While this may again encourage the use of phenytoin as prophylaxis against early PTS, it is important to note that the analysis was not powered to assess a mortality benefit and when corrected for severity of injury, the mortality benefit was no longer observed. Considering the risk-benefit ratio for 1 week of therapy and considering the two previous investigations, a recommendation limiting PTS prophylaxis to 7 days post injury was put forth.

Phenytoin, while potentially efficacious as prophylaxis against early PTS, is a potentially toxic medication. The side-effect profile of this drug is well documented and while these effects are rarely seen in a 7 day treatment period, they must be none-the-less considered. Severe, cutaneous hypersensitivity reactions associated with phenytoin are well documented and potentially life-threatening. [52, 59, 60] Fever, a significant confounder in the critically ill, and potential cause of secondary neurological injury, is reported frequently as well. [52, 53, 61] Phenytoin is an inducer of CYP450 and the UGT isozyme system potentially leading to multiple drug interactions involving absorption, metabolism, and protein binding which may drastically impact the effect of the drug on physiology. [52, 53] Phenytoin's enteric absorption and bioavailability can also be altered when exposed to a food bolus or continuous enteral tube feeds. [52] Bauer evaluated the impact of continuous tube feeds on phenytoin absorption in 53 neurosurgical patients when administered via enteric route. All patients were found to have subtherapeutic serum phenytoin concentrations and approximately 60% continued to be subtherapeutic even after dosage increase. He notes that hypermetabolism and binding of drug to tubing were unlikely as symptoms of phenytoin toxicity were observed following discontinuation of tube feed. [62] In response to these findings, the investigator held tube feedings for 2 hours prior to and following phenytoin administration and flushed the feeding tube with

60mL of water before restarting. With this intervention, serum phenytoin concentrations became therapeutic with only slight dosage increases. [62] Currently, this practice is widely implemented but also leads to significant nutritional issues. [63] With phenytoin typically requiring thrice daily dosing, continuous tube feeds could potentially be held for 12 hours daily. This strategy is met with much resistance as appropriate nutrition may be significantly hindered.

Fosphenytoin (Cerebyx) was approved by the Food and Drug Administration in 1996 as a potential replacement for phenytoin. Fosphenytoin is a pro-drug, fully converting via phosphatases in the liver, red blood cells, and tissue, to phenytoin within 20 minutes of administration. The most clinically significant benefit of fosphenytoin is the ability to infuse the medication as a more rapid rate. Phenytoin loading is often limited by the risk of extravasation and cardiovascular collapse (hypotenion, bradycardia) and due to these concerns, can only be infused at a maximum rate of 50mg/ min. Dosed in phenytoin equivalents (PE), the use of fosphenytoin allows for faster infusion (100-150mg PE/min) and IM administration when there is a lack of effective IV access. [79]

Due to the above mentioned concerns, much effort has been invested in finding an efficacious treatment alternative to phenytoin. The drug most commonly utilized in place of phenytoin is levetiracetam. Levetiracetam is available in both IV and PO formulations with equal bioavailability. Enteral absorption is rapid and predictable, with peak plasma concentrations occurring less than 1 hour following administration. Levetiracetam does not undergo any significant metabolism, avoiding the CYP system which drastically reduces the incidence of clinically relevant drug interactions. Levetiracetam is excreted primarily by the kidney and dosage reductions are recommended in patients with significant renal impairment. [64] Levetiracetam's mechanism of action is poorly understood, but it is thought that it may be novel in its activity. Animal data seems to suggest that levetiracetam may be protective against the development of epilepsy in certain clinical scenarios, yet this is unproven in human subjects. [52, 64, 65] Levetiracetam is very well tolerated and is associated with very few adverse drug events; however, in several patient populations, levetiracetam has been noted to induce non-psychotic behavioral disorders and mood instability. [64] Serum levetiracetam concentrations are not affected by enteric feeds and serum drug level monitoring is not recommended although there are some reports of increased clearance in TBI patients. [66, 67]

The first published trial assessing the use of levetiracetam for PTS was published by Jones et al in 2008. In this analysis, 32 patients with severe TBI (GCS 3-8) were given levetiracetam as PTS prophylaxis at a dosage of 500mg IV every 12 hours for the first 7 days following injury. These patients were compared with a historical control of 41 patients with similar injuries. If a clinical seizure was suspected, an EEG was performed and was subsequently interpreted by a blinded neurologist. The EEG results were classified as normal or abnormal, with abnormal being further stratified into status epilepticus, seizure, or seizure tendency. The patients receiving levetiracetam for prophylaxis had 15 EEG examinations with 53% being abnormal. Seizure activity was only seen in 1 patient, while seizure tendency was observed in the 7 other abnormal EEG's. Of the 41 patients receiving phenytoin for prophylaxis, 12 required EEG and of those 12, none were considered abnormal. The results of this small, non-randomized investigation led the authors to conclude that levetiracetam was as effective as phenytoin in prevention of early PTS. They noted that the observed trend of an increase in seizure tendency required further investigation. [61]

Szalflarski at al completed a prospective, randomized, placebo controlled trial investigating the use of levetiracetam versus phenytoin for PTS prophylaxis. Patients with subarachnoid hemorrhage (SAH) or TBI were randomized in a 2:1 ratio to receive levetiracetam or phenytoin for 7 days following injury. Levetiracetam was loaded at 20mg/kg followed by 1000mg IV q12 hours. Phenytoin was also loaded, followed by twice daily maintenance dosing but no mention of desired blood level or strategy of dose adjustment was noted. Patients were placed on continuous EEG monitoring until awake and following commands or for a maximum of 72 hours. Of the 52 patients enrolled, 34 received levetiracetam while 18 were managed with phenytoin. No difference was observed in the incidence of seizure or overall mortality. Phenytoin use was associated with an increase in the incidence of neurological status decline and gastrointestinal upset while those treated with levetiracetam were devoid of significant adverse drug reactions. In surviving patients, those treated with levetiracetam had significantly better functional outcomes via GOS and the Disability Rating Scale (DRS) at both 3 and 6 months. [68]

The largest investigation to date comparing levetiracetam to phenytoin for early PTS prophylaxis enrolled 813 patients with severe TBI secondary to blunt impact trauma. At the discretion of the providing physician, patients received levetiracetam at a dose of 1g every 12 hours or phenytoin titrated to a serum level of 10-20mcg/mL. No significant difference in the rate of clinical seizures was noted between groups, nor any difference in adverse drug reactions, complications of therapy, or mortality. More patients had therapy discontinue due to medication side effects in the phenytoin group; however, hospital length of stay was increased in the levetiracetam group. [69]

With neither therapy providing a distinct advantage in several individual clinical trials, Zafar at al conducted a meta-analysis attempting to identify any difference in early PTS incidence when levetiracetam or phenytoin were used for prophylaxis. Eight studies (6 observational/ 2 randomized controlled trials) were included, leading to a total patient population of 990. There was a trend toward increased efficacy with levetiracetam, but this difference did not reach statistical significance even when corrected for heterogeneity. It was noted that levetiracetam may have a more favorable side effect profile, but this meta-analysis was not designed to formally assess adverse drug events. As no difference in efficacy was noted, the authors conclude that cost should be the driving factor in the choice of agent for PTS prophylaxis. [70]

A cost-utility analysis by Cotton et al attempted to determine whether levetiracetam or phenytoin was more cost effective as an early PTS prophylaxis strategy. Using quality-adjusted life years (QALY) as the primary cost-utility determinant, phenytoin was found to be the more cost- effective management strategy. Phenytoin was reported to have a ratio of $1.58/ QALY versus levetiracetam which had a ratio of $20.72/QALY. It must be noted that at the time of this analysis, levetiracetam was not available as a generic product. Levetiracetam has been available via several generic manufactures since May 2010 and the subsequent cost reduction must be taken in consideration when interpreting these results. [71]

Several other treatment modalities have been investigated as preventive strategies for PTS with little benefit derived. Valproate was compared with phenytoin for prevention of PTS in high risk TBI patients. No difference in the incidence of either early or late PTS was noted, but mortality in the valproate group (13.4%) was almost double that seen in those managed with phenytoin (7.2%) leading to the early closure of the investigation. [72] Phenobarbital has been assessed both alone and in combination with phenytoin as a PTS prophylaxis strategy. When used as monotherapy for PTS prophylaxis in severe head injury, no benefit was observed and, due to adverse drug reactions, medication compliance was poor. [73] In combination with phenytoin, there was an observed reduction in seizures, but this difference could have been influenced by the use of phenytoin, and significant concern of toxicity was noted. [74] Magnesium was thought to be potentially neuroprotective, but when higher serum concentrations were targeted with continuous infusion there was an increase in the incidence of hypotension, reduced cerebral perfusion pressure, and a doubling of mortality. Lower magnesium target ranges also failed to provide any benefit. [75] In an observational series, corticosteroids were found to provide no PTS protection and were found to worsen excitotoxicity and oxidative neuronal damage in animal models. [76] There is a theoretic benefit with targeted temperature management as this therapy has several neuroprotective effects such as reduced metabolic rate, reduced inflammatory response, fewer epileptic discharges, and a reduction in the production of reactive oxygen species. This modality has not been formally evaluated for its impact on PTS, but offers a potential area of future research and potential benefit. [77]

As of 2007, the Brain Trauma Foundation guidelines for the management of severe traumatic brain injury consider the use of anti-epileptic medications for early PTS prophylaxis a Level II recommendation and note that prolonged prophylactic therapy (>7days) is not recommended. At the time of publication, phenytoin was the preferred agent for early PTS prophylaxis, but in the time since, a significant amount data surrounding the use of levetiracetam has been published. At this point, the two therapies should be considered equivalent from an efficacy standpoint, but consideration needs to be given to the individual characteristics of each medication and institutional costs associated with their administration. [78]

Traumatic brain injury is a devastating disorder having significant impact on patient morbidity and mortality. Seizures following TBI are a potentially preventable complication if the patients at highest risk are identified quickly and are initiated on a prophylactic regimen. The highest risk patients (penetrating injury, age <16, GCS <10, basilar skull fracture, intracerebral blood) should be started on prophylactic anticonvulsant therapy as soon as possible. Based on the latest evidence, there are two potentially efficacious strategies; phenytoin (or substituted fosphenytoin) and levetiracetam. Phenytoin appears most effective when loaded at a dosage of 10-15mg/kg followed by a regimen of 100mg every 8 hours and should be titrated to a trough total phenytoin concentration of 10-20 mcg/mL. Levetiracetam is an acceptable alternative regimen found to be effective when dosed at 1000mg every 12 hours with no serum drug monitoring being currently recommended. Both phenytoin and levetiracetam should be administered for 7 days following initial injury and when utilized in this manner a significant reduction in early PTS is observed, potentially improving patient outcomes.

Drug Name (Brand)	Phenytoin (Dilantin)	Levetiracetam (Keppra)
Mechanism of Action	Enhanced sodium efflux from neurons of the motor cortex, stabilizing the threshold against hyperexcitability. Posttetanic potentiation at synapses is then reduced preventing cortical seizure foci from detonating adjacent cortical areas	Inhibition of voltage-dependent N-type calcium channels; facilitation of GABA-ergic inhibitory transmission; reduction of delayed rectifier potassium current; and/or binding to synaptic proteins which modulate neurotransmitter release
Route of Administration	IV/ PO	IV/ PO
Typical Loading Dose	10-15mg/kg x1 ***Fosphenytoin:*** 10-20mg PE/kg	None recommended
Typical Maintenance Dose	100mg q8hr ***Fosphenytoin:*** 4-6mg PE/kg	500-1000mg q12hr
Elimination Half-Life	7-42 hours	6-8 hours (Metabolite =8.4 hr)
Metabolism/ Excretion	Metabolism: Hepatic via hydroxylation Excretion: Extensively excreted in bile as well as in urine following gastrointestinal reabsorption	Metabolism: enzymatic hydrolysis via liver Excretion: 66% unchanged in urine
Dosing Considerations	Metabolism and excretion may be impaired in renal and hepatic disease. Consider following unbound phenytoin levels for dose adjustment	Consider dosage reduction in patients with renal failure
Major Adverse Effects	Rash Nausea/ vomiting Ataxia Confusion Fever Stevens-Johnson Syndrome Myelosuppression Nephrotoxicity Hypotension Bradycardia Venous irritation	Pancytopenia Thrombocytopenia Liver Failure Personality disturbances
Monitoring/ Laboratory Considerations	Monitor trough concentration for efficacy. Toxicity is a clinical diagnosis and must be assess based on patient	No routine monitoring currently recommended

Drug Name (Brand)	Phenytoin (Dilantin)	Levetiracetam (Keppra)
	presentation. At times, patients may require blood concentrations outside therapeutic range	
	If rapid therapeutic levels are needed, a level may be drawn 2 hrs after completion of IV load or 24 hrs after administration of an oral loading dose	
	Draw within 5-8 days of therapy initiation with subsequent doses of phenytoin adjusted accordingly If complex patient free phenytoin concentration is desirable	
	Goal concentration 10-20 mcg/ml (Total)	
	1-2.5mcg/mL (Free)	
	In patients with hypoalbuminemia, phenytoin concentration needs to be corrected mathematically or free level should be drawn	
	CORRECTED PHENYTOIN= (Measured Phenytoin) 0.1 x Albumin +0.1	

Table 3. makinji caption

Author details

Matthew J. Korobey

Mercy Hospital St. Louis, St. Louis MO, USA

References

[1] Temkin O. The Falling Sickness: A History of Epilepsy from the Greeks to the Beginnings of Modern Neurology. The Johns Hopkins Press. Baltimore, MA. 1945

[2] Lowenstein DH. Epilepsy after Head Injury: An Overview. Epilepsia 2009; 50(Suppl. 2): 4-9

[3] Henry FP. A Notice of the Life and Writings of Valescus de Tarenta. Maryland Medical Journal 1901; 44(6): 237-251

[4] Spratling WP. Epilepsy and Its Treatment. WB Saunders and Company. Philadelphia, PA. 1904

[5] Elvidge AR. Remarks on Post-Traumatic Convulsive State. Transactions of the American Neurological Association 1939; 65: 125-129

[6] Hauser WA, Annegers JF, Kurland LT. Prevalence of Epilepsy in Rochester, Minnestoa: 1940-1980. Epilepsia 1991; 32(4): 429-445

[7] Jennett WB, Lewin W. Traumatic Epilepsy after Closed Head Injury. J Neurol. Neurosurg. Psychiat. 1960; 23:295-301

[8] Annegers JF, Grabow JS, Groover RV et al. Seizures after Head Trauma: A Population Study. Neurology 1980; 30:683-689

[9] Desai BT, Whitman S, Coonley-Hoganson R et al. Seizures and Civilian Head Injuries. Epilepsia 1983; 24: 289-296

[10] Annegers JF, Hauser WA, Coan SP, Rocca WA. A Population-Based Study of Seizures after Traumatic Brain Injuries. NEJM 1998; 338: 20-24

[11] Asikainen I, Kaste M, Sarna S. Early and Late Posttraumatic Seizures in Traumatic Brain Injury Rehabilitation Patients: Brain Injury Factors Causing Late Seizures and Influence of Seizures on Long-Term Outcome. Epilepsia 1999; 40(5): 584-589

[12] Salazar AM; Jabbari B, Vance S et al. Epilepsy After Penetrating Head Injury. I. Clinicla Correlates: a Report of the Vietnam Head Injury Study. Neurology 1985; 35: 1406-1414

[13] Caveness WF, Meirowsky AM, Rish BL et al. The Nature of Posttraumatic Epilepsy. J Neurosurg 1979; 50: 545-553

[14] Temkin NR. Risk Factors for Posttraumatic Seizures in Adults. Epilepsia 2003; 44(Suppl 10): 18-20

[15] Lee ST, Lui TN. Early Seizures after Mild Closed Head Injury. J Neurosurg 1992; 76: 435-439

[16] Gilad R, Boaz M, Sadeh M et al. Seizures After Very Mild Head or Spine Trauma. J Neurotrauma 2013; 30: 469-472

[17] Lee TS, Luie TN, Wong CW et al. Early Seizures After Severe Closed Head Injury. Can J Neurol Sci 1997; 24: 40-43

[18] Weiss GH, Caveness WF. Prognostic Factors in the Persistence of Posttraumatic Epilepsy. J Neurosurg 1972; 37: 164-169

[19] Haltiner AM, Temkin NR, Dikmen SS. Risk of Seizure Recurrence After the First Late Posttraumatic Seizure. Arch Phys Med Rehabil 1997; 78: 835-840

[20] Endlander J, Bushnik T, Duong TT et al. Analyzing Risk Factors for Late Posttraumatic Seizures: A Prospective, Multicenter Investigation. Arch Phys Med Rehabil 2003; 84: 365

[21] Christensen J, Pedersen MG, Pedersen CB,Sidenius P, Olsen J, Vastergaard M. Long-Term Risk of Epilepsy After Traumatic Brain Injury IN Children and Young Adults: A Population-Based Cohort Study. Lancet 2009; 373: 1105-1110

[22] Garga N, Lowenstein SH. Posttraumatic Epilepsy: A Major Problem in Desperate need of Major Advances. Epilepsy Currents 2006; 6(1): 1-5

[23] Hunt RF, Boychuck JA, Smith BN. Neural Circuit Mechanisms of Post-traumatic Epilepsy. Frontiers in Cellular Neuroscience 2013; 7 (Article 89): 1-14

[24] Bao, Y, Bramlett HM, Atkins CM et al. Post-Traumatic Seizures Exacerbate Histopathological Damage after Fluid-Percussion Brain Injury. J Neurotrauma 2011; 23: 35-42

[25] Willmore LJ. Post-Traumatic Epilepsy: Cellular Mechanism and Implications for Treatment. Epilepsia 1990; 31(Suppl 3): S67-73

[26] Zasler N, Katz D, Zafonte RD. Brain Injury Medicine: Principles and Practice. New York, NY: Demos Medical Publishing, LLC; 2012

[27] Goddard BS. Developmnet of Epileptic Seizures Through Brain Stimulation at Low Intensity. Nature 1967; 214: 1020-1021

[28] Cavalheiro EA, Leite JP, Bortolotto ZA et al. Long-Term Effects of Pilocarpine in Rats: Structural Damage of the Brain Triggers Kindling and Spontaneous Recurrent Seizures. Epilepsia 1991; 32: 778-782

[29] Temkin NR, Jarell AD, Anderson GD. Antiepileptic Agents: How Close are We?. Drugs 2001; 61: 1045-1055

[30] D'Ambrosio R, Fairbanks JP, Fender JS et al. Post-Traumatic Epilepsy Following Fluid Percussion Injury in the Rat. Brain 2004; 127: 304-314

[31] Lieth E, Barber AJ, Xu B et al. Glial reactivity and Impaired Glutamate Metabolism in Short-Term Experimental Diabetic Retinophaty. Penn State Research Group. Diabetes 1998; 47 (5): 815-820

[32] Lowenstein DH, Thomas MJ, Smith DH, McIntosh TK. Selective Vulnerability of Dentate Hilar Neurons Following Traumatic Brain Injury: A Potential Mechanistic Link Between Head Trauma and Disorders of the Hippocampus. J Neurosci 1992; 12: 4846-4853

[33] Levin HA. Neuroplasticity Following Non-Penetrating Traumatic Brain Injury. Brain Inj 2003; 8: 665-674

[34] Seitz RJ, Huang Y, Knorr U et al. Large-Scale Plasticity of the Human Motor Cortex. Neuroreport 1995; 6: 742-744

[35] Albensi B, Janigro D. Traumatic Brain Injury and its Effects on Synaptic Plasticity. Brain Inj 2003; 17: 653-656

[36] Sankar R, Shin D, Liu H, Wasterlain C, Mazarati A. Epileptogenesis During Development: Injury, Circuit Recruitment, and Plasticity. Epilepsia 2002; 43 Suppl 5: 47-53

[37] Prince DA, Connors BW. Mechanisms of Epileptogenesis in Cortical Structures. Ann Neurol 1984; 16 (Suppl): S59-S64

[38] Montanez S, Kline AE, Gasser TA, Hernandez TD. Phenobarbital Administration Directed Against Kindled Seizures Delays Functional Recovary Following Brain Insult. Brain Res 2000; 860: 29-40

[39] Cifu DX, Kreutzer JS, Marwitz JH et al. Etiology and Incidence of Rehospitalization after Traumatic Brain Injury: A Multicenter Analysis. Arch Phys Med Rehabil 1999; 80: 85-90

[40] Shavelle RM, Strauss D, Whyte J, Day SM, Yu YL. Long-term Causes of Death After Traumatic Brain Injury. Am J Phys Med Rehabil 2001; 80: 510-6

[41] Swanson SJ, Rao SM, Grafman J, Salazar AM, Kraft J. The Relationship Between Seizure Subtype and Interictal Personality. Results from the Vietnam Head Injury Study. 1995; 118: 91-103

[42] Schwab K, Grafman J, Salazar Am, Kraft J. Residual Impairments and Work Status 15 Years After Penetrating Head Injury: Report from the Vietnam Head Injury Study. Neurology 1993; 43: 95-103

[43] Mazzini L, Cossa FM, Angelino E et al. Neuroradiologic and Neuropsychological Assessmetn of Long-Term Outcome. Epilepsia 2003; 44:569-74

[44] Corkin S, Sullivan EV, Carr FA. Prognostic Factors for Life Expectancy After Head Injury. Arch Neurol 1984; 41: 975-977

[45] Walker AE, BLumer D. The Fate of World War II Veterans with Post-traumatic Seizures. Arch Neurol 1989; 46: 23-26

[46] Weiss GH, Caveness WF, Eisiedel-Lechtape H, McNeel M. Life Expectancy and Causes of Death in a Group of Head Injured Veterans of World War I. Arch Neurol 1982; 39: 741-743

[47] Walker AE, Erculei F. Post-traumatic Epilepsy 15 Years Later. Epilepsia 1970; 11:17-26

[48] Rish B, Caveness W. Relation of Prophylactic Medication to the Occurrence of Early Seizures Following Craniocerbral Trauma. J Neurosurg 1973;38: 155-158

[49] Rish BL, Dillon JD, Weiss GH. Mortality Following Penetrating Craniocerebral Injuries. J Neurosurg 1983: 59;775-80

[50] Rapport RL, Penry JK. A Survey of Attitudes Toward the Pharmacological Prophyaxis of Posttraumatic Epilepsy. J Neurosurg 1973; 38: 159-166

[51] Rang HP, Dale MM, Ritter JM, Moore PK. Pharmacology. 5th Ed. St. Louis: Churchill Livingstone. 2003

[52] DiPiro JT, Talber RL, Yee GL. Pharmacotherapy, A Pathophysiological Approach, 8th Ed. McGraw-Hill. 2011

[53] Parenteral Dilantin [Package Insert]. New York, NY: Pfizer; 2011

[54] Wohns RNW, Wyler AR. Prophylactic Phenytoin in Severe Head Injuries. J Neurosurg 1979; 51: 507-509

[55] Young B, Rapp RP, Norton JA et al. Failure of Prophylactically Administered Phenytoin to Prevent Late Posttraumatic Seizures. J Neurosurg 1983; 58: 236-241

[56] Temkin NR, Dikmen SS, Wilensky AJ et al. A Randomized, Double-Blind Study of Phenytoin for the Prevention for Post-Traumatic Seizures. NEJM 1990; 323(8): 497-502

[57] Dikmen SS, Temkin NR, Miller B, Machamer J, Winn HR. Neurobehavioral Effects of Phenytoin Prophylaxis of Posttraumatic Seizrues. JAMA 1991; 265:1271-1277

[58] Haltiner AM, Newell DW, Temkin NR, Kikmen SS, Winn HR. Side Effects and Mortality Associated with Use of Phenytoin for Early Posttraumatic Seizure Prophylaxis. J Neurosurg 1999; 91: 588-592

[59] Jones GL, Wimbish GH, McIntosh WE. Phenytoin: Basic and Clinical Pharmacology. Med Res Rev 1983; 3: 383-434

[60] Stern RS. Exanthematous Drug Eruptions. N Engl J Med 2012; 366:2492-2501

[61] Jones KE, Puccio AM, Harshman KJ et al. Levetiracetam Versus Phenytoin for Seizure Prophylaxis in Severe Traumatic Brain Injury. Neurosurg Focus 2008; 25(4): E3 15

[62] Bauer LA. Interference of oral phenytoin absorption by continuous nasogastric feedings. Neurology 1982;32: 570-2

[63] Chan LN. To Hold (Enteral Feeding) or Not to Hold: That IS the Question; A Commentary and Tutorial. Practical Gastroenterology 2012; January: 13-21

[64] Keppra [Package Insert]. Symrna, GA: UCB; 2011

[65] Loscher W, Honack D, Rundfeldt C. Antiepileptogenic Effects of the Novel Anticonvulsant Levetiracetam (ucb LO59) in the Kindling Model of Temporal Lobe Epilepsy. J Pharmacol Exp Ther 1998;284:474–479.

[66] Cook AM, Arora S, Davis J, Pittman T. Augmented Renal Clearance of Vancomycin and Levetiracetam in a Traumatic Brain Injury Patient. Neurocrit Care 2013; 19: 210-214

[67] Klein P, Herr D, Pearl PL et al. Results of Phase II Pharmacokinetic Study of Levetiracetam for Prevention of Post-Traumatic Epilepsy. Epilepsy & Behavior 2012; 24: 457-461

[68] Szaflarski JP, Sangha KS, Lidsell CJ, Shutter LA. Prospective, Randomized, Single-Blinded Comparative Trial of Intravenous Levetiracetam Versus Phenytoin for Seizure Prohylaxis. Neurocrit Care 2010; 12: 165-172

[69] Inaba K, Menaker J, Branco DC et al. A Prospective Multicenter Comparison of Levetiracetam Versus Phenytoin for Early Posttraumatic Seizure Prophylaxis. J Trauma Acute Care Surg 2013; 74(3): 766-773

[70] Zafar SN, Kahn AA, Ghuri AA, Shamim MS. Phenytoin Versus Leviteracetam for Seizure Prophylaxis after Brain Injury – A Meta Analysis. BMC Neurology 2012; 12: 30-38

[71] Cotton BA, Kao LS, Kozar R, Holcomb JB. Cost-Utility Analysis of Levetiracetam and Phenytoin for Posttraumatic Seizure Prophylaxis. J Trauma 2011; 71: 375-379

[72] Temkin NR, Kikmen SS, Anderson GD et al. Valproate Therapy for Prevention of Posttraumatic Seizures: A Randomized Trial. J Neurosurg 1999; 91: 593-600

[73] Manaka S. Cooperative Prospective Study on Posttraumatic Epilepsy: Risk Factors and the Effect of Prophylactic Anticonvulsant. The Japanese Journal of Psychiatry and Neurology 1992; 46(2): 311-315

[74] Servit Z, Musil F. Prophylactic Treatment of Posttraumatic Epilepsy: Results of a Lont-Term Follow-Up in Czechoslovakia. Epilepsia 1981; 22: 315-320

[75] Temkin NR, Winn HR, Ellenbogen RG et al. Magnesium Sulfate for Neuroprotection after Traumatic Brain Injury: A Randomised Controlled Trial. Lancet 2007; 6: 29-38

[76] Watson NF, Barber JK, Doherty MJ, Miller JW, Temkin NR. Does Glucocorticoid Administration Prevent Late Seizures after Head Injury?. Epilepsia 2004; 45(6): 690-694

[77] Christian E, Sada G, Sung G, Giannotta SL. A Review of Selective Hypothermia in the Management of Traumatic Brain Injury. Neurosurg Focus 2008; 25 (4): E9 1- 8

[78] Brain Trauma Foundation. Guidelines for the Management of Severe Traumatic Brain Injury. J Neurotrauma 2007; 42, Supplement 1: S1-S106

[79] Kirschbaum K, Gurk-Turner C. Phenytoin vs Fosphenytoin. BUMC Proceedings 1999; 12:168-172.

Permissions

All chapters in this book were first published by InTech Open; hereby published with permission under the Creative Commons Attribution License or equivalent. Every chapter published in this book has been scrutinized by our experts. Their significance has been extensively debated. The topics covered herein carry significant findings which will fuel the growth of the discipline. They may even be implemented as practical applications or may be referred to as a beginning point for another development.

The contributors of this book come from diverse backgrounds, making this book a truly international effort. This book will bring forth new frontiers with its revolutionizing research information and detailed analysis of the nascent developments around the world.

We would like to thank all the contributing authors for lending their expertise to make the book truly unique. They have played a crucial role in the development of this book. Without their invaluable contributions this book wouldn't have been possible. They have made vital efforts to compile up to date information on the varied aspects of this subject to make this book a valuable addition to the collection of many professionals and students.

This book was conceptualized with the vision of imparting up-to-date information and advanced data in this field. To ensure the same, a matchless editorial board was set up. Every individual on the board went through rigorous rounds of assessment to prove their worth. After which they invested a large part of their time researching and compiling the most relevant data for our readers.

The editorial board has been involved in producing this book since its inception. They have spent rigorous hours researching and exploring the diverse topics which have resulted in the successful publishing of this book. They have passed on their knowledge of decades through this book. To expedite this challenging task, the publisher supported the team at every step. A small team of assistant editors was also appointed to further simplify the editing procedure and attain best results for the readers.

Apart from the editorial board, the designing team has also invested a significant amount of their time in understanding the subject and creating the most relevant covers. They scrutinized every image to scout for the most suitable representation of the subject and create an appropriate cover for the book.

The publishing team has been an ardent support to the editorial, designing and production team. Their endless efforts to recruit the best for this project, has resulted in the accomplishment of this book. They are a veteran in the field of academics and their pool of knowledge is as vast as their experience in printing. Their expertise and guidance has proved useful at every step. Their uncompromising quality standards have made this book an exceptional effort. Their encouragement from time to time has been an inspiration for everyone.

The publisher and the editorial board hope that this book will prove to be a valuable piece of knowledge for researchers, students, practitioners and scholars across the globe.

List of Contributors

Tobias Wensing
Centre Interdisciplinaire de Recherche en Réadaptation et Intégration Sociale, Canada
Faculty of Psychology and Neuroscience, Maastricht University, Maastricht, The Netherlands

Jean Levasseur-Moreau
Centre Interdisciplinaire de Recherche en Réadaptation et Intégration Sociale, Canada
Centre de Recherche Universitaire en Santé Mentale de Québec, Quebec, Canada
Medical School, Laval University, Quebec, Canada

Alexander T. Sack
Faculty of Psychology and Neuroscience, Maastricht University, Maastricht, The Netherlands
Maastricht Brain Imaging Center, Maastricht University, Maastricht, The Netherlands

Shirley Fecteau
Centre Interdisciplinaire de Recherche en Réadaptation et Intégration Sociale, Canada
Centre de Recherche Universitaire en Santé Mentale de Québec, Quebec, Canada
Medical School, Laval University, Quebec, Canada

Narayan P. Verma
Oakland University William Beaumont School of Medicine, Oakland, USA

Shawn M. McClintock
Neurocognitive Research Laboratory, Division of Brain Stimulation and Neurophysiology, Department of Psychiatry and Behavioral Sciences, Duke University School of Medicine, Department of Psychiatry, UT Southwestern Medical Center, USA

Jesús Moreta and José Luis Martínez-de los Mozos
Department of Orthopaedic Surgery and Trauma, Hospital de Galdakao-Usansolo, Galdakao, Spain

Hans von Holst
Dept. of Neurosurgery, Karolinska University Hospital, Stockholm, Sweden
Division of Neuronic Engineering, Royal Institute of Technology, Stockholm, Sweden

Svein Kleiven
Division of Neuronic Engineering, Royal Institute of Technology, Stockholm, Sweden

Giovanna Mioni
École de Psychologie, Université Laval, QC, Canada
Department of General Psychology, Padova, Italy

Franca Stablum
Department of General Psychology, Padova, Italy

Arunima Verma Jayakar
BG Tricounty Neurology and Sleep Clinic PC, USA

Wafa Al Yazeedi, Loganathan Venkatachalam, Somaya Al Molawi and Fatma Al Kuwari
Department of Physical Medicine & Rehabilitation, Hamad Medical Corporation, Doha, Qatar

Farid Sadaka, Tanya M Quinn, Rekha Lakshmanan and Ashok Palagiri
Mercy Hospital St. Louis/St. Louis University, Critical Care Medicine/Neurocritical Care, St. Louis, USA

Fernando Salierno, María Elisa Rivas, Pablo Etchandy, Verónica Jarmoluk, Diego Cozzo, Martín Mattei, Eliana Buffetti, Leonardo Corrotea and Mercedes Tamashiro
Physical Therapy Department, FLENI Rehabilitation Institute, Escobar, Prov. de Buenos Aires, Argentina

Birgitta Johansson and Lars Rönnbäck
Department of Clinical Neuroscience and Rehabilitation, Institute of Neuroscience and Physiology, Gothenburg University, Sweden

Matthew J. Korobey
Mercy Hospital St. Louis, St. Louis MO, USA

Index

www.ingramcontent.com/pod-product-compliance
Lightning Source LLC
LaVergne TN
LVHW080614210926
848485LV00003B/158

* 9 7 8 1 6 3 9 2 7 8 4 3 5 *